Biopsy Pathology of the Lymphoreticular System

BIOPSY PATHOLOGY SERIES

Biopsy Pathology of the Lymphoreticular System

DENNIS H. WRIGHT
B.Sc., M.D., F.R.C.Path.
Professor of Pathology, The University of Southampton,
and Honorary Consultant Pathologist,
Southampton and South-West Hampshire District Health Authority

and

PETER G. ISAACSON
D.M., M.R.C.Path.
Reader in Pathology, The University of Southampton,
and Honorary Consultant Pathologist,
Southampton and South-West Hampshire District Health Authority
Now Professor of Morbid Anatomy, School of Medicine,
University College, London

LONDON
CHAPMAN AND HALL

First published 1983
by Chapman and Hall Ltd
11 New Fetter Lane, London EC4P 4EE

Phototypeset by
Wyvern Typesetting Ltd, Bristol
Printed in Great Britain at the
University Press, Cambridge

ISBN 0 412 16050 1

British Library Cataloguing in Publication Data

Wright, Dennis H.
Biopsy pathology of the lymphoreticular system.
1. Reticulo——endothelial system
2. Biopsy
I. Title   II. Isaacson, Peter G.
616.4′207′58   QR180.3

ISBN 0–412–16050–1

Contents

Preface

Biopsy pathology of the lymphoreticular system has been written primarily for diagnostic histopathologists although we hope that other workers in the field of lymphoreticular disease will find it of interest and value. With our primary readership in mind we have generously illustrated most sections of the book. All illustrations are of haematoxylin and eosin stained sections unless otherwise specified.

Conceptual understanding of the histogenesis and interrelationship of non-Hodgkin's lymphomas has been in a state of turmoil for over a decade. In more recent years immunological and immunocytochemical studies have clarified some problems although in other areas such as the T-cell lymphomas histogenetic interrelationships are still far from clear. We are aware, therefore, that in writing this book we have been aiming at a moving target; nevertheless, we feel that the need for such a book, particularly amongst diagnostic histopathologists, outweighs the advantage of waiting until all the t's are crossed and all the i's dotted.

No doubt some pathologists remembering the limited categories of malignant lymphoma recognized in the past, will be dismayed at the complexity of present-day classifications. This complexity reflects the functional diversity and interrelationship of cells of the lymphoreticular system recognized in recent years. Our understanding of malignant lymphoma is now based on a more secure scientific basis and the study of these tumours is consequently more rewarding. The histopathologist must, however, recognize the need for the highest standards of histological technique and that other techniques are necessary for the accurate categorization of some types of lymphoma. We hope that this book will help him or her through the maze.

Soon after we completed the manuscript for this book the findings and conclusions of the National Cancer Institute sponsored study of classifications of non-Hodgkin's lymphomas was published (*Cancer*, **49**, 2112–35, 1982). We have written a brief addendum including the 'Working Formulation' that evolved from this study, to be found in the Appendix.

Acknowledgements

We would like to acknowledge the co-operation of many pathologists, particularly in the Wessex Region, who have provided us with biopsy material from patients with lymphoreticular disease and who have allowed us to use this material to illustrate this book. The laboratory staff at Southampton General Hospital have provided us with high quality histological preparations. We are particularly indebted to Brian Mepham, Mary Judd, Karen Britton and Najat Al-Safar for the immunohistochemical preparations. Karen Britton also earns our gratitude for many hours spent in the dark room developing and printing the illustrations for this book. We are grateful to Maureen Bathard for typing much of the manuscript and to Olive Huber for taking over when the arrival of Helen stilled Maureen's keys. Finally, we would like to thank Barry Shurlock of Chapman and Hall for his patience and tact in extracting this book from us only three years after the original deadline.

1 The normal lymph node and spleen

1.1 Lymph node

An appreciation of normal lymph node histology is essential to the understanding of non-Hodgkin's lymphomas since each malignant cell type has its benign analogue in the non-neoplastic lymph node. The localization of a malignant lymphomatous infiltrate within a lymph node is also influenced by the position that the equivalent benign cells occupy in the node and can be a valuable diagnostic aid. To appreciate the morphology of normal lymph node cells it is best to study reactive or hyperplastic lymph nodes since it is only in this type of node that there are sufficient numbers of each cell type fully to reflect the morphological range.

The overall structure of lymph nodes is well illustrated in reticulin preparations (Fig. 1.1). The lymph node is surrounded by a thin fibrous capsule from which fibrous trabeculae penetrate the node. These are most prominent at the hilum of the node. Afferent lymphatics penetrate the capsule at various points and efferent lymphatics leave at the hilum. Beneath the fibrous capsule is the marginal or subcapsular sinus which sends branches into the cortical lymphoid tissue (Fig. 1.2). Many more interconnecting sinuses are present in the medulla of the node where they are separated by broad trabeculae of lymphoid tissue, the medullary cords. The sinuses of the lymph node are divided by multiple reticulin fibres forming a sponge-like structure and contain macrophages (sinus histiocytes) as well as variable numbers of lymphocytes and occasionally other cells such as plasma cells and polymorphs (Fig. 1.3).

The lymphoid tissue of the node can be conveniently divided into B- and T-lymphocyte regions (Figs 1.1 and 1.4) although there is some overlap. The B-cell regions of lymph nodes comprise discrete follicles (Figs 1.4 and 1.5). These consist of a mantle of small lymphocytes, which is broadest towards the capsule of the node, and a follicle centre. The size of the follicle centre reflects the reactivity of the node and it is within the reactive follicle centre that the cells from which most B-cell lymphomas are derived can best be seen. The majority of the cells have irregular

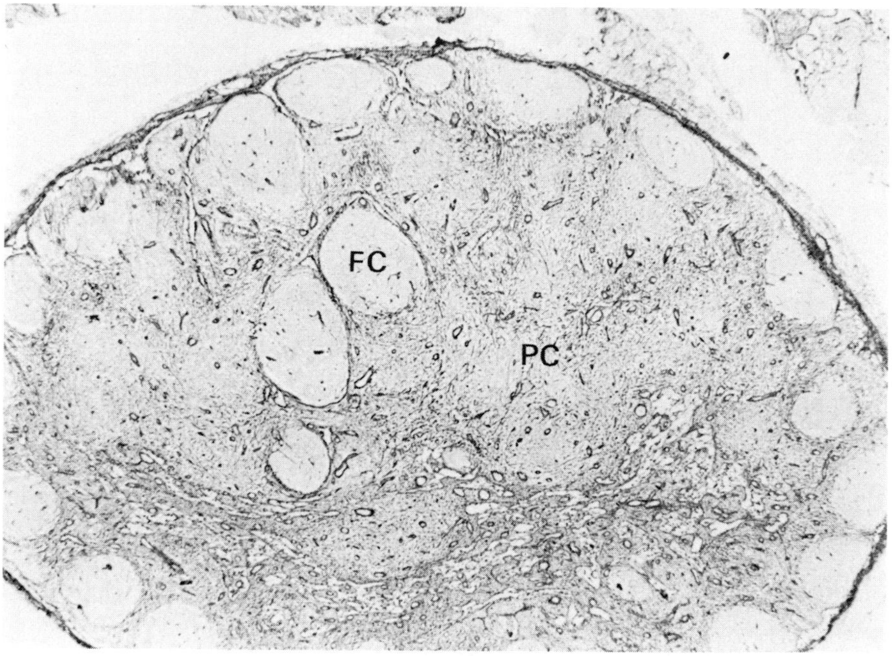
FC
PC

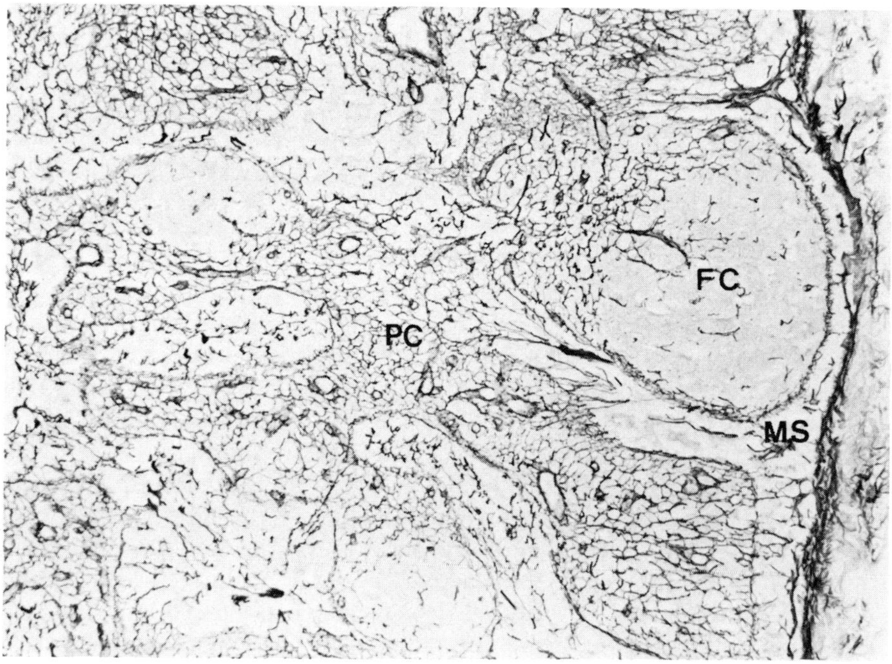
FC
PC
MS

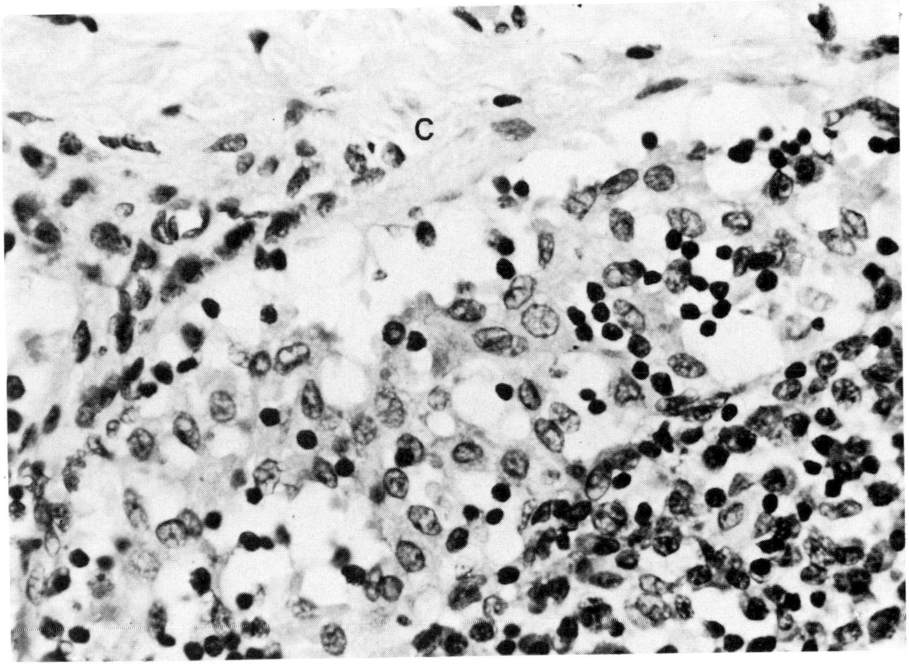

Fig. 1.3 The marginal sinus beneath the lymph node capsule (C) contains numerous macrophages (sinus histiocytes) together with lymphocytes and occasional plasma cells, × 400.

indented nuclei resulting in a deformed or tortuous appearance (Figs 1.6 and 1.7). These cells, termed centrocytes, vary in size from a little larger than a small lymphocyte, as seen in the mantle zone, to about twice that size. The nuclei, which stain more lightly than those of small lymphocytes, may show small centrally-placed nucleoli. In paraffin sections, the cytoplasm is pale staining and indistinct. Centroblasts are found in the follicle centre, usually in smaller numbers than centrocytes. These cells have round, pale-staining nuclei which are not indented and which usually contain several prominent nucleoli often approximating the nuclear membrane. The distribution of centroblasts and centrocytes is

---

Fig.1.1 Reticulin stain of a reactive lymph node. Hyperplastic follicle centres (FC) are outlined and numerous thick wall blood vessels are evident in the paracortex (PC). Interconnecting sinuses characterize the medulla of the node, × 20.

Fig. 1.2 Reticulin fibres can be seen traversing the marginal sinus (MS) and deeper sinuses of the lymph node. The almost reticulin free follicle centre (FC) contrasts with the fine reticulin network of the paracortical T-zone (PC), × 80.

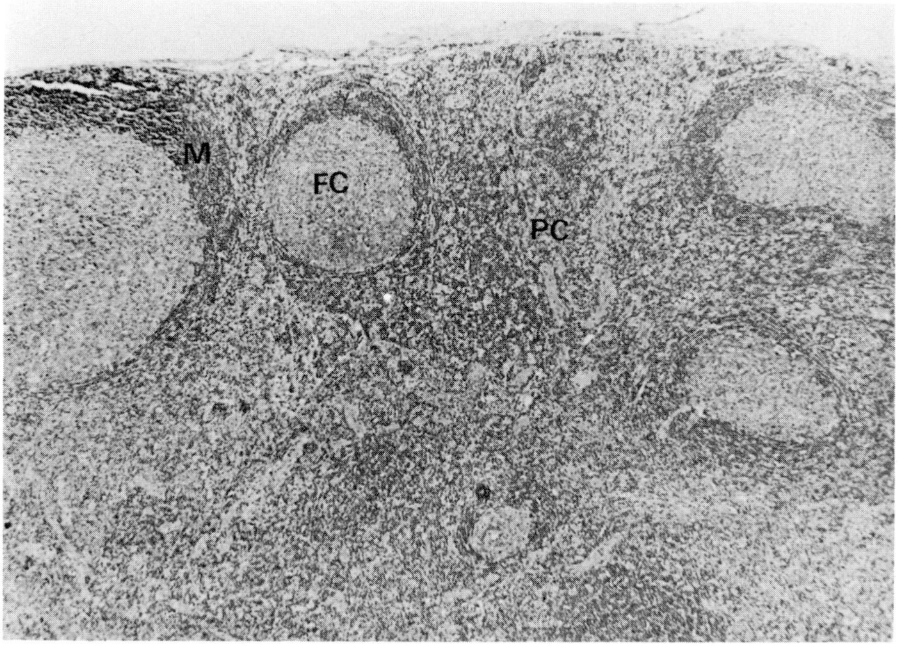
M
FC
PC

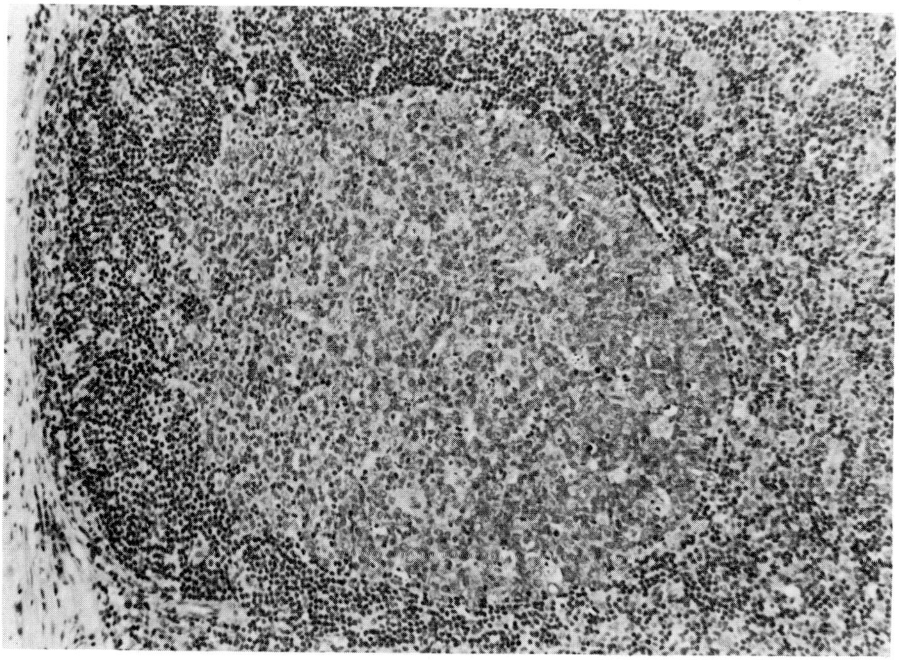

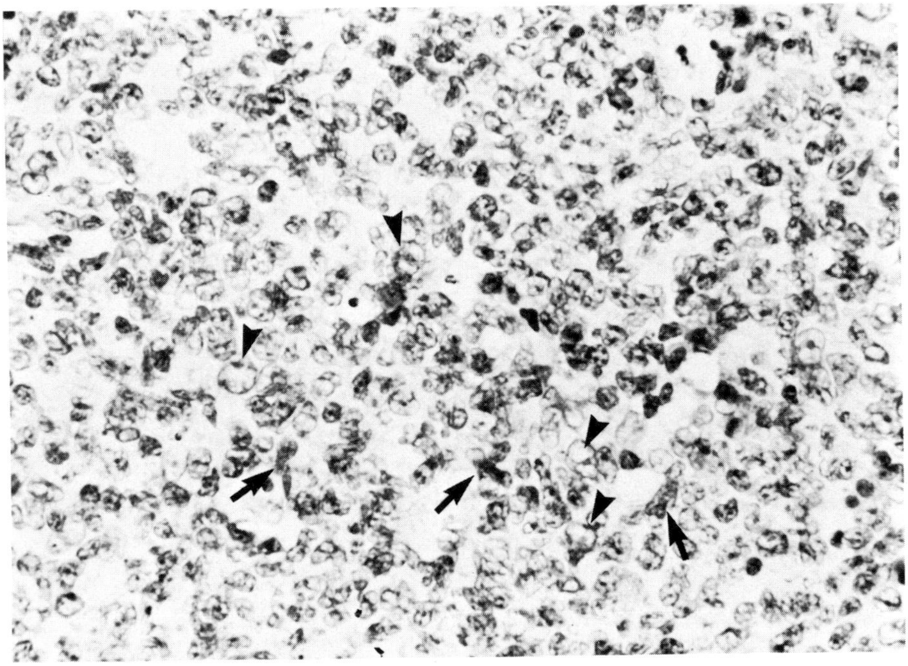

Fig. 1.6 Lymph node follicle centre containing both centrocytes (arrows) and centroblasts (arrowheads), × 400.

uneven within the follicle and this divides the follicle into so-called light and dark zones (Fig. 1.5). Centroblasts are concentrated in the dark zone and centrocytes in the light zone (Figs 1.8 and 1.9). The third cell type which can be distinguished in follicle centres is the large pale-staining phagocytic histiocyte which usually contains ingested cell debris (tingible bodies) (Fig. 1.10). T-cells are also present within the follicle but these small lymphocytes are not conspicuous unless specifically demonstrated (see below). Although an important component of the follicle centre, the dendritic reticulum cell cannot be identified in routine paraffin sections and is only recognizable following silver impregnation techniques or in electron micrographs.

Fig. 1.4 Low power view of a reactive lymph node. The B-lymphocyte region consists of follicle centres (FC) and their mantle zones (M). The T-lymphocyte region or paracortex (PC) has a slightly mottled appearance and the thick-walled postcapillary venules can be discerned, × 40.
Fig. 1.5 A lymph node follicle comprising the mantle zone of small lymphocytes at left and the follicle centre. The 'light zone' of the follicle centre is adjacent to the mantle and the 'dark zone' is at the opposite pole, × 80.

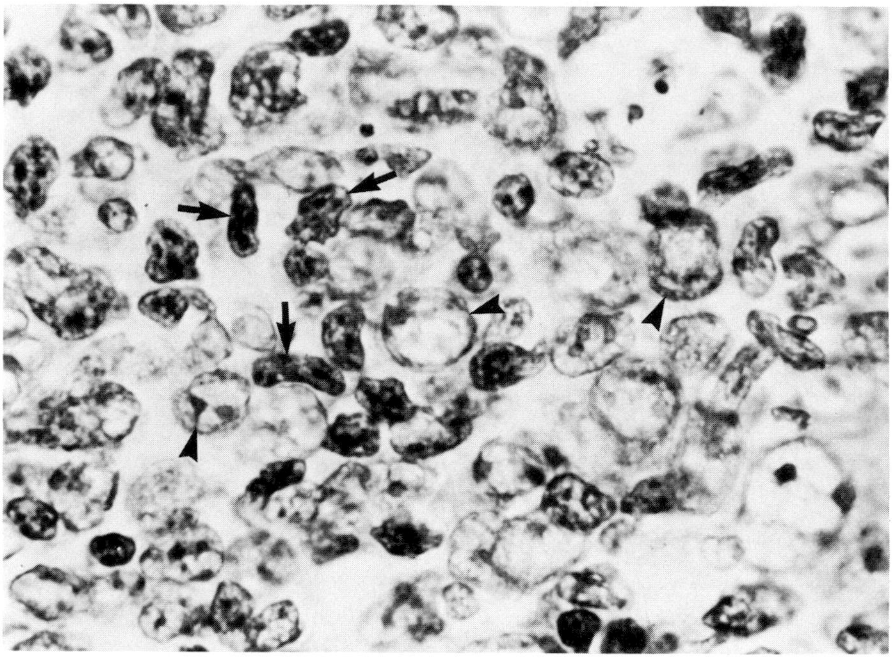

Fig. 1.7 Follicle centre seen under high (oil immersion) magnification. Centrocytes (arrows) and centroblasts (arrowheads) can be clearly distinguished, × 1000.

Plastic embedded sections (Figs 1.11 and 1.12) highlight the detailed morphology of follicle centre cells and the strong resemblance between these cells and those of many of the non-Hodgkin's lymphomas. In this type of preparation the morphology of centroblasts and centrocytes is more clearly shown and gradations between the two cell types can be seen. The irregular outline and heterochromatic centrocytic nuclei, which often contain multiple small nucleoli, are sharply contrasted with the leptochromatic large smooth contoured centroblastic nuclei with from 1–3 large nucleoli usually apposed to the nuclear membrane but occasionally centrally placed. The cytoplasm of centroblasts is abundant and pale and in well-fixed preparations organelles such as strands of rough endoplasmic reticulum can be identified (Fig. 1.13).

In Giemsa-stained imprint preparations the nuclei of centrocytes are

---

Fig. 1.8 The 'light zone' of the follicle centre consisting predominantly of centrocytes as seen with high power (a) and oil immersion (b) objectives, × 400 (a), × 1000 (b).

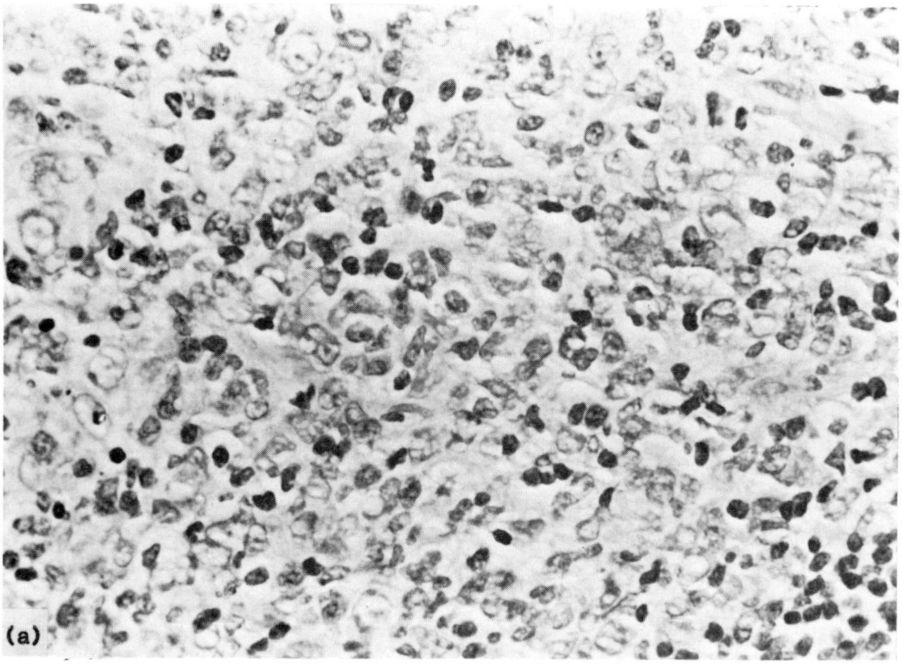
(a)

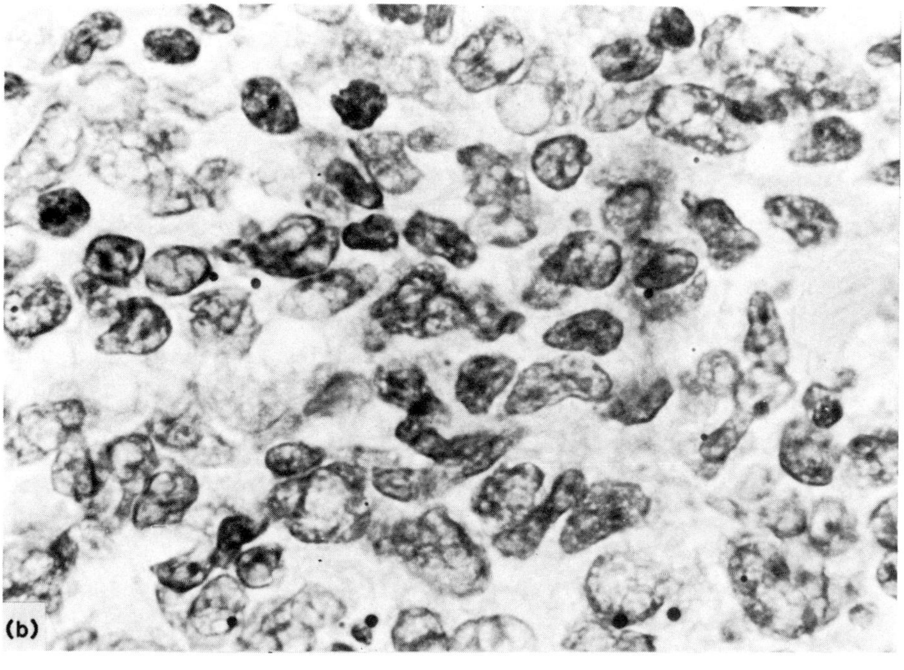
(b)

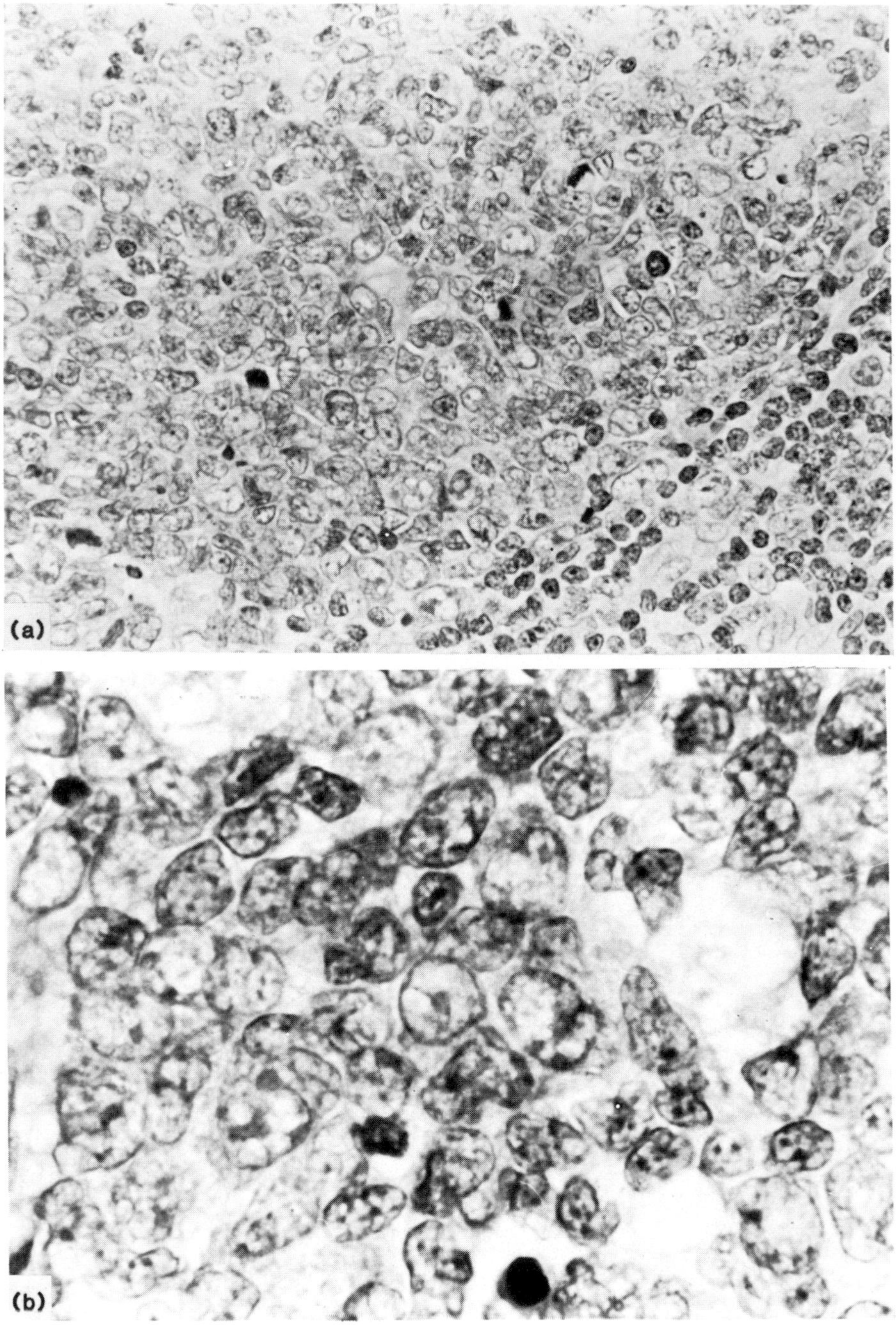

Fig. 1.9 The 'dark zone' of the follicle centre which consists almost entirely of centroblasts seen under high power (a) and oil immersion (b), × 400 (a), × 1000 (b).

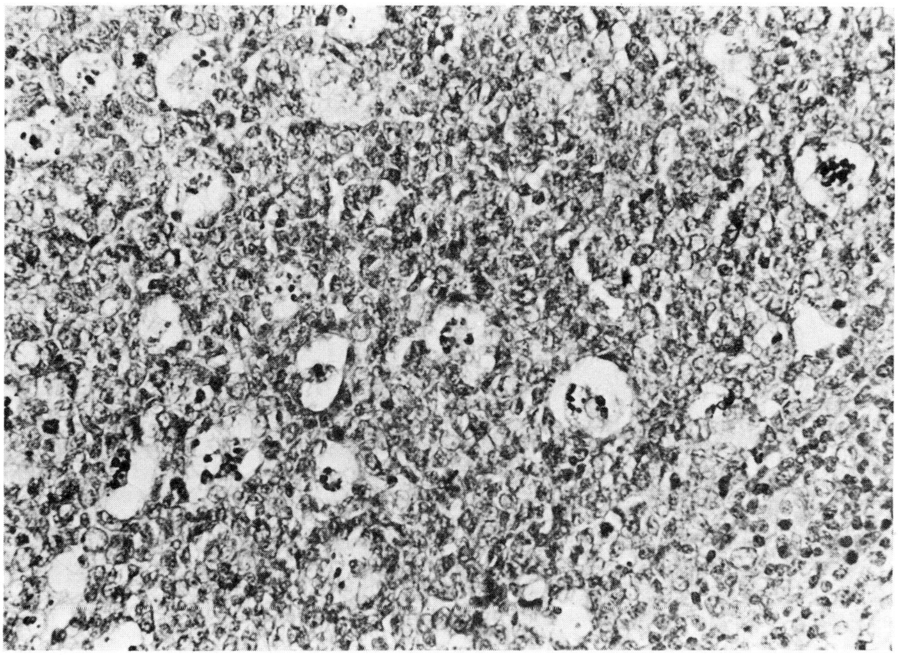

Fig. 1.10 A reactive follicle centre in which there are numerous macrophages with clear cytoplasm containing phagocytosed cell debris; so-called tingible body macrophages, × 250.

less irregular than they appear in tissue sections. They have pale-staining cytoplasm and coarsely aggregated nuclear chromatin. Centroblasts are 4–6 times larger than small lymphocytes with well-defined basophilic cytoplasm. The rounded nucleus contains three or more large nucleoli each surrounded by condensed heterochromatin (Fig. 1.14).

Studies of T-cell deficient patients and thymectomized animals have shown that the T-cell or thymus dependent zone extends from the mid-cortex between the follicles, to the level of the medullary cords (Fig. 1.4). This is variable, however, and the zone may extend up into the outer cortex and also more deeply towards the hilum. A range of lymphocytes is present in the T-zone (Figs 1.15–1.18) with small cells containing round, uncomplicated nuclei predominating. In a stimulated node many larger cells are evident and a proportion of these are characterized by a large open nucleus with a prominent central nucleolus and abundant dark-staining cytoplasm – the so-called immunoblasts. Other large cells with rather pale-staining irregular nuclei and more abundant clear cytoplasm are the interdigitating reticulum cells. The T-cell zone is characterized by the presence of postcapillary venules.

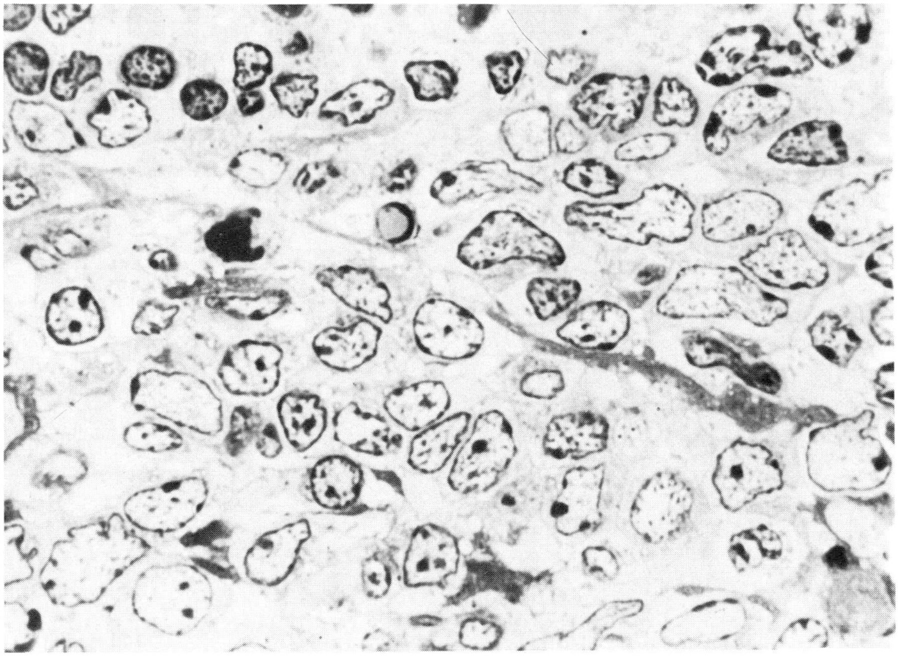

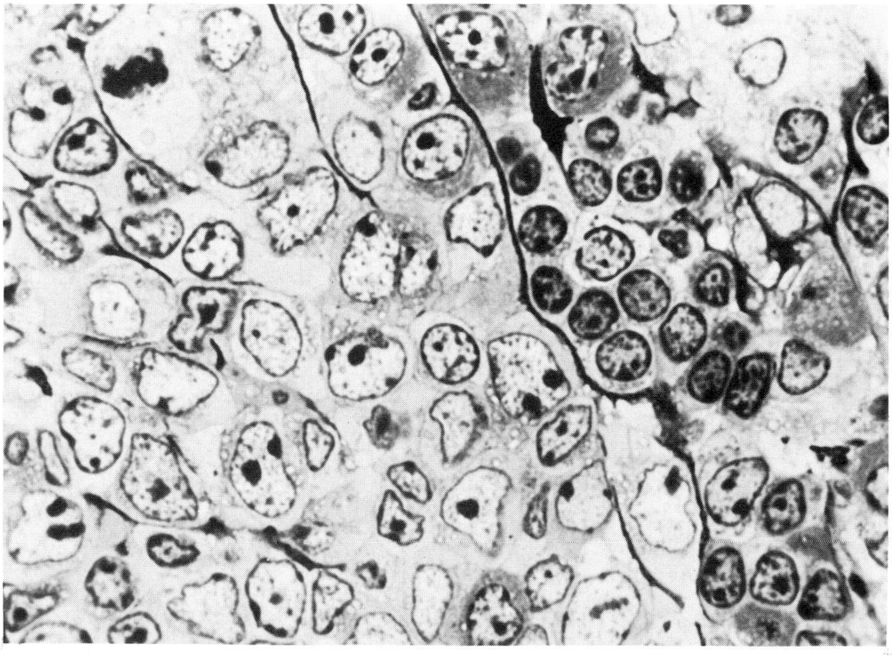

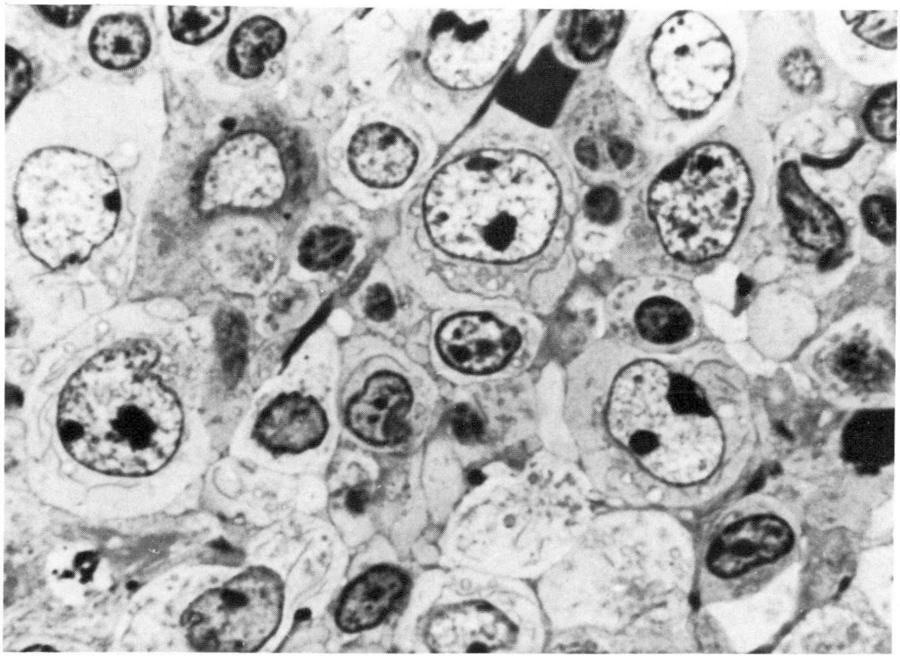

Fig. 1.13 Plastic embedded section demonstrating the abundant cytoplasm of centroblasts within which strands of rough endoplasmic reticulum can be distinguished. Toluidine blue, × 1200.

These blood vessels are lined by tall, plump endothelial cells and are well seen in paraffin sections particularly when stained for reticulin (Fig. 1.1).

In sections embedded in plastic the postcapillary venules are conspicuous structures and lymphocytes can be seen passing between the endothelial cells (Fig. 1.19). The interdigitating reticulum cells are also best seen in plastic sections (Fig. 1.20). These cells with their complex folded nuclei, abundant clear cytoplasm and closely interdigitating cell membranes, contrast with the surrounding small T-lymphocytes.

Within the medullary cords (Fig. 1.21) there is a mixed population of B- and T-cells and it is here that the greatest number of plasma cells is found

---

Fig. 1.11 Plastic embedded section of follicle centre. This section is from the 'light zone' and shows the irregular outline and heterochromatic nuclei of centrocytes, many of which contain small nucleoli. Toluidine blue, × 1000.

Fig. 1.12 Plastic embedded section of the 'dark zone' of the follicle centre showing centroblasts with their characteristic leptochromatic smooth contoured nuclei. The prominent nucleoli are mostly situated on the nuclear membrane. Toluidine blue, × 1000.

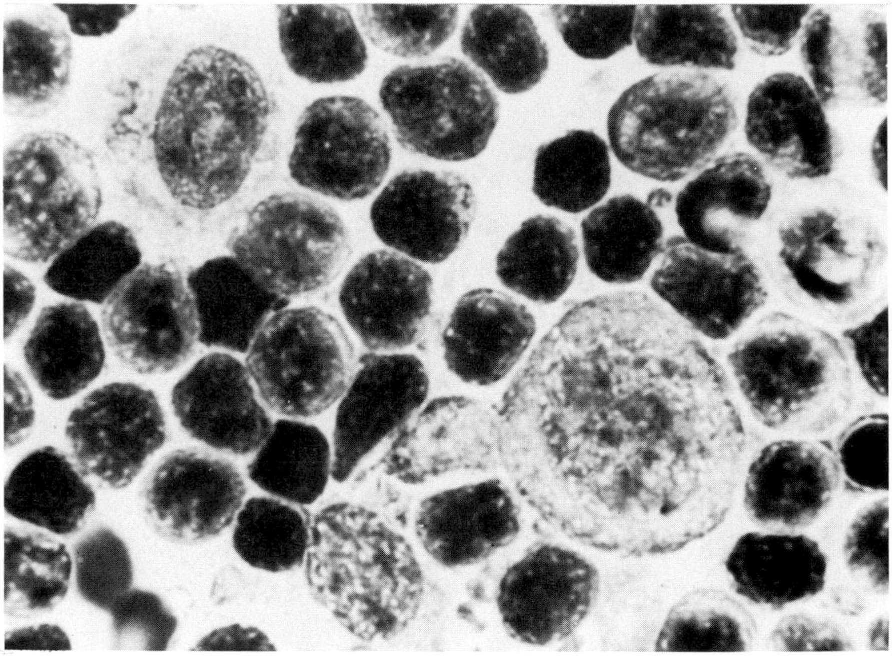

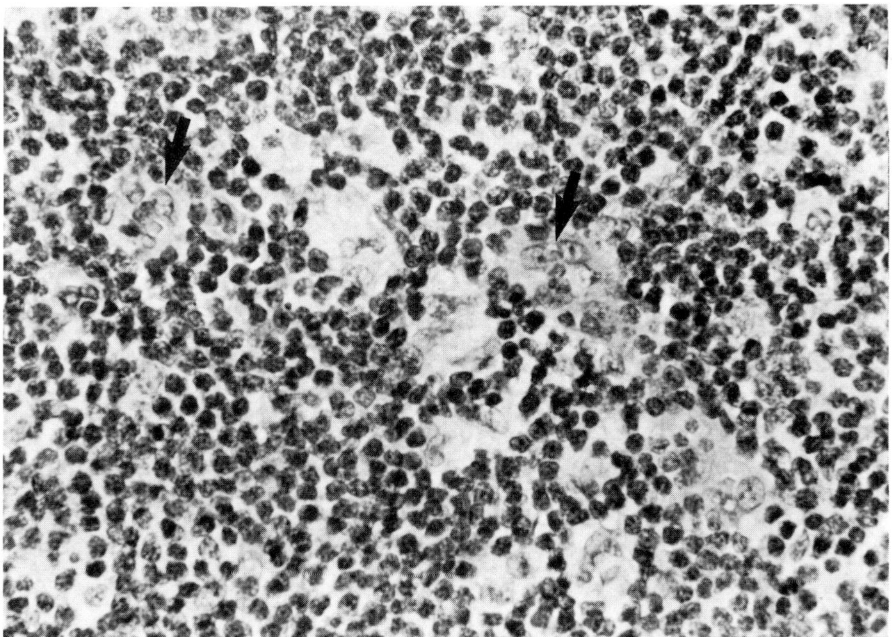

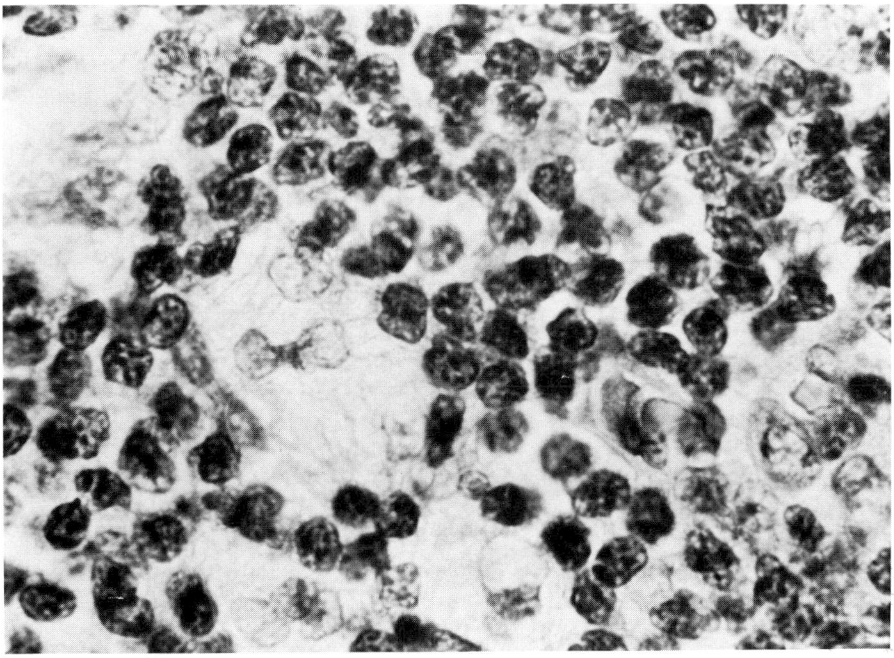

Fig. 1.16 Interdigitating reticulin cells of the T-zone seen under oil immersion. Note their irregular nuclei and abundant pale-staining cytoplasm, × 1000.

(Fig. 1.22).

The special stains that we apply routinely to lymph node biopsies highlight certain features of the reactive lymph node. The reticulin stain as shown in Fig. 1.1 delineates the general structure of the node. The follicles contain few reticulin fibres. They are to a variable degree sharply defined by surrounding reticulin fibres which enclose the whole follicle, that is the follicle centre and the mantle zone. This appearance is in contrast to neoplastic follicles where compressed reticulin may surround the neoplastic follicle alone (see Chapter 7). The reticulin stain also outlines the sinusoidal pattern of the node, which may be obscured by the intrasinusoidal accumulation of cells. The T-cell areas are also well

---

Fig. 1.14 Giemsa stained imprint from a reactive lymph node. Smaller centrocytes with coarsely aggregated nuclear chromatin contrast with large centroblast which contains abundant cytoplasm and prominent nucleoli. The cell at top left is a histiocyte, × 1200.

Fig. 1.15 The T-cell zone (paracortex) of the lymph node showing postcapillary venules with their high endothelial lining (arrows) and scattered interdigitating reticulum cells distinguished by their clear cytoplasm, × 400.

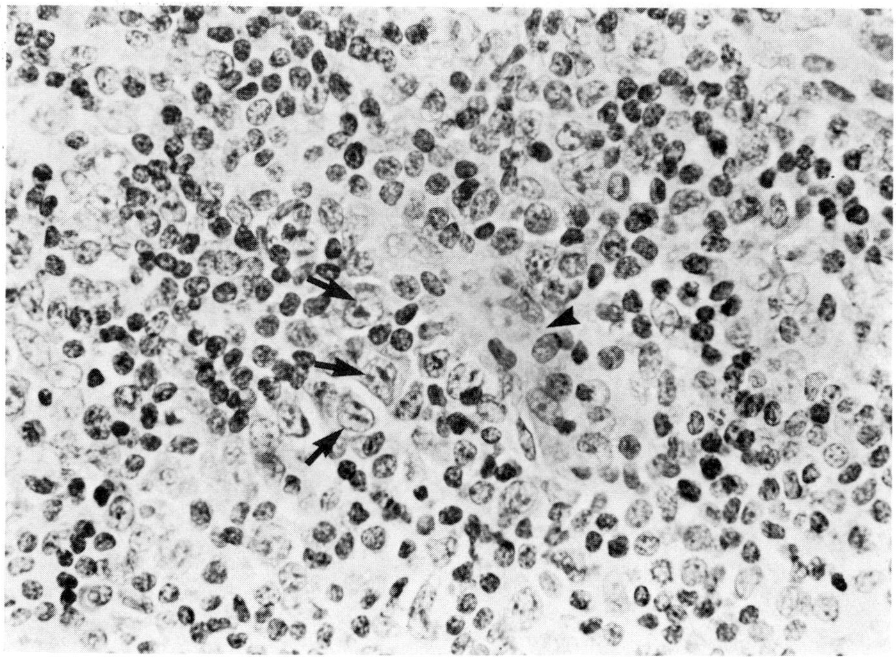

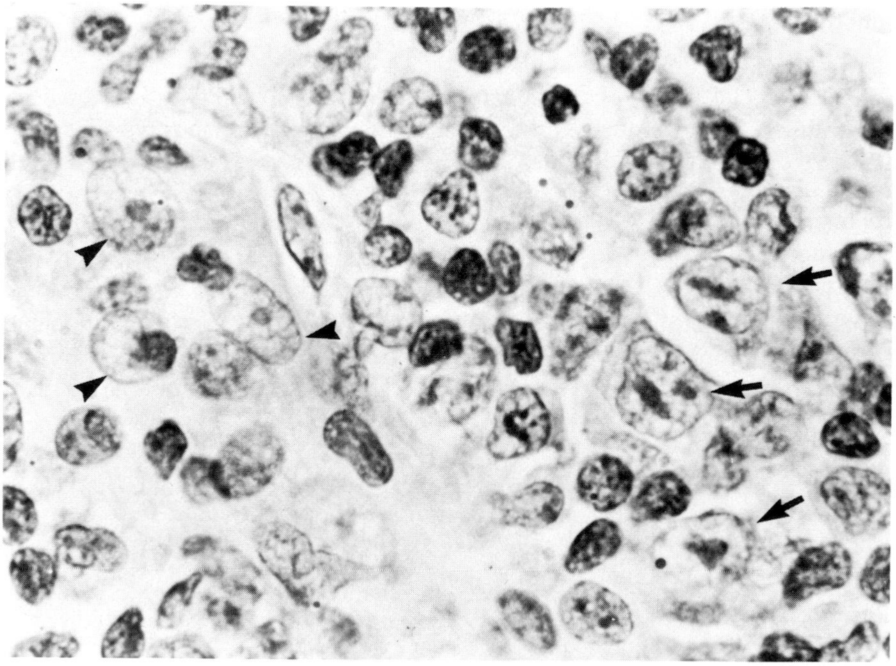

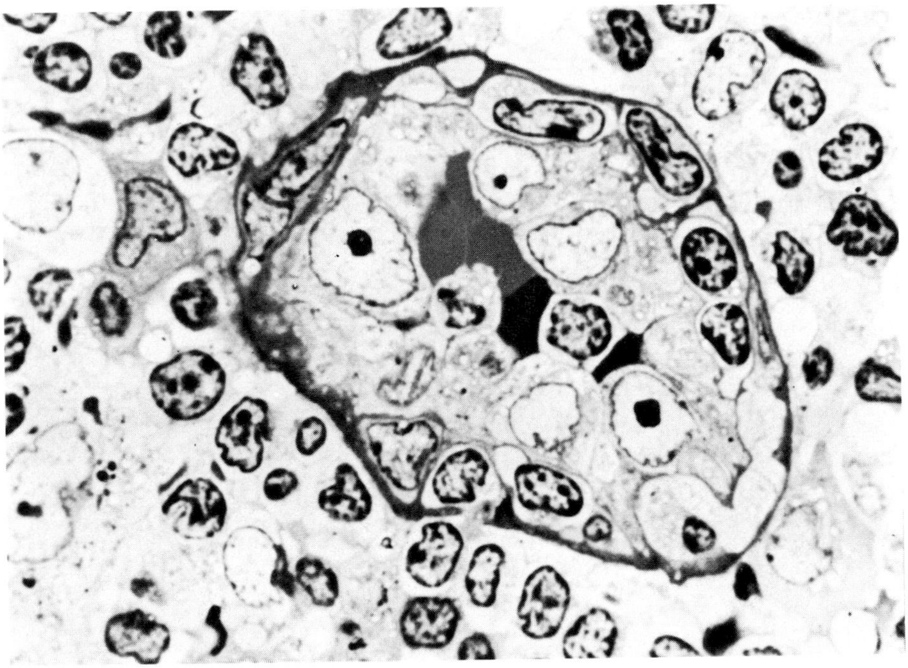

Fig. 1.19 Plastic embedded section of lymph node T-zone showing a postcapillary venule. Lymphocytes are present in the lumen and between the tall endothelial cells and the basement membrane. Toluidine blue, × 1200.

outlined by the reticulin stain which shows a fine reticulin network punctuated by postcapillary venules. Staining with PAS highlights the thick basement membrane of postcapillary venules and often stains material within follicle centre cell macrophages. Immunoglobulin inclusions within cells may also be PAS positive. The methyl green pyronin (MGP) stain shows up the strongly pyroninophilic cytoplasm of plasma cells, especially in the medullary cords. Follicle centre cells also have pyroninophilic cytoplasm, although less so than plasma cells, with centroblasts showing more pyroninophilia than centrocytes. This variation in pyroninophilia highlights the different zones within the follicle centre, a feature that is absent in neoplastic follicles. Within T-cell areas T-immunoblasts may also be strikingly pyroninophilic. Lennert

---

Fig. 1.17 T-immunoblasts (arrows) adjacent to a postcapillary venule (arrowhead) in the lymph node T-zone, × 400.
Fig. 1.18 T-immunoblasts (arrows) seen under oil immersion. Their defined cytoplasm and dark nucleoli contrast with endothelial cells (arrowheads), × 1000.

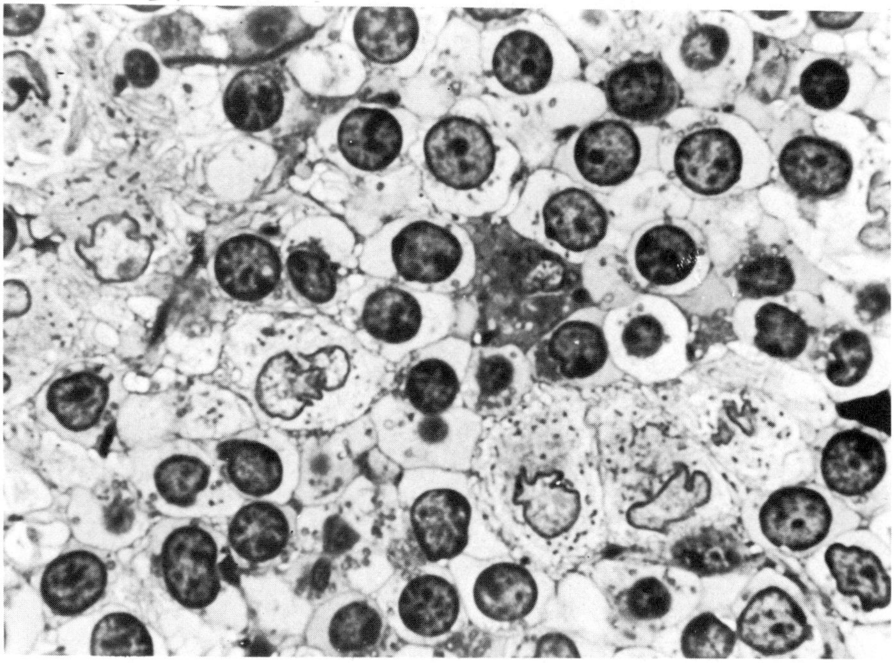

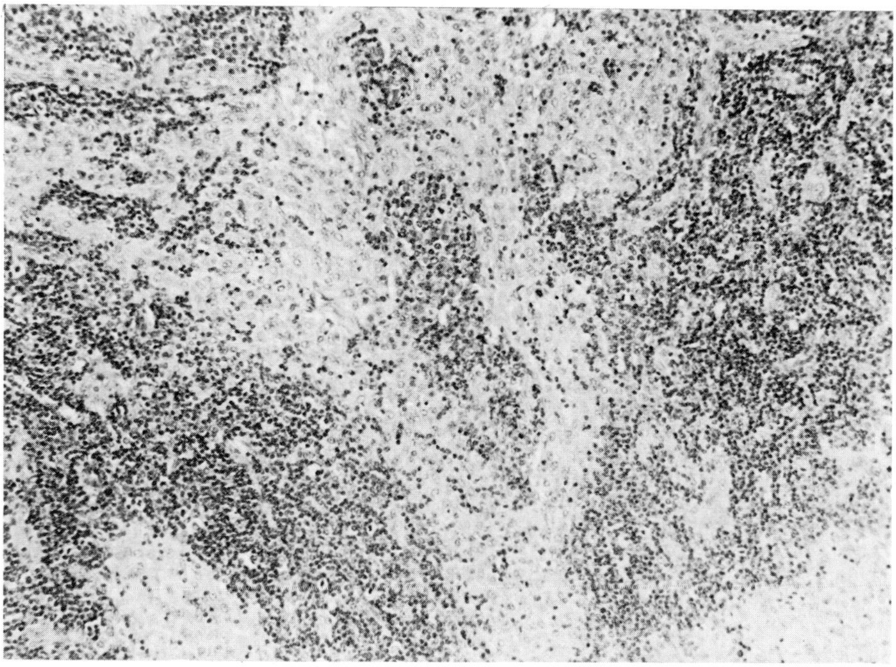

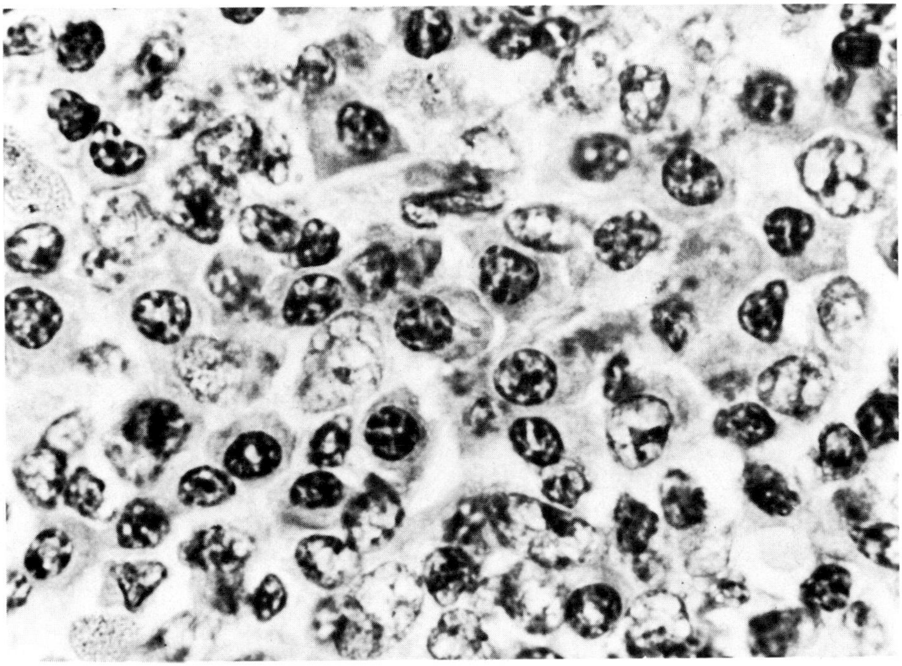

Fig. 1.22 Lymph node medulla seen under oil immersion. There are numerous plasma cells, × 1000.

(1981) strongly advocates the use of the Giemsa stain for the study of lymphoid tissues. The basic dye in this stain has an affinity for ribonucleic acid similar to that shown by pyronin. Thus cells that show cytoplasmic pyroninophilia with the methyl green pyronin stain will be basophilic in Giemsa-stained sections.

There is some variation of lymph node structure according to the anatomical site of the node. Resting axillary and inguinal lymph nodes consist largely of an adipose tissue core with only a narrow marginal zone of lymphoid tissue (Fig. 1.23). Inguinal nodes, especially, may show distortion of their normal architecture by bands of fibrous tissue resulting from previous inflammation. In mesenteric lymph nodes (Fig. 1.24), sinuses and medullary cords are particularly prominent and follicles may be inconspicuous.

Fig. 1.20 Plastic embedded section of the lymph node T-zone showing interdigitating reticulum cells amidst small lymphocytes. Toluidine blue, × 1200.
Fig. 1.21 Section of medulla of lymph node showing cords of cells separated by sinuses filled with histiocytes, × 100.

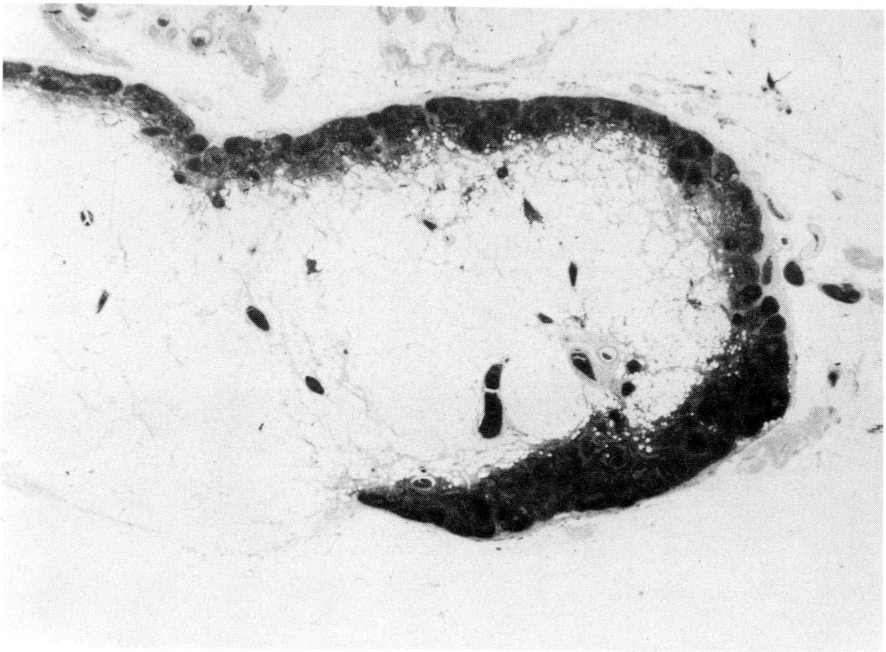

Fig. 1.23 Section of resting axillary lymph nodes showing a rim of lymphoid tissue surrounding fat, × 12.

The relationship between the structure and the function of the lymph node merits a brief review. Antigen enters the node through the afferent lymphatics and depending on the nature and the quantity of the antigen some will be taken up by sinusoidal histiocytes and possibly degraded and some will enter the follicles. Here it is trapped and processed by dendritic reticulum cells which, together with appropriate T-lymphocytes, appear to instruct and select clones of antibody-producing B-cells. In nodes undergoing intense antigenic stimulation antibody (immunoglobulin) producing centroblasts and centrocytes may be seen in the germinal follicles but it is more usual for B-cells to leave the follicle and to mature into antibody-producing plasma cells either in the medullary cords or at other sites in the body. Stimulated lymphocytes leave the lymph node through the efferent lymphatics and enter the circulation by way of the thoracic duct. The lymph node is repopulated by T- and B-lymphocytes from the peripheral blood. These cells enter the node between the tall endothelial cells of the postcapillary venules and thence migrate to thc appropriate area of the node. Antigens that stimulate an antibody response will cause follicular hyperplasia in which the follicles become more numerous and larger and show centroblast

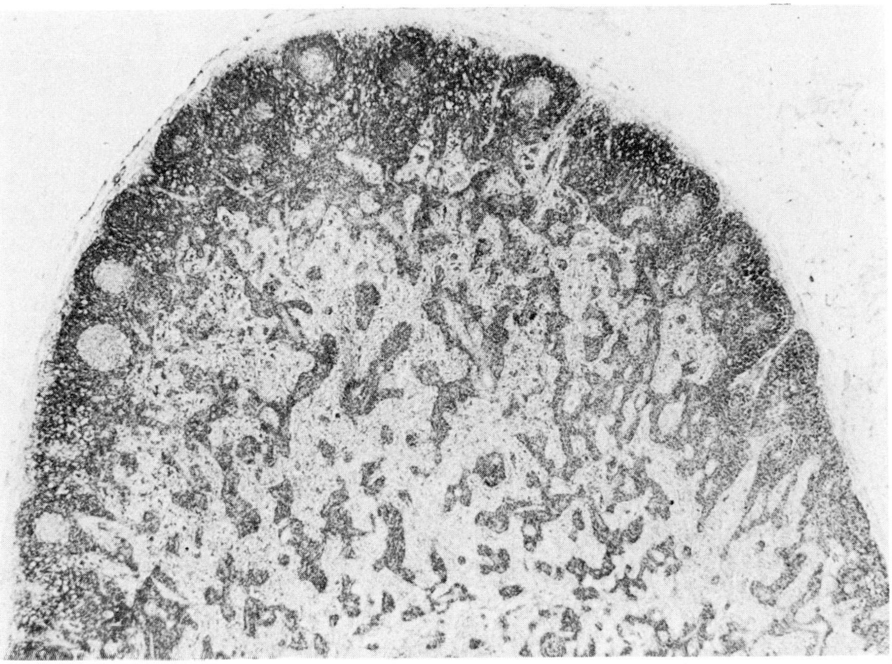

Fig. 1.24 A mesenteric lymph node. The bulk of a node consists of medullary cords and sinuses, × 20.

proliferation. Stimuli that elicit a T-cell response result in expansion of the paracortex of the lymph node usually with increased prominence of the postcapillary venules and, in some circumstances, accompanied by a proliferation of interdigitating reticulum cells. T-cell stimulation also leads to a proliferation of T-immunoblasts in the paracortex, a reaction typically seen in a number of virus infections.

The relationship between the structure and function of the lymph node is particularly well illustrated by the staining of specific cells using immunohistochemical techniques on frozen sections (Stein *et al.*, 1980). Monoclonal antibodies specific for T-cell subsets stain most of the cells of the paracortex. Scattered (helper and suppressor) T-cells can be demonstrated within the follicle and within the mantle (Fig. 1.25). Most of the cells in the mantle can be distinguished by the presence of surface IgM and IgD (Fig. 1.26). These 'virgin' cells are recruited into the follicle following antigenic stimulation. In reactive lymph nodes a lace-work pattern of IgM staining, presumably on the surface of dendritic reticulum cells, can be seen in the outer zone of the germinal follicles (Fig. 1.27).

The histology of malignant lymphomas, both architecturally and cytologically, relates closely to the histology of the normal or reactive

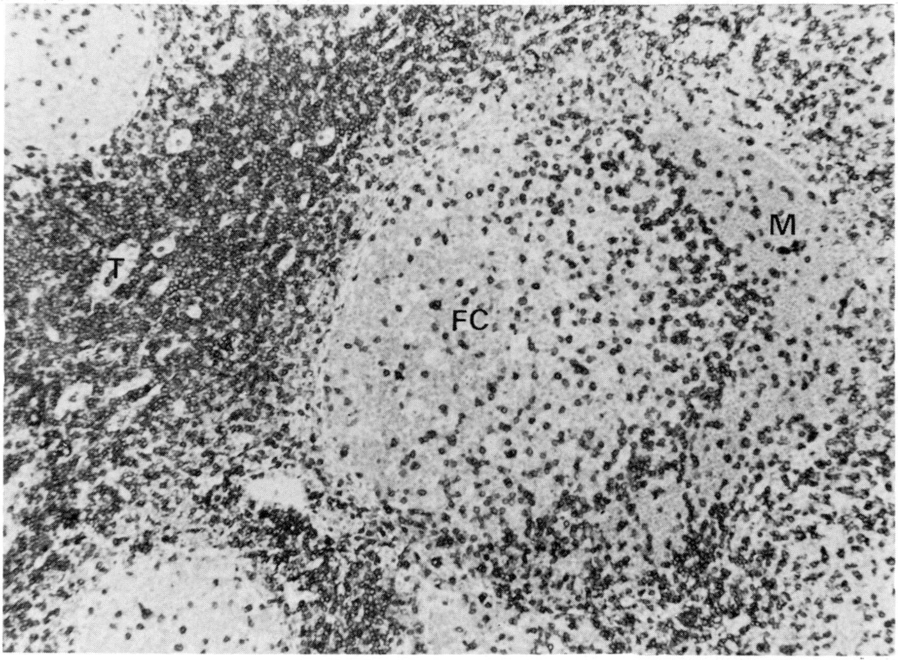

Fig. 1.25 A frozen section of a reactive lymph node stained with a monoclonal antibody to T-cells using an immunoperoxidase technique. There is positive staining of most cells in the T-zone (T) within which the postcapillary venules stand out as negative staining structures. Within the follicle centre (FC) T-cells are concentrated towards the mantle (M) in the 'light zone', × 80.

lymph node. Lymphomas derived from follicle centre cells often themselves form follicles both within and outside lymph nodes and cytologically are composed of mixtures of centroblasts and centrocytes in varying proportions. Recognition of this fact has, perhaps, been the most significant recent advance in the classification of non-Hodgkin's lymphomas. Dendritic reticulum cells can be demonstrated by electron microscopy in neoplastic follicles; further evidence of their relationship to normal follicles.

T-cell lymphomas usually arise in the paracortical area of the lymph nodes, often with sparing of the follicles which survive in a sea of

---

Fig. 1.26 A frozen section of a reactive lymph node follicle stained by an immunoperoxidase technique for IgD. There is positive staining of the surfaces of most of the small lymphocytes of the mantle zone, × 80.

Fig. 1.27 In this frozen section stained for IgM a lacework pattern of positive staining is evident in the follicle centre concentrated towards the mantle in the 'light zone'. The mantle lymphocytes show positive surface staining, × 80.

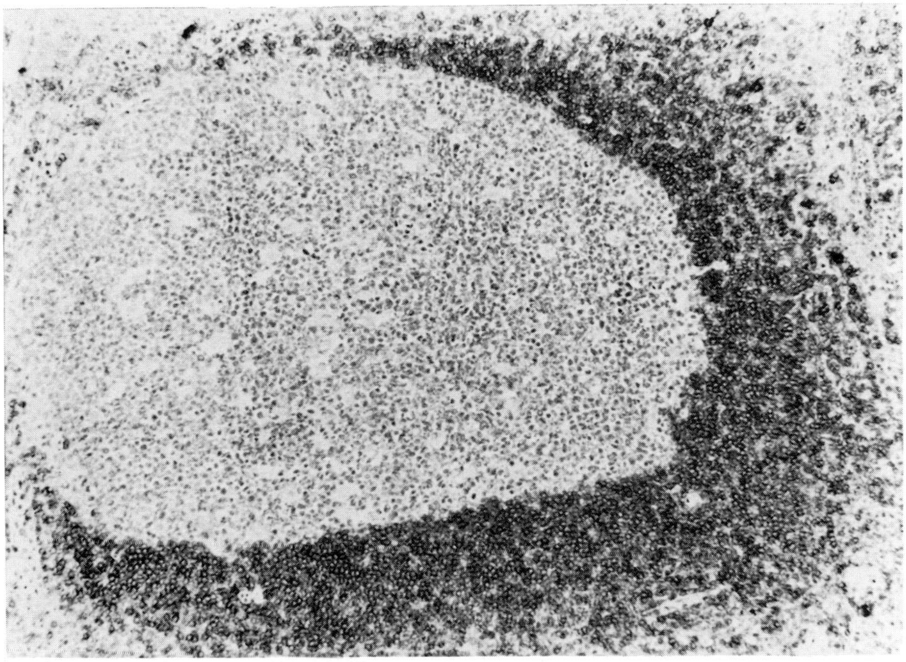

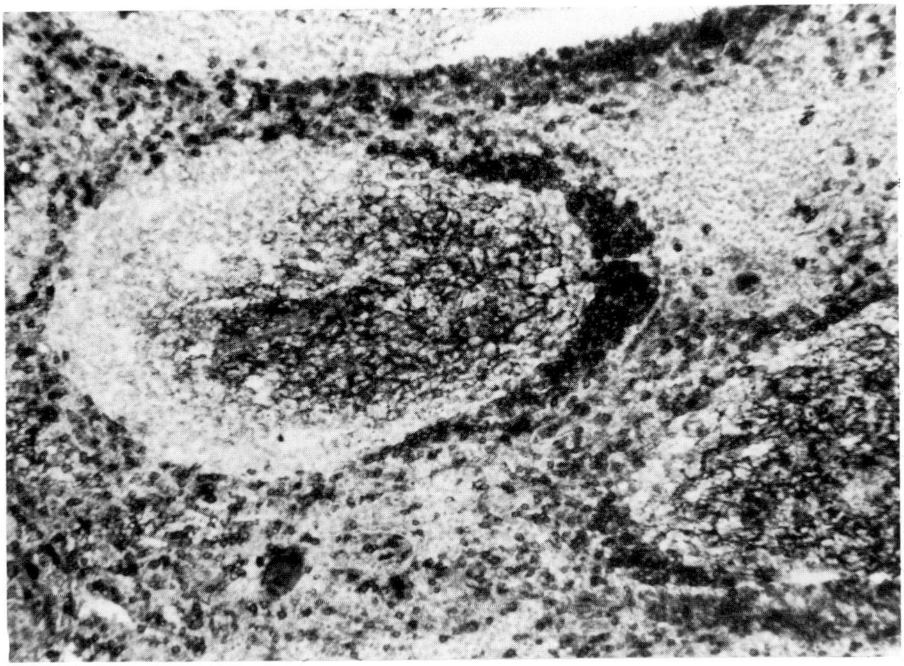

lymphoma cells. They are often accompanied by a marked proliferation of blood vessels with high endothelium resembling normal postcapillary venules. Some T-cell lymphomas are characterized by the presence of large numbers of epithelioid histiocytes, a feature that may be related to the production of lymphokines by the tumour cells.

Neoplastic involvement of the sinuses as a predominant feature usually excludes either B- or T-cell lymphoma but is characteristic of some true histiocytic malignancies as well as being a feature of metastatic neoplasms.

1.2 The spleen

Splenectomy either for diagnostic or therapeutic purposes or as part of a staging procedure is now a fairly common undertaking in patients with malignant lymphoma. As with the lymph node an appreciation of the normal histology of the spleen is essential if the changes that occur in lymphoma, are to be understood. Again the normal morphology is seen to advantage in sections stained for reticulin. The spleen (Fig. 1.28) is surrounded by a capsule of fibroelastic tissue from which trabeculae extend into the parenchyma. These meet up with arborizing fibrous trabeculae extending from the hilum. Arteries and veins are situated within these trabeculae and it is by following the circulation from the trabeculae that the more detailed histology of the spleen can best be understood. As the small arteries or arterioles leave the trabeculae they become ensheathed with T-lymphocytes. Focally these sheaths expand to form reticulin-rich lymphoid nodules of periarteriolar T-cells with an adjacent reticulin-depleted follicle centre comprised of B-cells (Figs 1.29 and 1.30). These nodules form the white pulp of the spleen. As the arterioles of the white pulp fade into the red pulp, linking with the sinusoids, the lymphoid tissue gradually decreases in density and consists of a mixture of T-cells, B-cells and immunoblasts. It is here, in the so-called marginal zone, that lymphocytes are thought to enter the spleen before migrating to T- and B-cell areas. The red pulp of the spleen consists of 'pulp cords' separated by sinusoids (Fig. 1.31). Within the cords are

---

Fig. 1.28 Section of spleen stained for reticulin. Fibrous trabeculae extend into the spleen from the capsule. The red pulp (R) consists of anastamosing sinusoids. The white pulp consists of reticulin free B-cell areas (B) and reticulin rich T-cell areas (T) around arteriolar branches, × 25.

Fig. 1.29 T-cell areas of the spleen (T) follow arteriolar branches and contain a fine reticulin network similar to that seen in the lymph node T-zone (Fig. 1.2). B-cell areas (B) with follicle centres (FC) form expanding nodules adjacent to the T-zones, × 40.

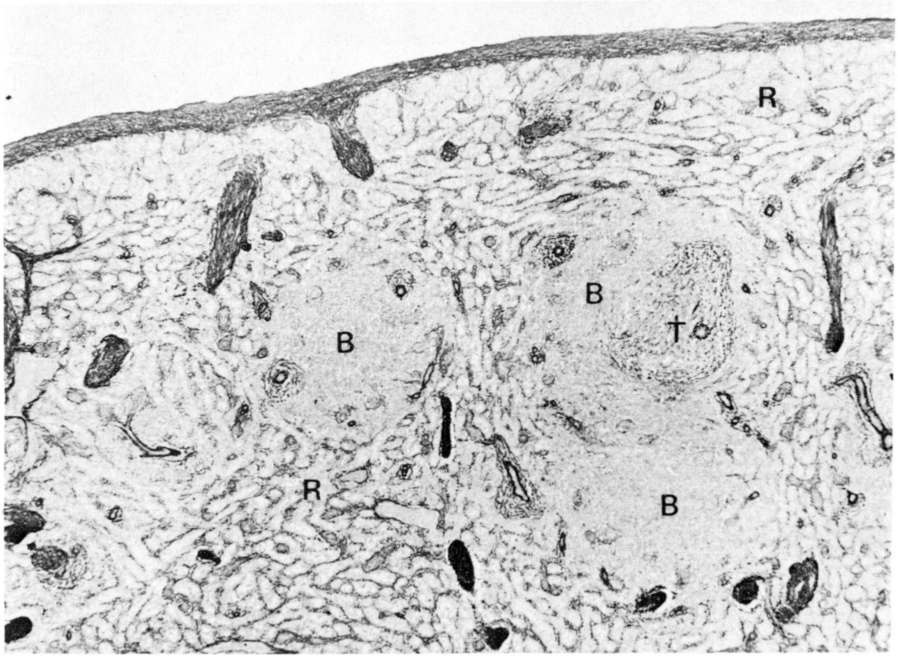
R
B
B
T
R
B

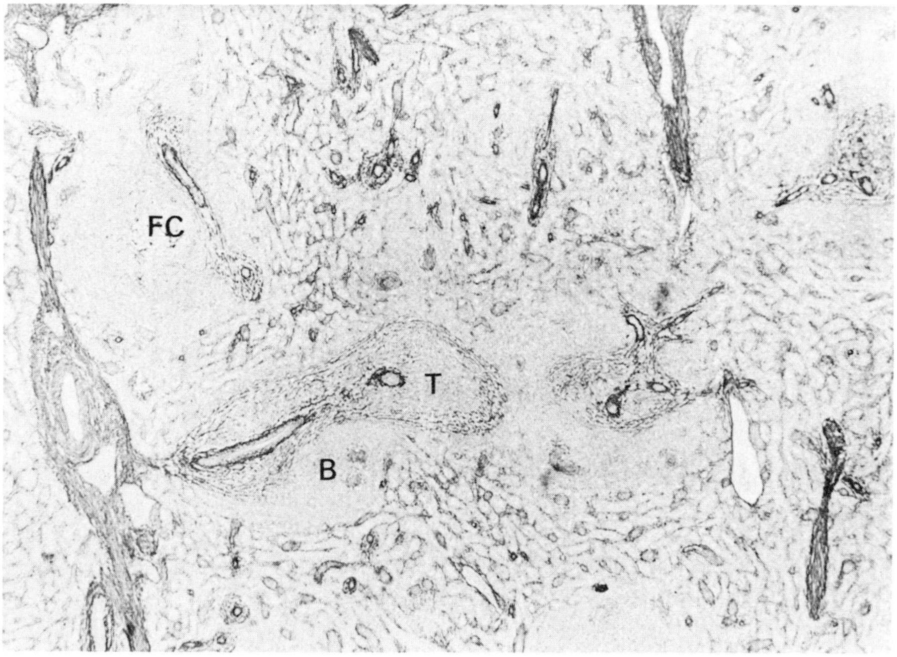
FC
T
B

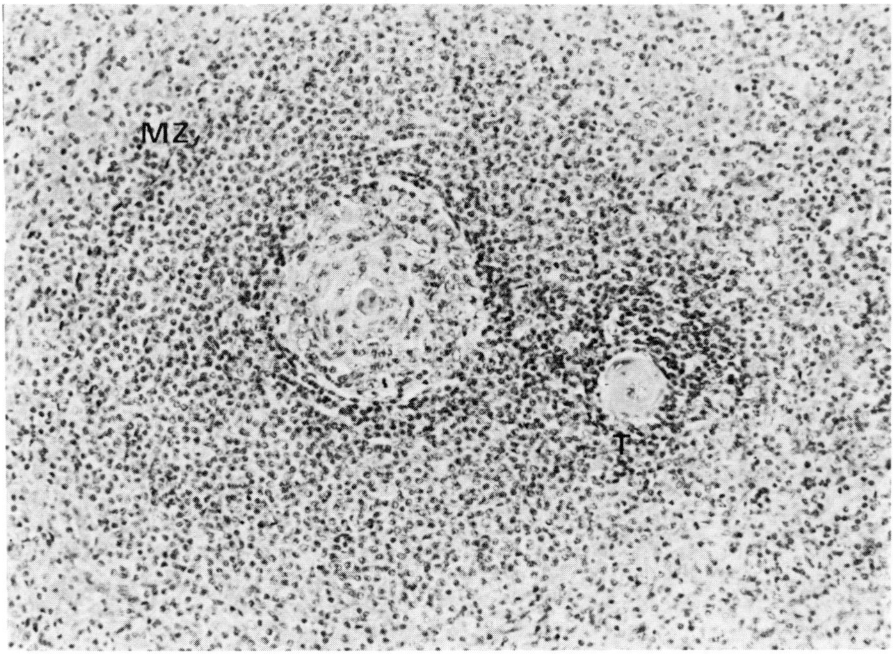
MZ
T

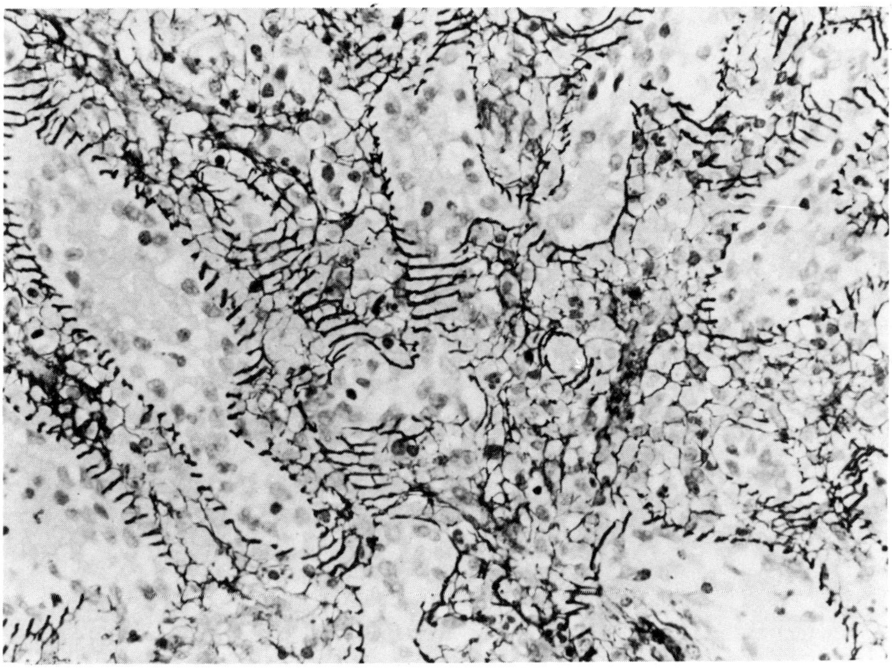

macrophages, red blood cells and plasma cells. The sinusoids are surrounded by characteristic hoop fibres and are lined by discontinuous endothelial cells and hence their lumens communicate directly with the pulp cords. Exactly how the blood passes from arterioles to sinusoids, whether directly or indirectly via the pulp cords, is controversial but once in the sinusoids the blood drains into trabecular veins and so into the splenic vein.

As in the lymph nodes, follicle centre cell lymphomas in the spleen characteristically involve the B-cell areas of the white pulp while T-cell malignancies localize around the arterioles. Diffuse infiltration of the red pulp occurs in a number of conditions, including malignant histiocytosis, small lymphocytic lymphomas, lymphoplasmacytic lymphomas and hairy cell leukaemia.

References

Lennert, K. (1981) *Histopathology of Non-Hodgkin's Lymphomas (Based on the Kiel Classification)*, Springer-Verlag, Berlin, Heidelberg, New York.

Stein, H., Bonk, A., Tolksdorf, G. *et al.* (1980) Immunohistologic analysis of the organisation of normal lymphoid tissue and non-Hodgkin's lymphomas. *J. Histochem. Cytochem.*, **28**, 746–60.

Fig. 1.30 Section of spleen showing the periarteriolar T-zone (T) with an adjacent B-area containing a follicle centre. The marginal zone (MZ) is at the interface between the red and white pulp, × 120.

Fig. 1.31 A section of splenic red pulp stained with methanamine silver. The characteristic hoop fibres that surround the sinusoids are well seen in this type of preparation, × 400.

2 Infectious and granulomatous conditions of lymph nodes

A wide variety of infectious agents may cause lymphadenopathy and only the most common will be considered here. Amongst these are the viral lymphadenopathies which, since they produce relatively similar histological appearances in lymph nodes, are conveniently considered as a group. A number of non-viral infectious lymphadenopathies are characterized by granulomatous inflammation and this is also true of some non-infectious conditions. In practical terms the histopathologist is faced with the differential diagnosis of granulomatous inflammation in the lymph node biopsy and for this reason most types of granulomatous inflammation, whether due to infection or not, are considered in this chapter.

2.1 Viral infections of lymph nodes

Lymphadenopathy due to infectious mononucleosis is of importance since both clinically and histologically it may closely simulate malignant lymphoma. Many other viral infections result in lymphadenopathy but lymph node biopsy is rarely performed in these conditions. Enlarged lymph nodes which occur in association with *Herpes zoster* infection are, however, occasionally biopsied and the histological appearances of these two conditions will be described here.

Infectious mononucleosis is predominantly a disease of adolescents and young adults. It follows infection with the Epstein–Barr (EB) virus which appears usually to be transmitted by oral secretions. Exposure to the virus in childhood results in a trivial or inapparent clinical response. The virus specifically infects B-lymphocytes, which have receptors for EB virus, and causes lymphoproliferation. The infected B-lymphocytes elicit a vigorous T-lymphocyte response with the production of killer T-cells. It is at this stage of T-lymphocyte response that the patient becomes symptomatic. In the early stages of the disease B-lymphoblasts are found in the peripheral blood to be replaced as the disease progresses by

T-blasts. Various apparently inappropriate antibodies are produced during the disease including autoantibodies and a heterophile antibody to sheep red cells that forms the basis of the diagnostic heterophile antibody test.

2.1.1 *Histology*

Lymph node biopsy is not performed as a deliberate diagnostic procedure in infectious mononucleosis so the experience of any one pathologist is likely to be very limited. Carter and Penman (1969) described the most striking morphological feature of this condition as 'the wild hyperplasia of lymphoreticular elements'. Unless the pathologist is aware of this hyperplasia there is a danger that he will categorize these lesions as malignant lymphoma. There is variable follicular hyperplasia but, as the disease progresses, the follicles become widely separated by expanding paracortical tissue (Fig. 2.1) and they may become gradually replaced by amorphous eosinophilic material (Fig. 2.2). A more constant feature is an intense proliferation of blast cells in the paracortex (Figs 2.2 and 2.3) accompanied by a marked increase in the vascularity of this area. There is

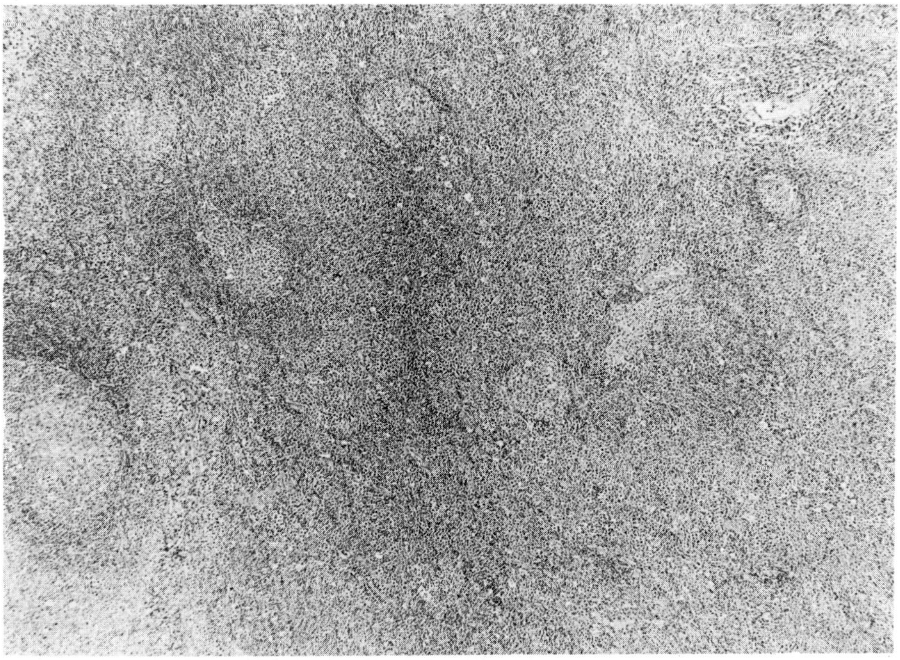

Fig. 2.1 Lymph node in infectious mononucleosis showing follicles widely separated by expanding paracortical tissue, × 20.

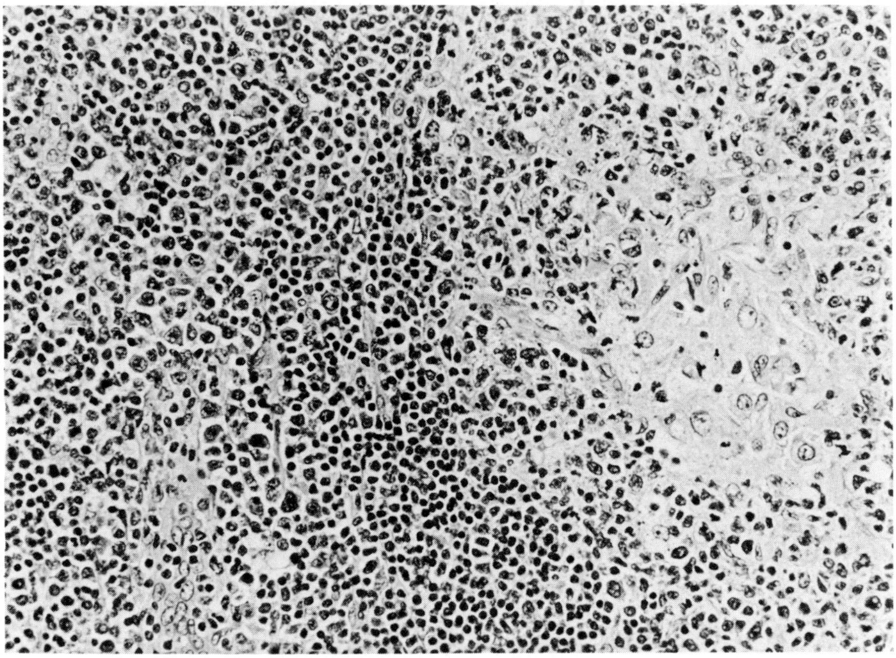

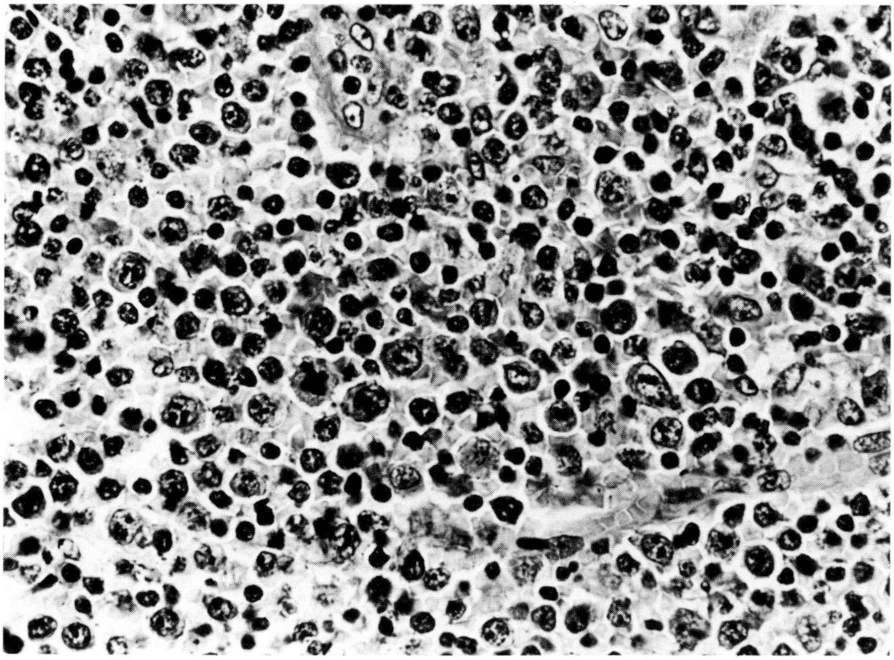

a concomitant proliferation of blast cells in the medullary cords. Carter and Penman (1969) remarked on the paucity of plasma cells in infectious mononucleosis even in the late stages of the disease. The florid blast cell proliferation induced by infectious mononucleosis may extend into the sinuses and partially obliterate the lymph node structure giving rise to an appearance resembling diffuse large cell lymphoma. This proliferative process may extend into perinodal tissues (Fig. 2.4) and may invade the

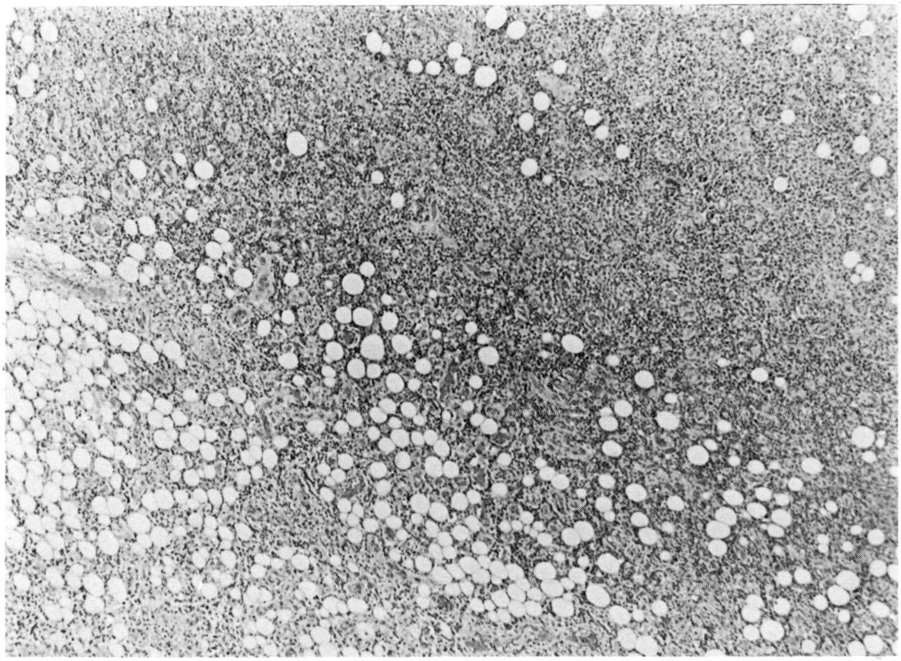

Fig. 2.4 Infiltration of perinodal fat in a case of infectious mononucleosis, × 32.

walls of large veins (Fig. 2.5). The presence of such a proliferation predominantly in the paracortex with the persistence of some residual nodal architecture, particularly in a young patient, should suggest the possibility of infectious mononucleosis and initiate the appropriate serological investigations. Reed–Sternberg-like cells are sometimes seen

---

Fig. 2.2 Follicle centre in infectious mononucleosis showing replacement by amorphous material. Atypical cells are readily apparent in the adjacent paracortex, × 250.
Fig. 2.3 Proliferating cells in the paracortex of a lymph node from a patient with infectious mononucleosis. Numerous 'blast' forms are present, × 400.

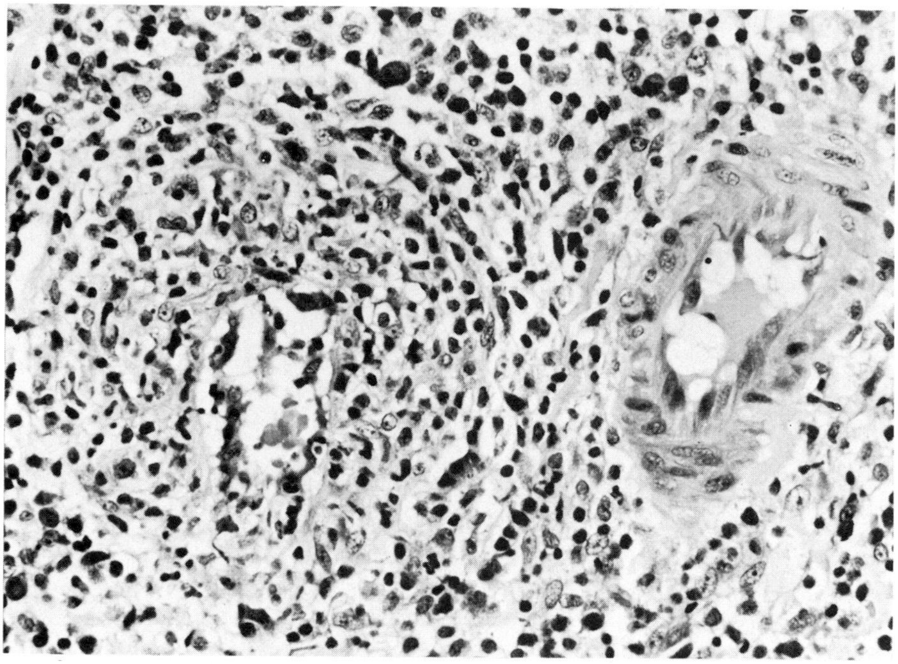

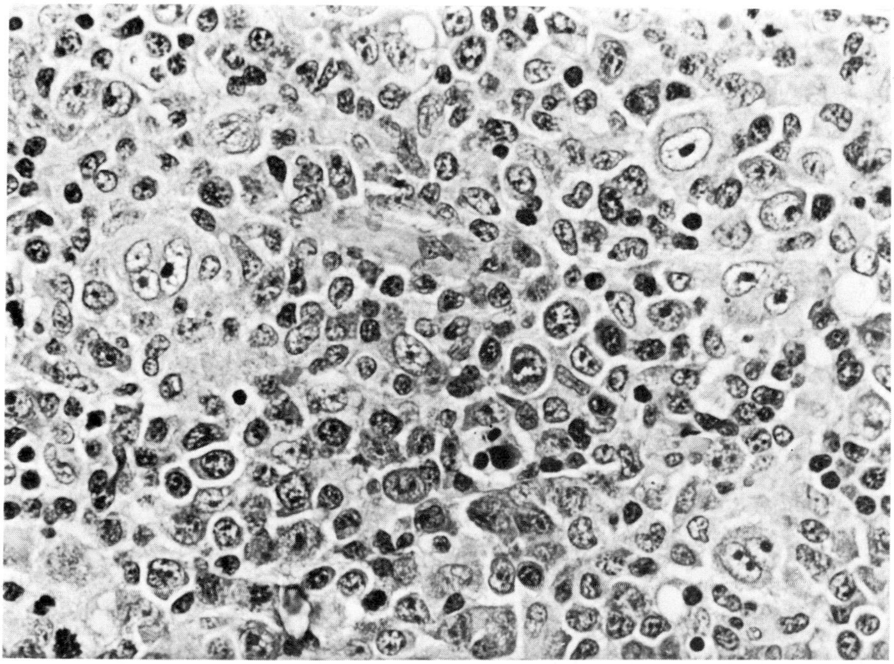

(Tindle *et al.*, 1972) in the lymph nodes of patients with infectious mononucleosis (Fig. 2.6). Vascular proliferation with engorged thin-walled vessels predominantly in the paracortex (Fig. 2.7) is a characteristic feature of infectious mononucleosis. These vessels do not show the complex arborization patterns typically seen in angioimmunoblastic lymphadenopathy.

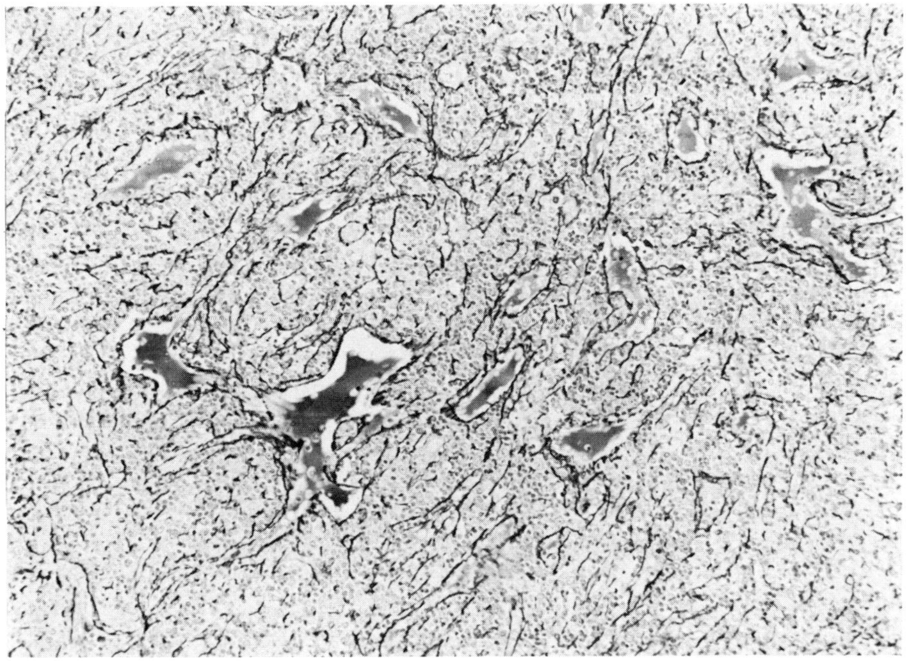

Fig. 2.7 Reticulin stain of a section of lymph node from a case of infectious mononucleosis. Numerous thin-walled blood vessels are present in the paracortex, × 100.

The tendency of the spleen to rupture in infectious mononucleosis makes this organ available for histopathological examination. The lymphoid follicles are not conspicuous but there is a marked proliferation of lymphoid cells in the splenic cords, sometimes leading to obliteration

---

Fig. 2.5 Proliferating cells in infectious mononucleosis invading the wall of a large vein, × 250.

Fig. 2.6 Numerous cells resembling Reed–Sternberg and mononuclear Hodgkin's cells may be present in infectious mononucleosis. Note the 'setting' of these cells in a sea of blasts which is wholly untypical for Hodgkin's disease, × 400.

of the sinusoids. Small areas of necrosis and of subcapsular and intrasplenic haemorrhage are frequently seen.

Hepatitis may occur during the course of infectious mononucleosis. This is probably mediated by immunological mechanisms since the EB virus is not known to be hepatotrophic. Liver biopsy may show portal and focal lobular infiltrates of lymphoid cells with increased numbers of plasma cells as the disease progresses. Focal necrosis and evidence of cellular regeneration may be present.

2.1.2 *Differential diagnosis*

The intense blast cell proliferation that occurs in infectious mononucleosis may mimic malignant lymphoma. Its distribution in the T-dependent paracortex with residual lymphoid follicles is not consistent with a B-cell lymphoma and the main differential diagnosis is T-immunoblastic sarcoma. The residual follicles in T-cell lymphomas are often active and do not show the degenerative effete changes seen in infectious mononucleosis. Vascular proliferation is prominent in both conditions but in infectious mononucleosis the vessels are usually dilated and congested whereas in T-cell lymphomas the high endothelial cells often appear to obliterate the lumen of the vessel. In general the proliferation in infectious mononucleosis is more polymorphic than in malignant lymphoma; however it would be wise to take into account clinical and immunological data before diagnosing T-immunoblastic sarcoma in a young patient.

The presence of Reed–Sternberg-like cells in infectious mononucleosis should not cause confusion with Hodgkin's disease since the background population of blast cells is not consistent with any of the recognized subtypes of Hodgkin's disease.

When enlarged lymph nodes are associated with *Herpes zoster* biopsy may be undertaken in the impression that the *Herpes zoster* is present as a complication of lymphoma (Patterson *et al.*, 1980). The histological appearances of the lymph nodes are not unlike those of infectious mononucleosis, with proliferation of lymphocytes in the T-areas of the nodes (paracortex) and variable follicular hyperplasia. Proliferating immunoblasts in the paracortex give the node a 'mottled' appearance but there is seldom the degree of lymphoproliferation that is seen in infectious mononucleosis. These appearances are common to many 'viral lymphadenopathies' and give no clue to the particular virus involved.

2.2 Granulomatous inflammation of lymph nodes

A wide variety of infective and non-infective non-neoplastic conditions are characterized by granulomatous inflammation within lymph nodes. It is important to be familiar with these both for their own sake and to avoid confusion with certain malignant lymphomas which themselves are characterized by the presence of granulomas; in particular Hodgkin's disease and malignant lymphoma with epithelioid histiocytes (Lennert's lymphoma). Although there is considerable overlap, granulomatous conditions of lymph nodes can be usefully divided according to the type of granulomatous inflammation produced. This may take the form of classical epithelioid granulomas, granulomas with central abscesses, often stellate in shape, or scattered aggregates of epithelioid cells without distinctive granuloma formation. It should be emphasized that in the early stages of their evolution these small epithelioid cell aggregates are found in all granulomatous conditions of lymph nodes.

Classical epithelioid granulomas are found in lymph nodes involved by tuberculosis, sarcoidosis, Crohn's disease and sometimes in nodes draining the site of a malignant tumour. Epithelioid granulomas may be seen in uninvolved lymph nodes and the spleen in Hodgkin's disease. They are also present in a rare but important condition, chronic granulomatous disease of childhood. The all too familiar histology of tuberculosis (Fig. 2.8) hardly needs description here. While caseation

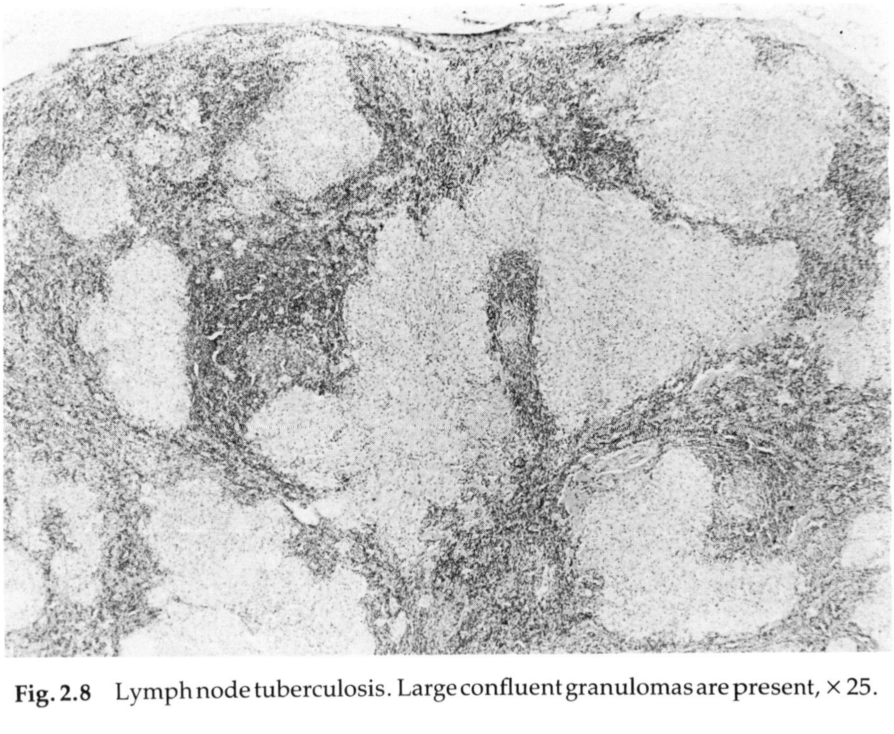

Fig. 2.8 Lymph node tuberculosis. Large confluent granulomas are present, × 25.

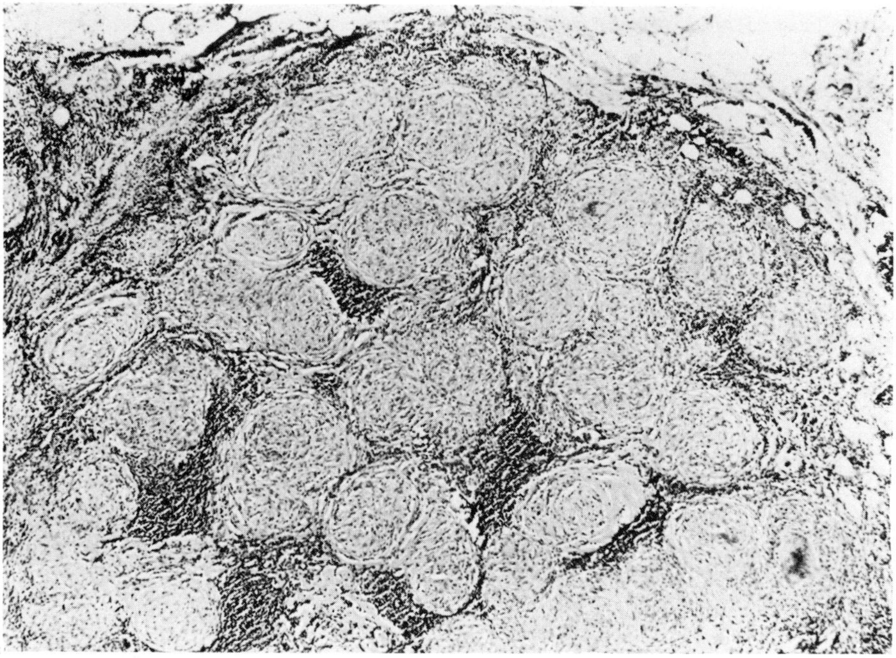

Fig. 2.9 Sarcoidosis of lymph node. The tightly packed non-caseating granulomas tend not to fuse as they do in tuberculosis, × 25.

necrosis is an important distinguishing feature of this disease, it is by no means always present and tuberculosis should be considered when granulomas of any description are found in a lymph node. The granulomas of sarcoidosis (Fig. 2.9) are usually small and multiple and whilst they efface much of the normal nodal tissue, tend to remain discrete, not fusing into larger lesions as occurs in tuberculosis; multinucleated giant cells are also not as frequent and there is often considerable fibrosis around the granulomas. Necrosis of sarcoid granulomas occurs infrequently (Fig. 2.10). The mesenteric lymph node granulomas in Crohn's disease vary from small epithelioid cell clusters to multiple well-formed epithelioid granulomas with central multinucleated giant cells. Necrosis, while infrequent, may occur but, as in sarcoidosis, is never as florid as in tuberculosis. Generalized lymphadenopathy may occur in chronic granulomatous disease of childhood (Figs 2.11 and 2.12).

Fig. 2.10 Central necrosis in sarcoid granulomas. The necrotic areas remain small and unobtrusive as compared with caseation necrosis in tuberculosis, × 80.
Fig. 2.11 Granulomatous disease of childhood. Necrotizing epithelioid granulomas are characteristic, × 80.

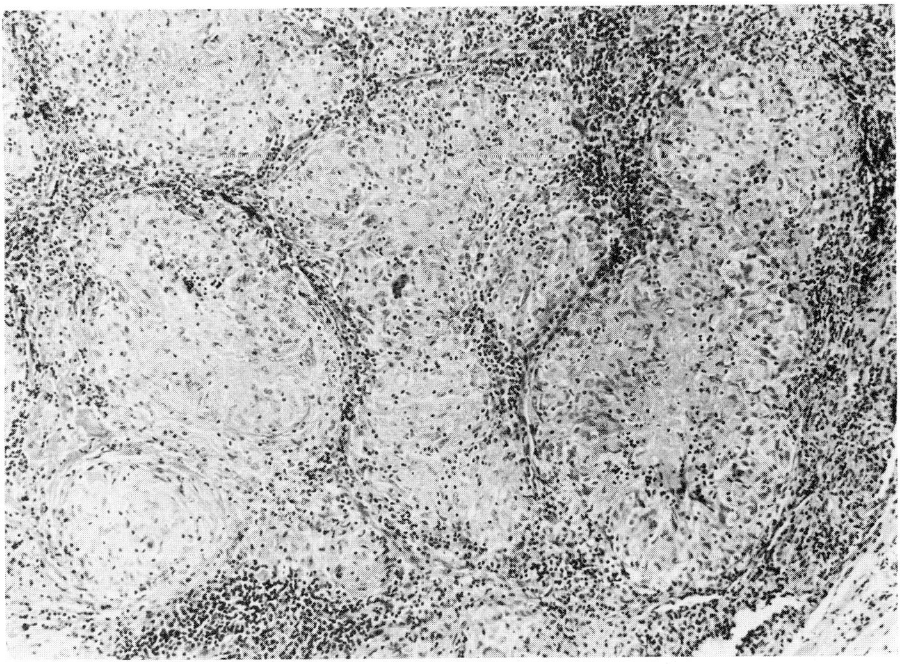

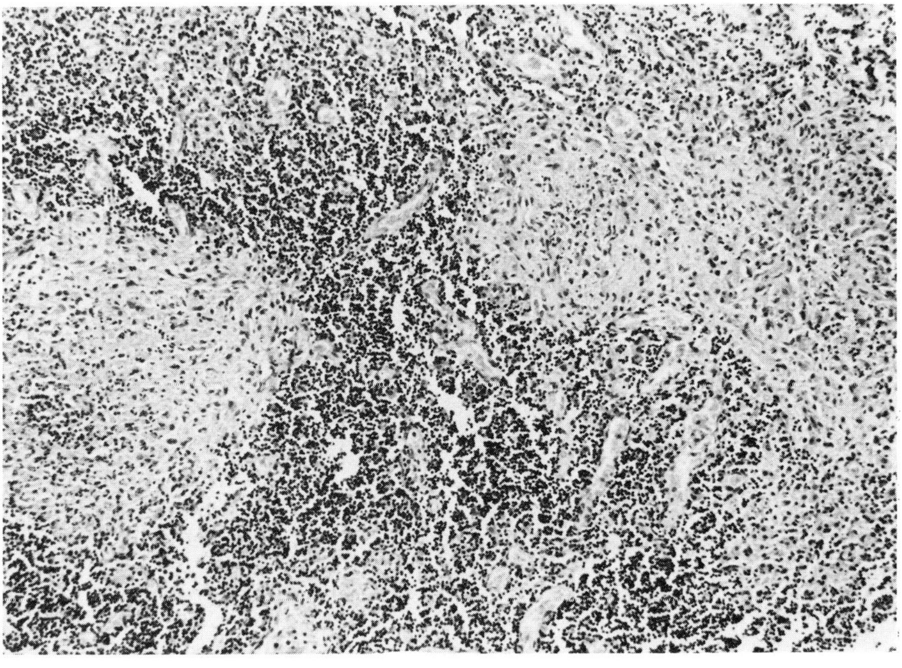

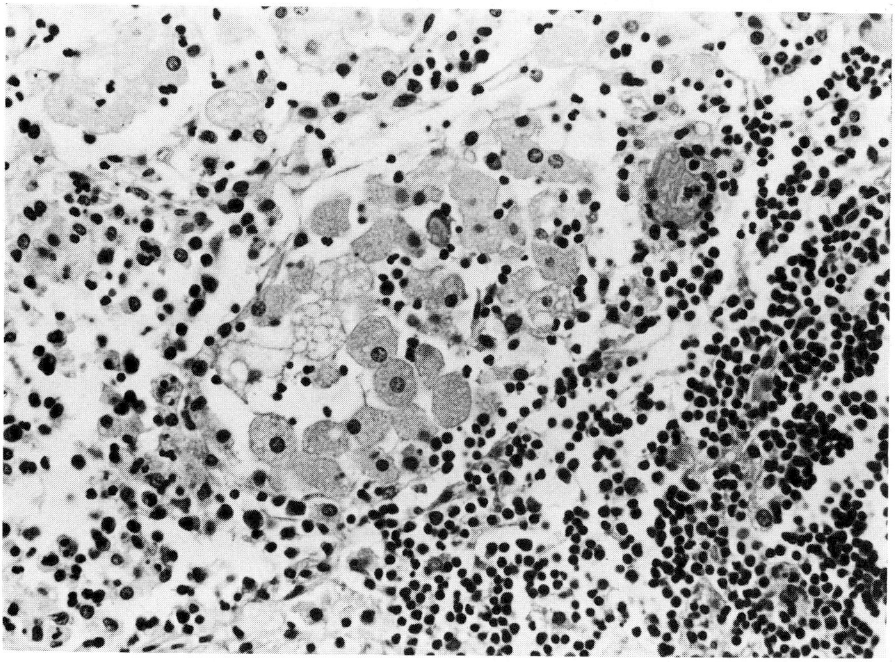

Fig. 2.12 Granulomatous disease of childhood. Sheets of large macrophages are present in addition to granulomas. These macrophages contain brown lipofuscin pigment, × 250.

The biopsy in this condition shows necrotizing epithelioid granulomas which may be indistinguishable from those seen in tuberculosis. Between the granulomas, however, numerous large macrophages containing variable amounts of lipofuscin pigment are present and it is this finding that distinguishes this disease from tuberculosis.

Granulomas with central abscess formation are usually associated with diseases of acute onset and rapid course, which is quite different from the chronic disorders considered in the previous paragraph. A variety of infections can produce this histological picture but the most common are cat-scratch disease, lymphogranuloma venereum and *Yersinia* infection.

Cat-scratch disease (Naji *et al.*, 1962) occurs in patients of all ages giving rise to rapid enlargement of axillary, cervical or inguinal lymph nodes. There is usually a definite history of a cat scratch in the relevant area of lymph node drainage but the lesion produced at the site of the scratch may be trivial and has usually disappeared by the time the lymph nodes start to enlarge some four or more weeks later. The histological appearances of the lymph node biopsy vary with the stage of the disease. Initially there are small clusters of epithelioid histiocytes (similar to those seen in toxoplasmosis) which soon coalesce to form granulomas in the centre of which there is necrosis with pus formation (Fig. 2.13). Histiocytes around the central suppurative core become arranged in pallisades (Fig. 2.14) and the abscesses take on a stellate appearance.

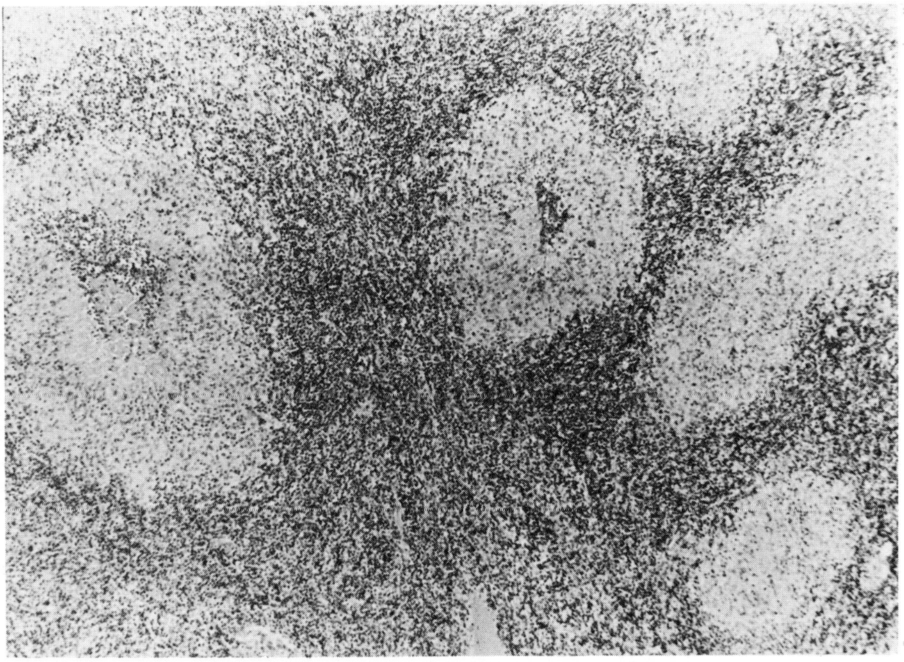

Fig. 2.13 Cat scratch disease. The granulomas, composed of epithelioid histiocytes, show a variable degree of central necrosis and suppuration, × 40.

Later in the disease the central necrotic and suppurative debris becomes converted to homogeneous eosinophilic material which may be surrounded by a zone of fibrosis (Fig. 2.15). Multinucleated giant cells are often scattered amongst the epithelioid histiocytes but true tuberculoid granulomas are not characteristic.

Lymphogranuloma venereum is an uncommon disorder in temperate parts of the world and, being a venereal disease, usually involves the inguinal nodes. The histology is identical to that of cat-scratch disease. The aetiological agent of lymphogranuloma venereum is a member of the bacterial genus *Chlamidiae* and thus it is assumed that a similar agent may be responsible for cat-scratch disease, although there is no evidence to support this assumption.

Yersinial infections also result in epithelioid granulomas with central areas of suppurative necrosis. The disease is confined to mesenteric

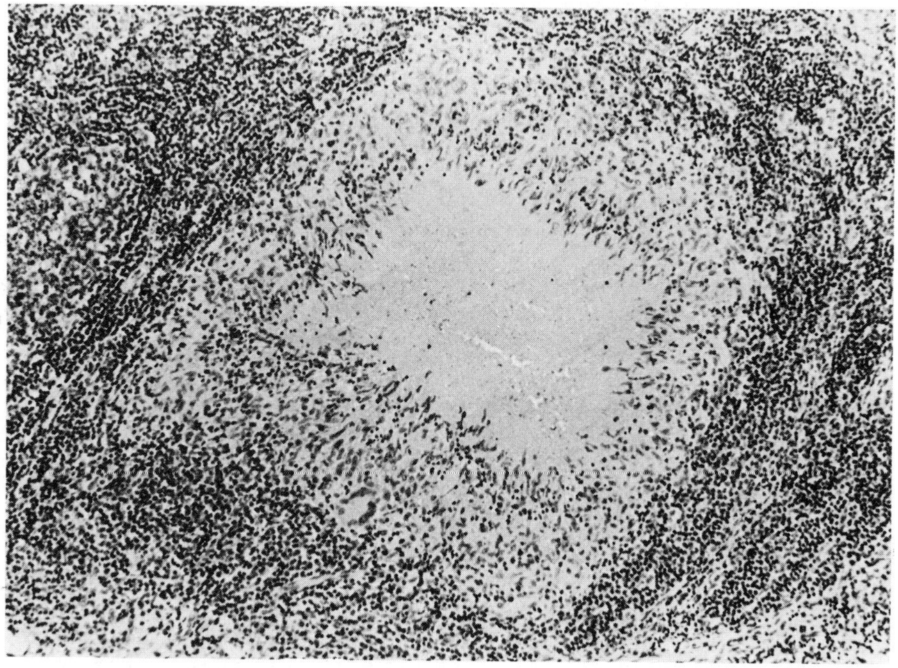

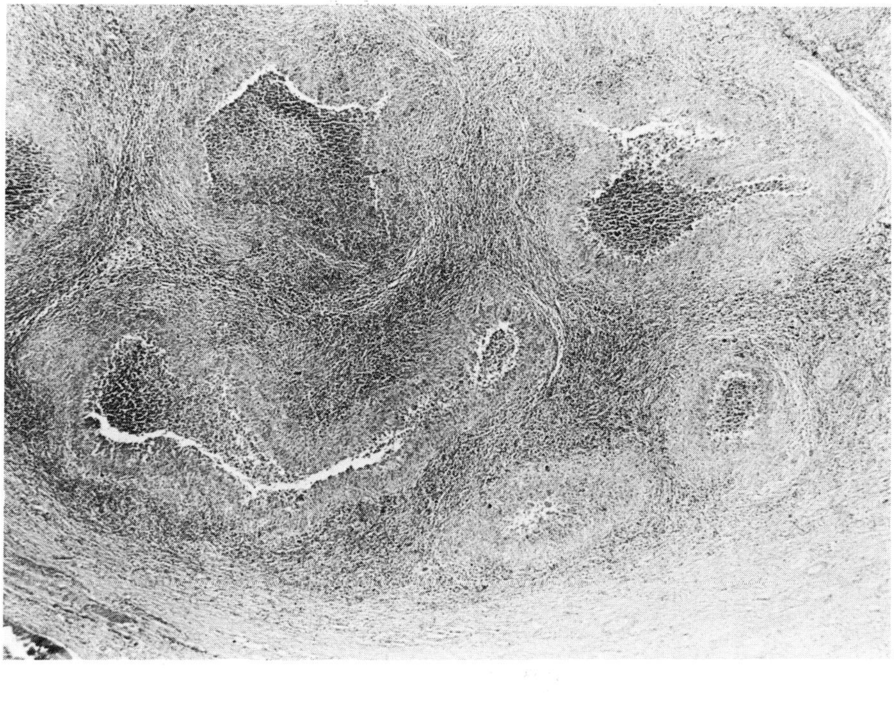

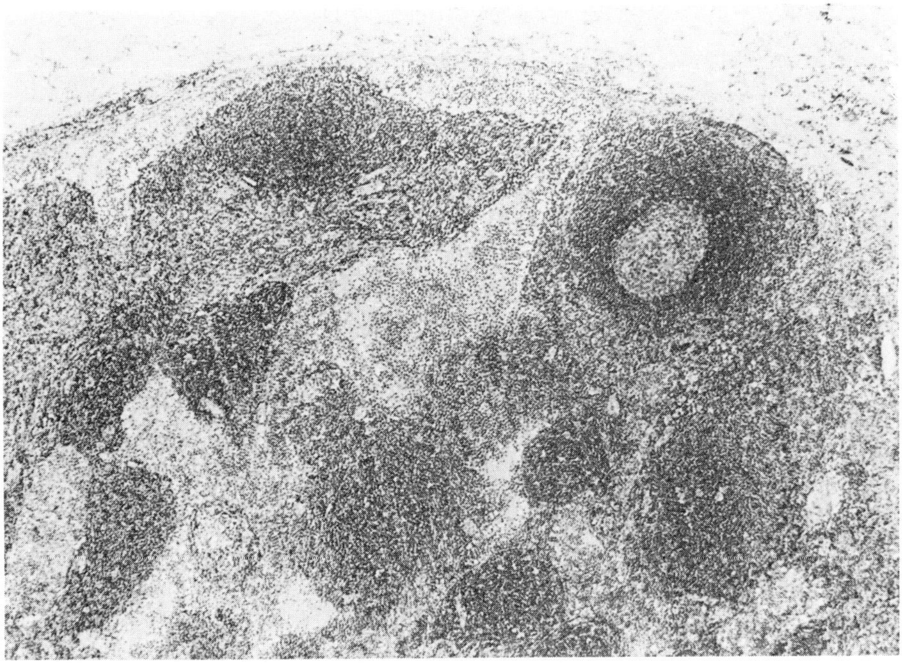

Fig. 2.16 Mesenteric lymph node from a case of *Yersinia* infection. There is follicular hyperplasia as well as expansion of the paracortex and dilatation of the sinuses. The paracortex in mesenteric nodes is normally very poorly developed, × 40.

lymph nodes and is associated with inflammation of the terminal ileum or appendix. The organism responsible is either *Yersinia entercolitica* or *Yersinia pseudotuberculosis* and in either case the presentation is of acute terminal ileitis or mesenteric adenitis (Bradford *et al.*, 1974; El-Maraghi and Mair, 1979). Although it has been suggested that the lymph node pathology differs according to which species of *Yersinia* is involved (Schapers *et al.*, 1981) there is enough overlap of the appearances to consider the yersinial infections as a whole. Characteristic appearances include oedema of the lymph node capsule, follicular hyperplasia, expansion of the paracortex and sinusoidal dilatation (Fig. 2.16). Increased numbers of transformed lymphocytes are seen within the paracortex and sinuses (Fig. 2.17). Neutrophil infiltration of follicle

---

Fig. 2.14 Characteristic granuloma from a case of cat scratch disease. Palisading histiocytes surround a central necrotic core. Giant cells are few in number, × 80.
Fig. 2.15 Serpiginous areas of amorphous material surrounded by epithelioid histiocytes and fibrosis are characteristic of the late phase of cat scratch disease, × 20.

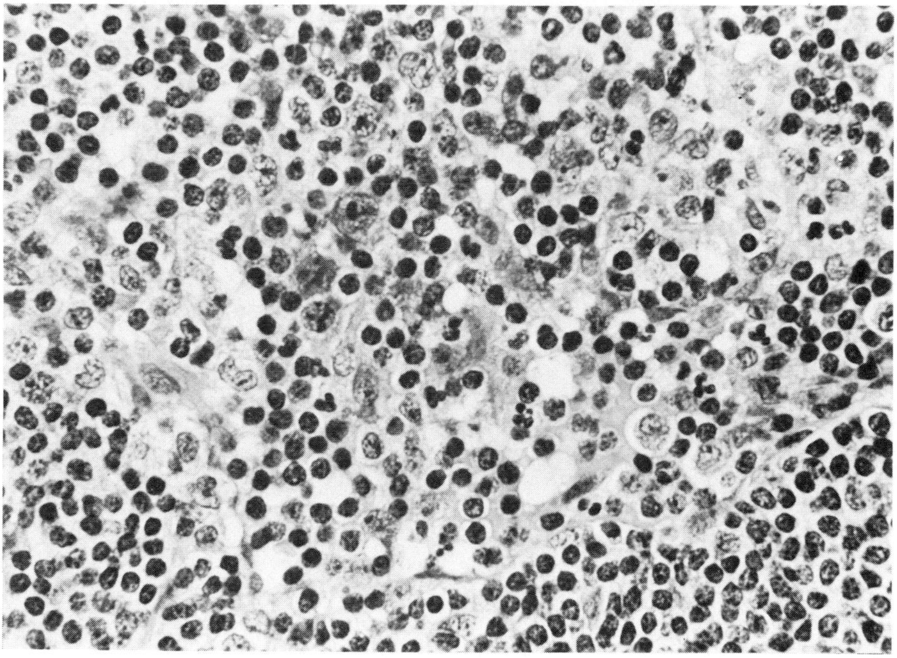

Fig. 2.17 High power of lymph node illustrated in Fig. 2.16 showing intrasinusoidal lymphocytes together with numerous nucleolated blasts, × 400.

centres may be evident (Winblad *et al.*, 1966) and epithelioid granulomas with central suppurative necrosis are characteristic (Ahlquist *et al.*, 1971) in more longstanding cases (Fig. 2.18).

Scattered aggregates of epithelioid histiocytes may be present in the lymph nodes in the early stages of most granulomatous conditions but when present in established lymphadenopathy a diagnosis of toxoplasmosis should be considered (Dorfman and Pennington, 1973). Toxoplasmosis, caused by the parasite *Toxoplasma gondii* is a common cause of cervical lymphadenopathy, often involving nodes in the posterior triangle of the neck. The histological appearances of the lymph nodes in toxoplasmosis are characterized by irregular clusters of epithelioid cells scattered throughout the paracortical areas of the node and encroaching on hyperplastic follicle centres (Fig. 2.19). Multinucleated giant cells are

---

Fig. 2.18 Epithelioid granuloma with central supperative necrosis from a case of *Yersinia* infection, × 100.

Fig. 2.19 Toxoplasmosis involving a lymph node. Small clusters of epithelioid cells are present in the paracortex and within the hyperplastic follicle centres. A dilated sinus filled with pale-staining cells is present at lower left, × 40.

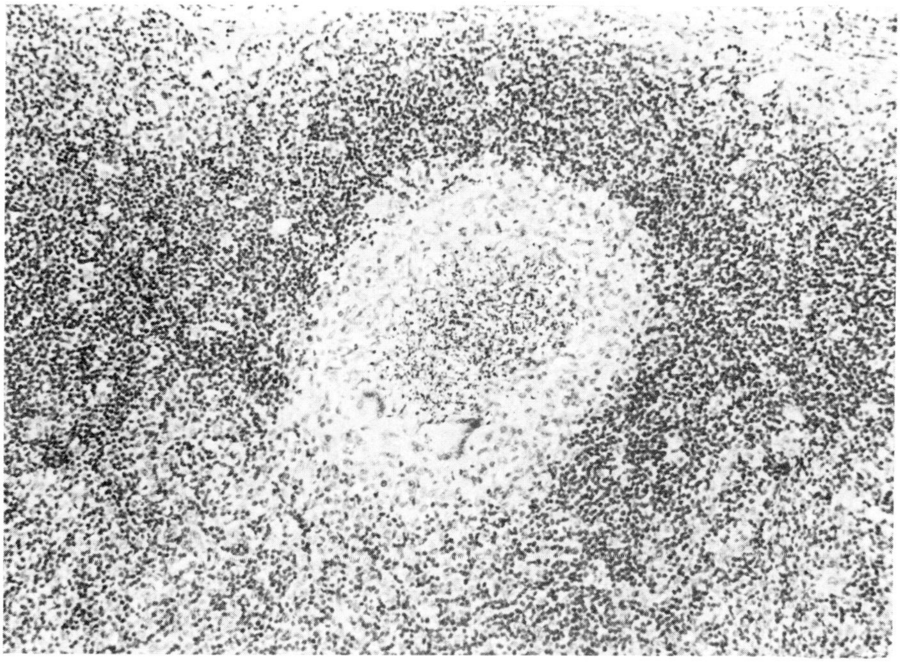

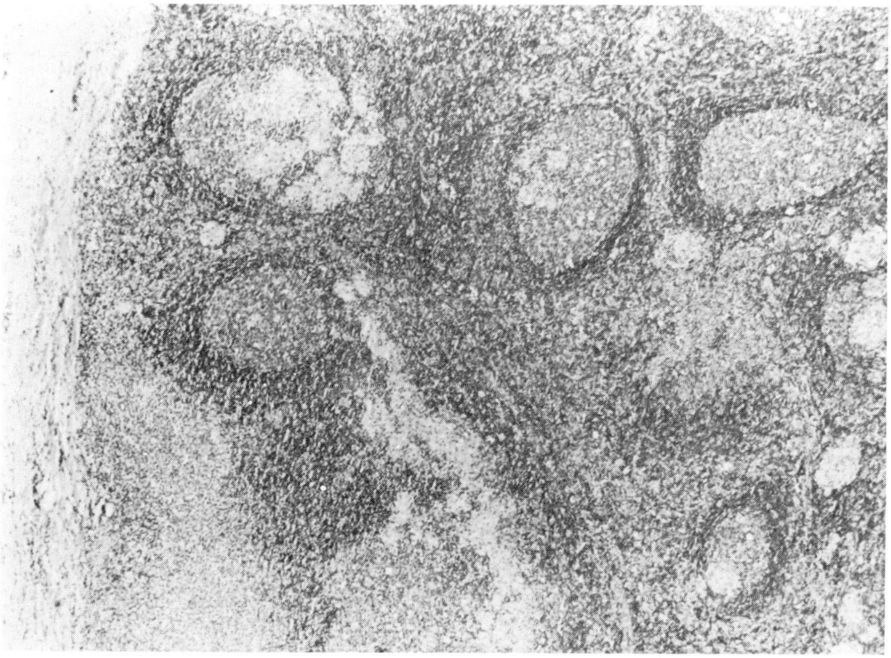

rare. Other features are the distention of the sinuses by small (monocytoid) macrophages (Fig. 2.20) and the presence of proliferating immunoblasts in the paracortex (Fig. 2.21). Large numbers of plasma cells and immunoblasts may be present in the medullary cords. The toxoplasma parasites themselves are only very rarely demonstrable in lymph nodes where they are contained within enlarged macrophages forming so-called parasitic cysts.

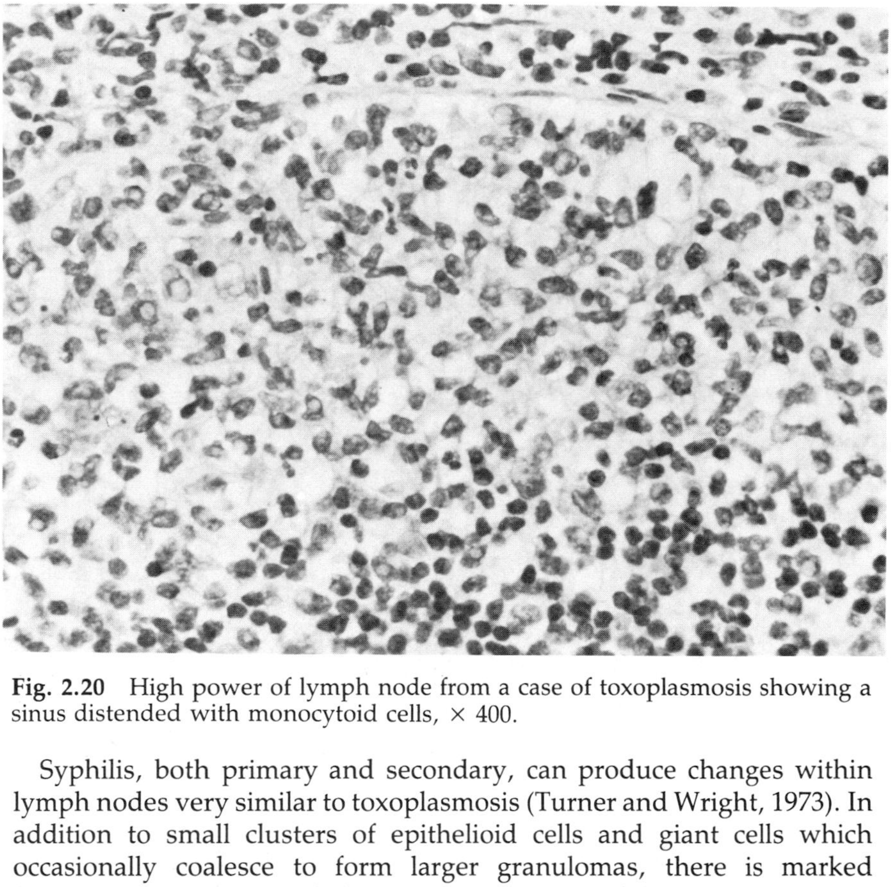

Fig. 2.20 High power of lymph node from a case of toxoplasmosis showing a sinus distended with monocytoid cells, × 400.

Syphilis, both primary and secondary, can produce changes within lymph nodes very similar to toxoplasmosis (Turner and Wright, 1973). In addition to small clusters of epithelioid cells and giant cells which occasionally coalesce to form larger granulomas, there is marked follicular hyperplasia and plasma cell infiltration of the node (Fig. 2.22).

Fig. 2.21 Lymph node paracortex in toxoplasmosis showing a small cluster of epithelioid macrophages at left and scattered pale-staining immunoblasts, × 400.
Fig. 2.22 Lymph node from a case of syphilis showing follicular and paracortical hyperplasia. Small clusters of pale-staining epithelioid cells are present in the paracortex in addition to confluent sheets at right. Epithelioid cell clusters are not seen within follicle centres, × 40.

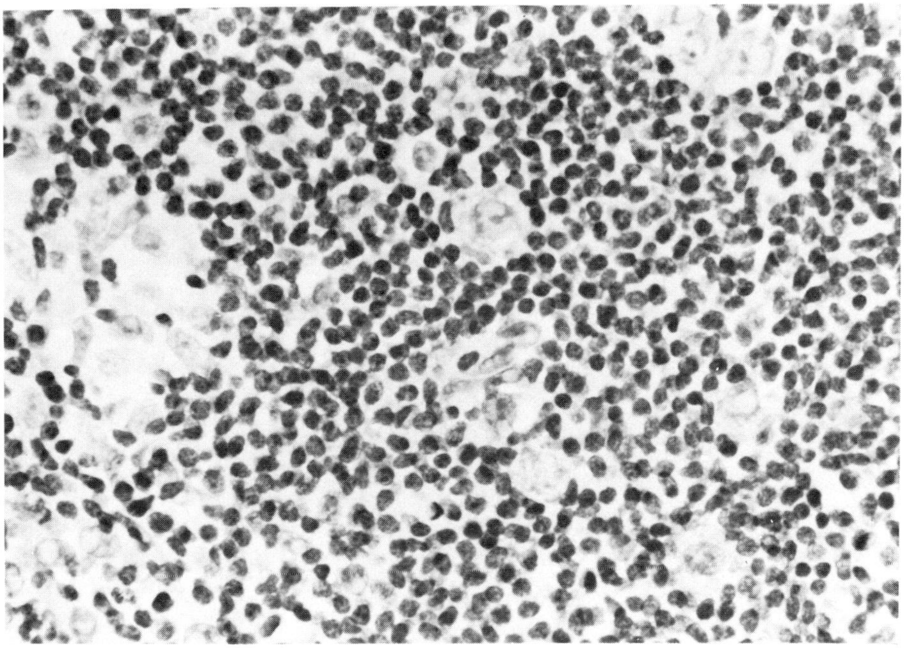

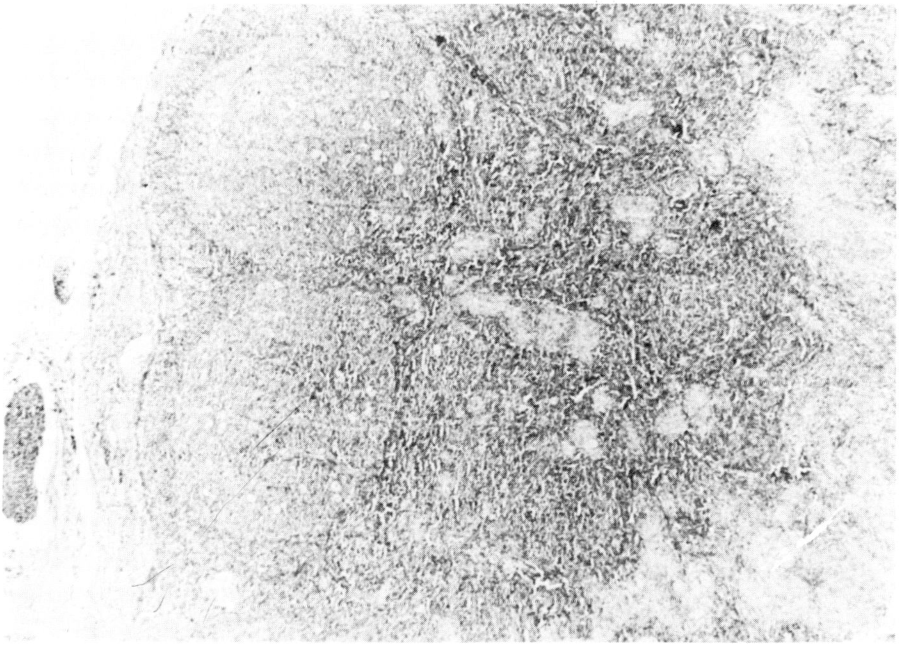

In contrast to toxoplasmosis, the epithelioid cell and giant cell clusters are mostly found in the paracortex and do not impinge on follicle centres. Vascular changes, consisting of endothelial swelling or a true vasculitis may occur in syphilis (Fig. 2.23).

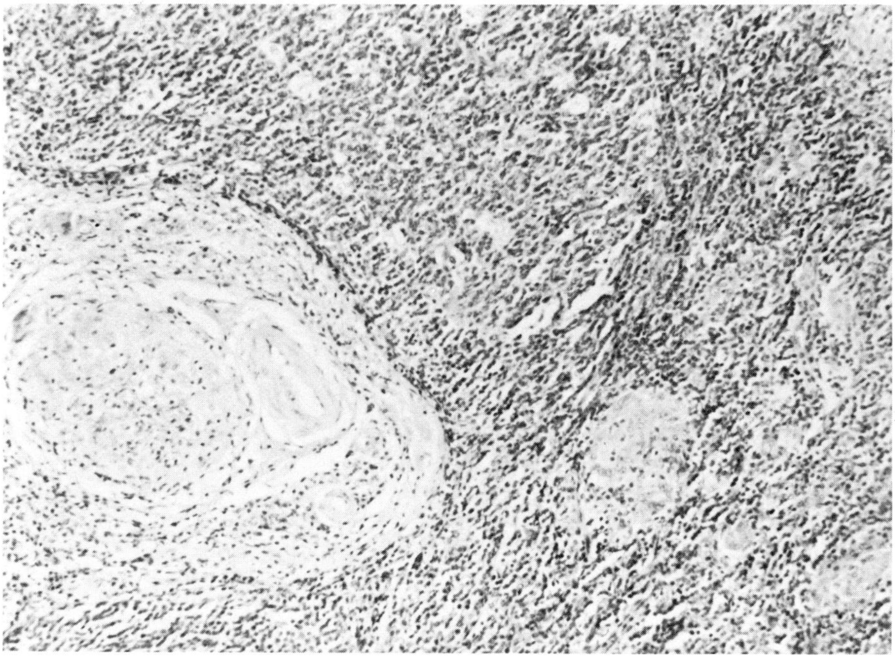

Fig. 2.23 Syphilitic involvement of lymph node showing granulomatous inflammation of a vein (left). A small giant cell granuloma is present below a hyperplastic follicle centre, × 100.

Clusters of histiocytes, but not true epithelioid cells, are also seen in lymph nodes from patients with typhoid or paratyphoid where there may also be marked plasmacytic infiltration. The histiocytes may have abundant cytoplasm and exhibit phagocytosis of red cells and other material. Extensive necrosis is usually present in lymph nodes involved by typhoid. Striking histiocytosis of lymph nodes is seen in lepromatous leprosy (Fig. 2.24) where the large, often rounded cells, with clear cytoplasm are present singly or in clusters. Ziehl–Neelsen stain will reveal aggregates of lepra bacilli within these cells (Fig. 2.25).

Fig. 2.24 Lymph node from a case of lepromatous leprosy showing numerous foamy macrophages, most abundant in the paracortex, × 30.
Fig. 2.25 Ziehl–Neelsen stain of the lymph node illustrated in Fig. 2.24. The histiocytes are stuffed with acid fast lepra bacilli, × 300.

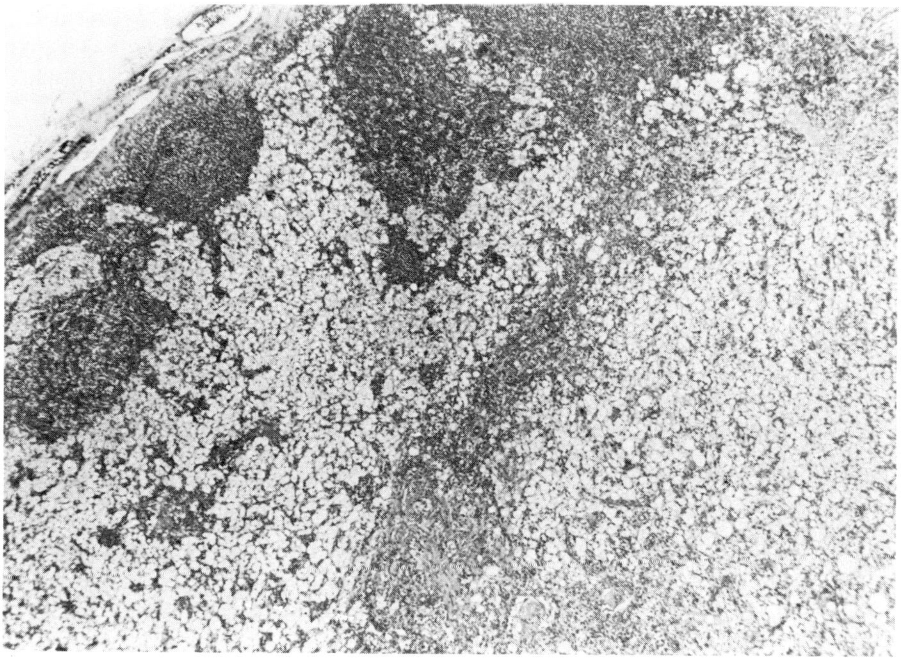

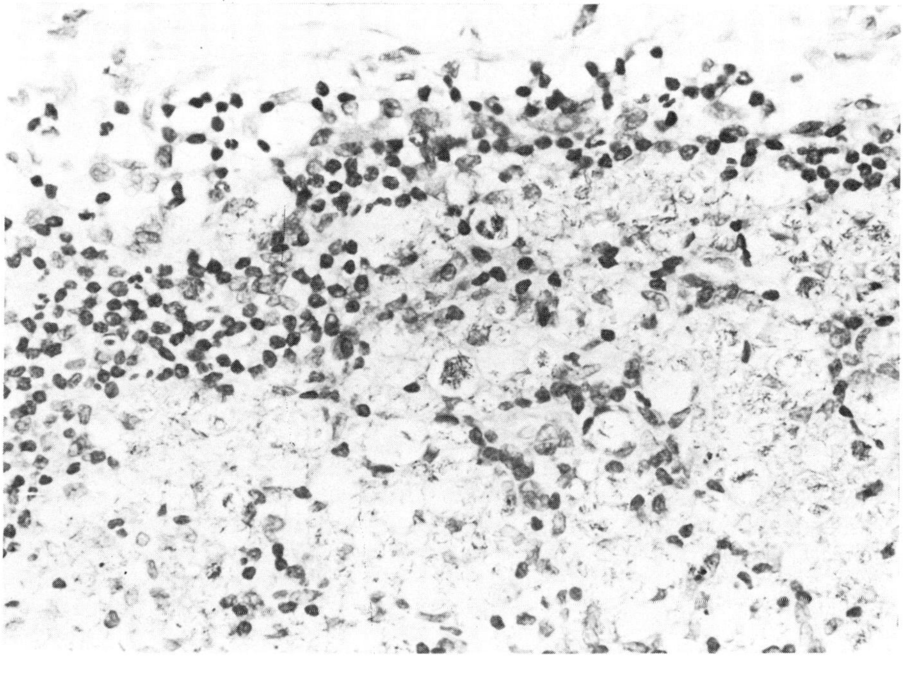

2.2.1 *Differential diagnosis*

Just as the possibility of tuberculosis must always be kept in mind whenever there is granulomatous inflammation of a lymph node so must the possibility of a granulomatous reaction occurring within a malignant lymphoma. Epithelioid histiocytes are frequently present in Hodgkin's disease where they may be distributed in much the same pattern as is seen in toxoplasmosis except that they do not encroach on any residual follicles that may be present. Large epithelioid granulomas sometimes form and occupy the major part of the node. Careful attention to the overall architecture of the node and the tissue between the granulomas will usually reveal the features of Hodgkin's disease with effacement of nodal architecture and the presence of Reed–Sternberg cells and mononuclear Hodgkin's cells. In toxoplasmosis care must be taken not to confuse immunoblasts in the medullary cords with Reed–Sternberg cells. The lymph nodes in non-Hodgkin's lymphomas may also contain granulomas and, in some instances, clusters of epithelioid cells may dominate the histological picture.

References

Ahlquist, J., Alivonen, P., Rasanan, J. A. and Wallgren, G. R. (1971), Enteric infections with *Yersinia enterocolitica*. *Acta Pathol. Microbiol. Scand. (Sect. A)*, **79**, 109–22.

Bradford, W. D., Noce, P. S. and Gutman, L. T. (1974), Pathological features of enteric infection with *Yersinia enterocolitica*. *Arch. Pathol.*, **98**, 17–22.

Carter, R. L. and Penman, H. G. (1969), Histopathology of infectious mononucleosis. In *Infectious Mononucleosis* (eds R. L. Carter and H. G. Penman), Blackwell Scientific Publications, Oxford, ch. 9.

Dorfman, R. F. and Pennington, J. S. (1973), Histological diagnosis of toxoplasmosis. *New Engl. J. Med.*, **289**, 878–81.

El-Maraghi, R. R. H. and Mair, N. S. (1979), The histopathology of enteric infection with *Yersinia pseudotuberculosis*. *Am. J. Clin. Pathol.*, **71**, 631–9.

Naji, A. F., Cabonell, B. and Barker, H. J. (1962), Cat scratch disease. *Am J. Clin. Pathol.*, **38**, 513–21.

Patterson, S. D., Larson, E. B. and Corey, L. (1980), Atypical generalised zoster with lymphadenitis mimicking lymphoma. *New Engl. J. Med.*, **302**, 848–51.

Schapers, R. F. M., Reif, R., Lennert, K. and Knapp, W. (1981), Mesenteric lymphadenitis due to *Yersinia enterocolitica*. *Virchows. Arch. (Pathol, Anat.)*, **390**, 127–38.

Tindle, B. H., Parker, J. W. and Lukes, R. J. (1972), Reed–Sternberg-like cells in infectious mononucleosis. *Am. J. Clin. Pathol.*, **58**, 607–17.

Turner, R. R. and Wright, D. J. M. (1973), Lymphadenopathy in early syphilis. *J. Pathol.*, **110**, 305–8.

Winblad, S., Nilehn, B. and Sternby, N. H. (1966), *Yersinia enterocolitica* ('Pasteurella X') in human enteric infections. *Br. Med. J.*, **2**, 1363–6.

3 Lymphadenopathy simulating malignant lymphoma

We include in this chapter a miscellaneous group of conditions which cause lymphadenopathy and which may simulate malignant lymphoma clinically and sometimes pathologically. Similar conditions that have a recognized infective cause have been included in Chapter 2. Following previous custom (Butler, 1969; Dorfman and Warnke, 1974; Robb-Smith, 1947) we have divided these conditions into three groups according to the basic histologic pattern observed in the affected lymph node (Table 3.1).

Table 3.1 Lymphadenopathy simulating malignant lymphoma

Follicular pattern
Reactive follicular hyperplasia
Non-specific
Rheumatoid disease
Angiofollicular hyperplasia
Hyaline vascular type
Plasma cell type
Sinus pattern
Histiocytosis X
Sinus histiocytosis with massive lymphadenopathy
Lymphangiogram effect
Kaposi's sarcoma and vascular transformation of sinuses
Mixed and diffuse patterns
Angioimmunoblastic lymphadenopathy
Dermatopathic lymphadenopathy
Metastatic neoplasms
Silicone lymphadenopathy
Diphenylhydantoin induced lymphadenopathy
Lupus erythematosus
Infarction of lymph nodes
Amyloidosis

3.1 Follicular pattern

3.1.1 Reactive follicular hyperplasia

The usual response by the lymph node to antigenic stimulation is one of follicular hyperplasia. Most cases of reactive hyperplasia are due to non-specific causes but a proportion of cases are associated with rheumatoid disease. In these patients there may be widespread and substantial lymphadenopathy which clinically simulates malignant lymphoma. When follicular hyperplasia is restricted to the lower cervical region and there is no apparent cause Hodgkin's disease should always be considered. In these cases a careful search for Reed–Sternberg cells and other features of Hodgkin's disease should be made in the interfollicular paracortical tissue (see Chapter 4; Fig. 4.1).

The distinction between reactive follicular hyperplasia and follicular lymphoma is one of the most common, and at times, most difficult diagnostic problems in lymphoreticular pathology and is discussed in detail in Chapter 7. None of the morphological features used to differentiate reactive from neoplastic follicles is, however, absolutely reliable and in a small number of biopsies this distinction cannot be made with certainty. The term atypical hyperplasia (Schroer and Fransilla, 1979) has been applied to this type of case in which close follow-up and repeat biopsies, sometimes over a period of years, may be necessary before a definitive diagnosis is possible.

Immunological and marker studies on fresh unfixed material may be of particular value in cases of atypical hyperplasia but are not always conclusive especially since a number of these cases eventually turn out to be Hodgkin's disease (Shroer and Fransilla, 1979). From the point of view of the patient's welfare it is better, if in doubt, to err on the side of a diagnosis of reactive hyperplasia.

3.1.2 Angiofollicular hyperplasia

This condition which can occur at any age most commonly presents as an asymptomatic mediastinal mass which is detected by routine chest X-ray. It may, however, involve lymph nodes at any site and multicentric cases have been recorded (Bartoli *et al.*, 1980; Gaba *et al.*, 1978). Angiofollicular hyperplasia has also been described in unusual sites such as the broad ligament and soft tissues of the shoulder (Dorfman and Warnke, 1974). The plasma cell variant of this disease is associated with systemic manifestations including fever anaemia and hyperglobulinaemia (Keller *et al.*, 1972) which disappear following excision of the lesion. The pathogenesis of angiofollicular hyperplasia is unknown and suggestions

include an immune reaction to undefined antigens (Keller *et al.*, 1972) and that the lesion is a lymphoid hamartoma (Lattes and Pachter, 1962). There is a need to study the lymphoid cells from these lesions by functional means and by using cell marker techniques (Diamond and Braylan, 1980).

The lymphoid masses in angiofollicular hyperplasia may attain a considerable size, and usually have a homogeneous tan-coloured cut surface.

(a) *Histology*

In the hyaline vascular type (Fig. 3.1) the tumour has a follicular structure, the nodules being composed predominantly of small lymphocytes arranged in an orderly concentric 'onion-skin' array (Fig. 3.2). Usually there is no discernible underlying lymph node structure although we have seen residual sinuses at the edge of some specimens. The centre of some of the nodules, presumably those cut through the equator, contain a few cells resembling centrocytes, amorphous hyaline material and a single small blood vessel with hyaline material in its wall. The resemblance of these structures to Hassal's corpuscles (Castleman *et al.*, 1956) is only superficial. Large numbers of blood vessels with plump endothelial cells and showing varying degrees of hyalinization occupy

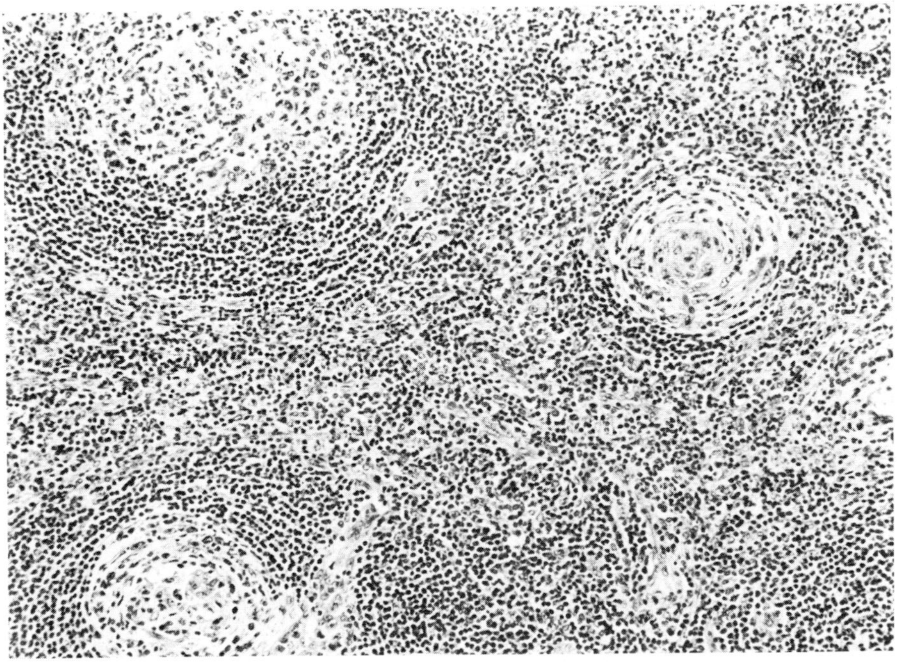

Fig. 3.1 Angiofollicular hyperplasia, hyaline vascular type. Atypical follicles are separated by vascular lymphoid tissue, × 160.

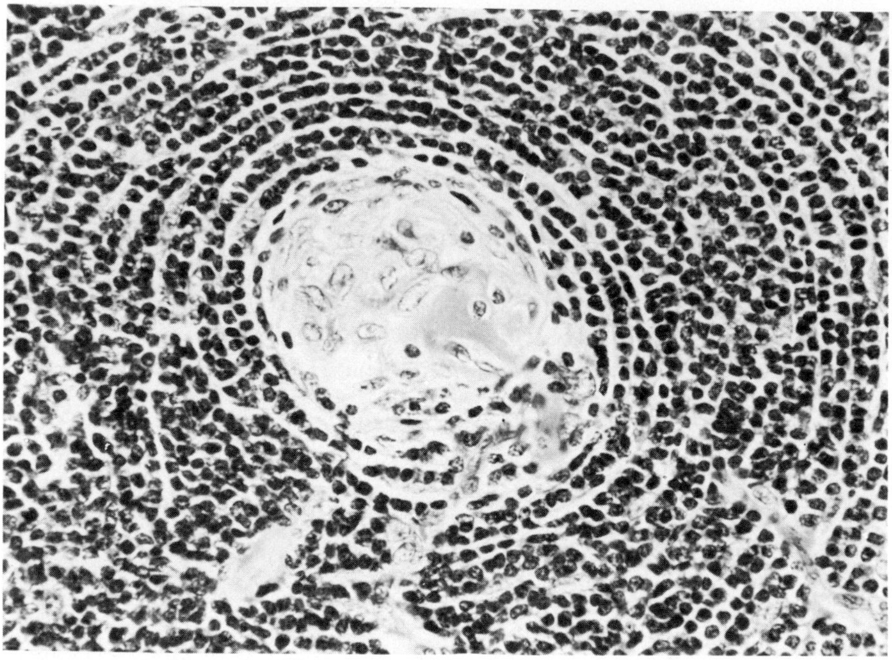

Fig. 3.2 Amorphous hyaline material is present in this follicle from a case of angiofollicular hyperplasia together with a few cells resembling centrocytes and dendritic reticulum cells. The follicle is surrounded by small lymphocytes in a concentric onion skin arrangement, × 300.

the interfollicular areas and are highlighted by the reticulin stain (Fig. 3.3).

The plasma cell type (Figs 3.4 and 3.5) differs from the hyaline vascular type in that there are large numbers of plasma cells in the interfollicular areas. The follicles appear more reactive with a higher content of controcytes and centroblasts.

(b) *Differential diagnosis*

Angiofollicular hyperplasia can be differentiated from reactive hyperplasia by the lack of normal lymph node architecture; in particular the absence of sinuses between the follicles. This feature will not serve to distinguish it from follicular lymphoma which may exhibit a similar interfollicular structure. Here differentiation must be made on the basis of

---

Fig. 3.3 The large numbers of blood vessels between the follicles in angiofollicular hyperplasia are well outlined by the reticulin stain, × 100.

Fig. 3.4 Angiofollicular hyperplasia, plasma cell type. The follicles are more cellular in this variant of the disease, × 100.

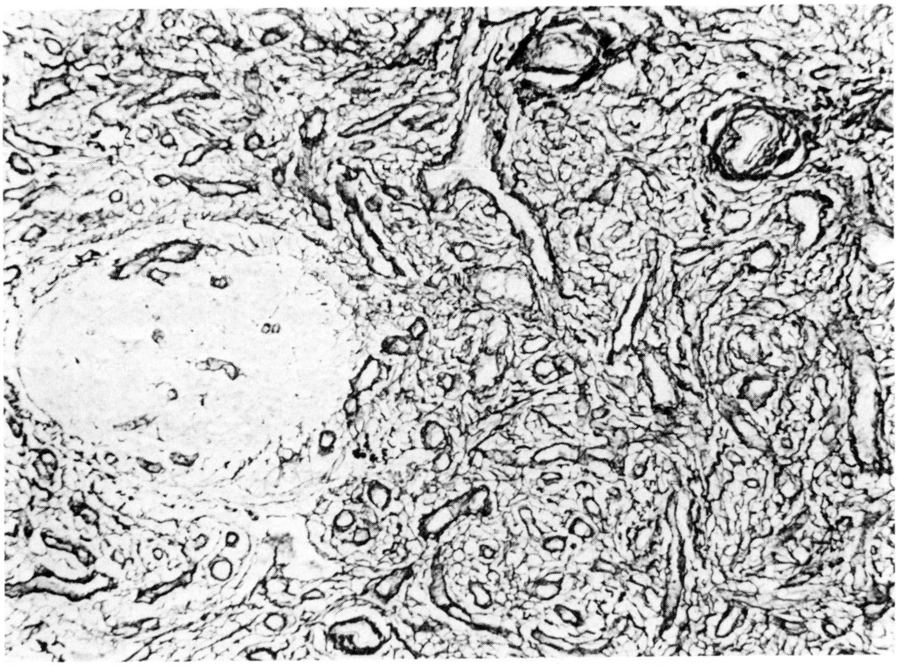

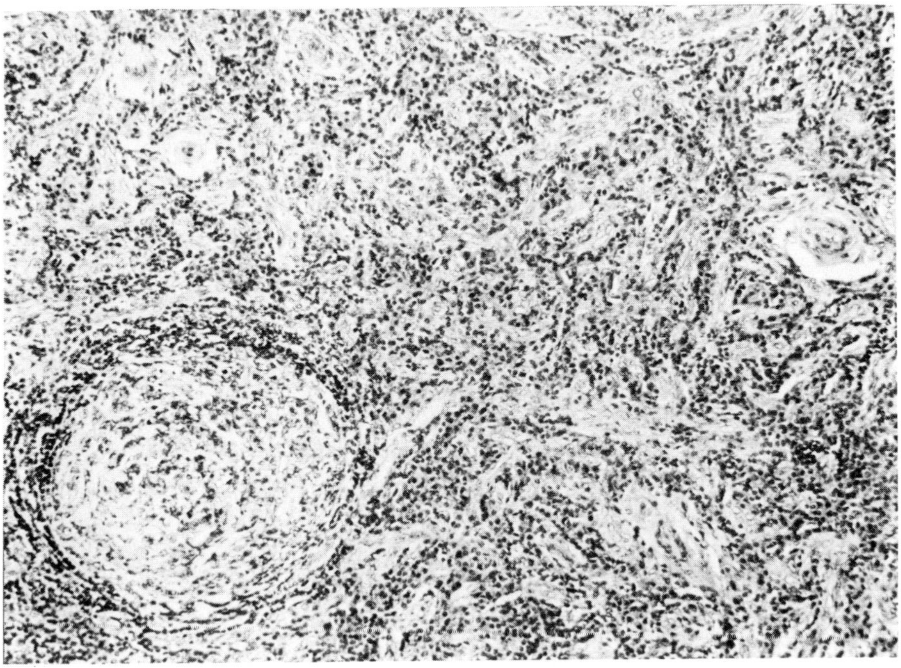

the cytology and size of the follicle centres. In angiofollicular hyperplasia these are small and contain few follicle centre cells whereas in follicular lymphoma the bulk of the lesion consists of centrocytes and centroblasts without the sharply defined 'onion-skin' arrangement of small lymphocytes.

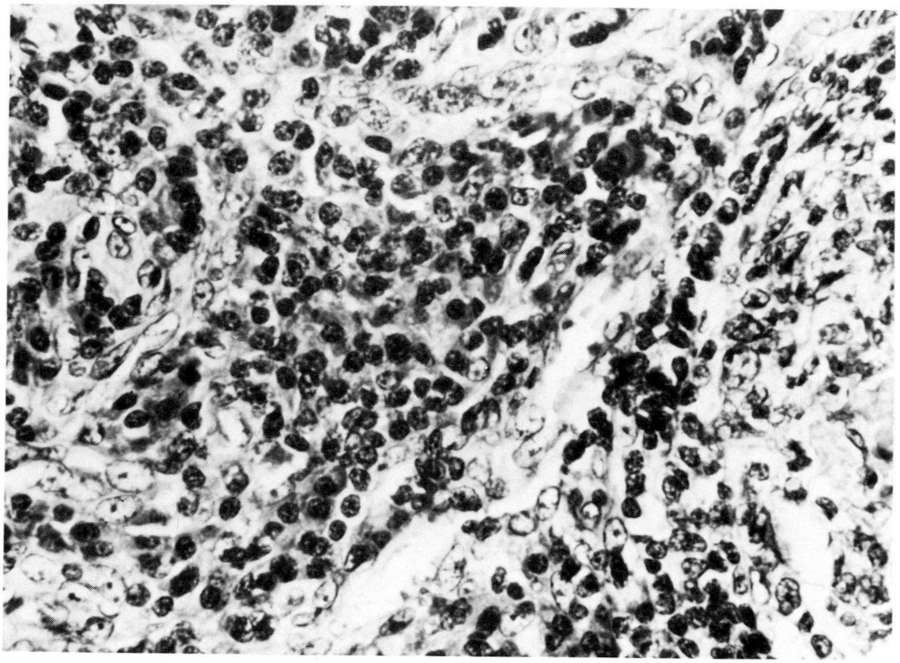

Fig. 3.5 The interfollicular areas of the plasma cell variant of angiofollicular hyperplasia contain a dense plasma cell infiltrate, × 400.

The plasma cell type must be differentiated from lymphoplasmacytic lymphoma, which often contains residual lymphoid follicles within a broad expanse of plasma cells. The presence of a prominent blood vessel component in this area would favour angiofollicular hyperplasia. Immunoperoxidase studies will clearly distinguish the monotypic proliferation of lymphoplasmacytic lymphoma from the polytypic proliferation of angiofollicular hyperplasia (Fig. 3.6).

Fig. 3.6 An example of the plasma cell type of angiofollicular hyperplasia stained by the immunoperoxidase technique for kappa light chain (a) and lambda chain (b). The presence of a mixture of cells producing both light chains indicates a polyclonal, non-neoplastic plasma cell infiltrate, × 100.

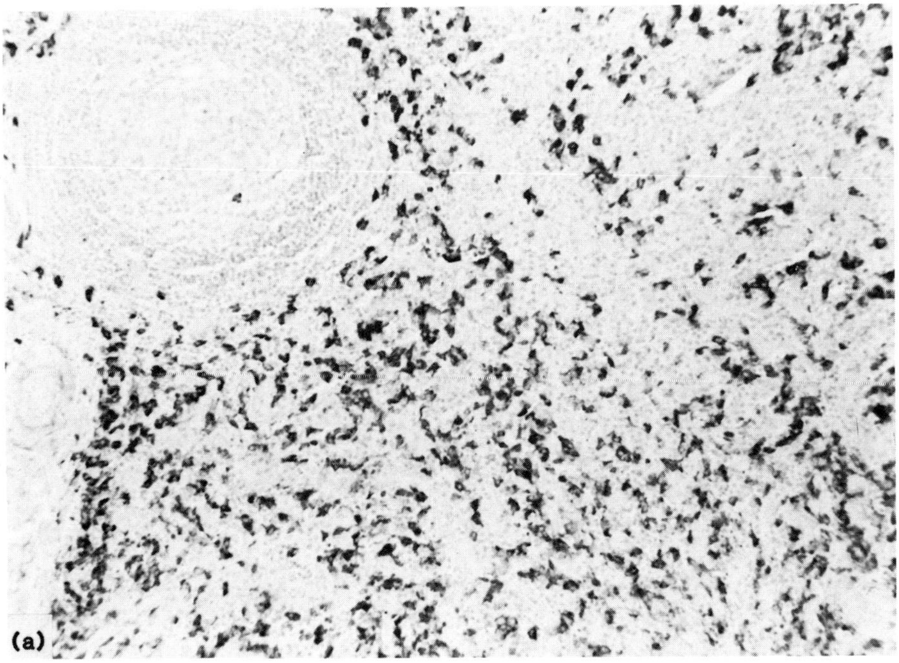
(a)

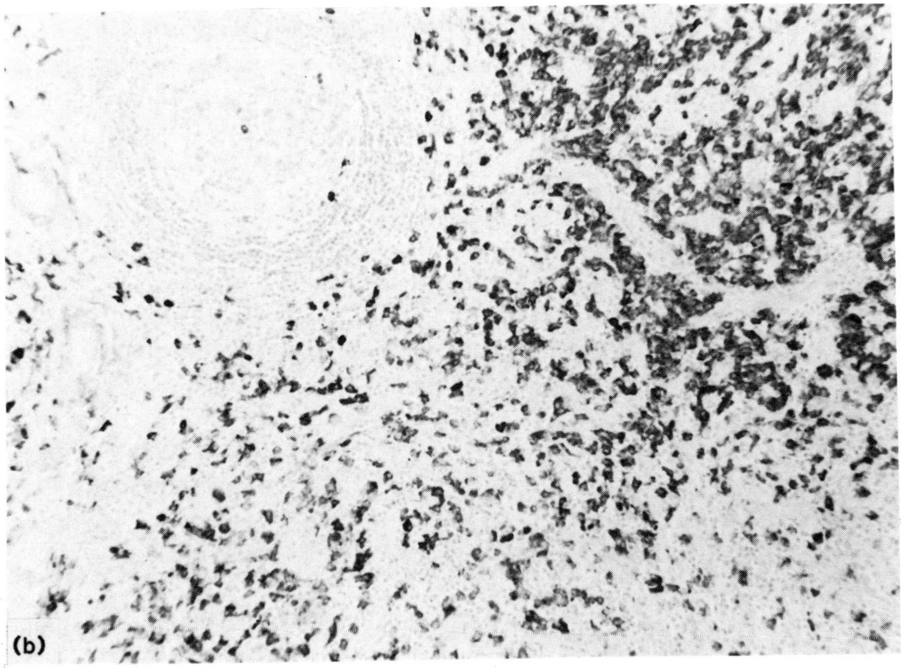
(b)

3.2 Sinus pattern

3.2.1 Histiocytosis X presenting with lymphadenopathy

Synonyms: Eosinophilic granuloma of lymph nodes
Hand–Schuller–Christian disease
Letterer–Siwe disease

The clinical spectrum of histiocytosis X as it affects the lymphoreticular system is well reviewed by Williams and Dorfman (1979). The age range of their 17 cases was 8 months to 33 years with two-thirds of the cases presenting in the first decade. Many patients experience fever, night sweats and malaise and have some degree of anaemia. Lymphadenopathy may be massive and tends to be generalized in the very young patients with predominantly cervical lymphadenopathy in the older age group. Hepatosplenomegaly and skin rashes are commonly found in the very young patients. Approximately two-thirds of the cases have concomitant or sequential osteolytic bone lesions. Various treatment regimes including the use of steroids, chemotherapy and radiation have been used with success. All the patients reported by Williams and Dorfman (1979) were alive at follow-up periods ranging from a few months to 12 years with a mean of 3.5 years. Our experience with older children is similar, but two of the three children less than one year old at presentation that we have observed have died within a few months.

We agree with the view that eosinophilic granuloma, Hand–Schuller–Christian syndrome and Letterer–Siwe disease are parts of a single disease spectrum, and can be regarded as clinical syndromes encompassed within the single pathological entity of histiocytosis X.

Histiocytosis X appears to be a non-neoplastic proliferation of Langerhan's cells. These cells normally reside in the epidermis and have a role in antigen trapping. Morphologically they closely resemble the interdigitating reticulum cell of the T-dependent areas of lymph nodes and can be distinguished from these cells only by the demonstration of Langerhan's granules with the electron microscope (Fig. 3.7). Langerhan's cells are derived from bone marrow monocytes which might account for the frequent occurrence of bone lesions in histiocytosis X.

(a) *Histology*

The essential feature of the lymph node form of histiocytosis X is the filling out and distention of sinuses by characteristic histiocytes (Fig. 3.8).

Fig. 3.7 Electron micrograph of a histiocyte from histiocytosis X showing typical Langerhan's (Birbeck) granules (arrows). Photograph by courtesy of Dr Carmen Rivas, Madrid, × 4200.

Fig. 3.8 Histiocytosis X. The sinuses of this lymph node are distended by an infiltrate of histiocytes amongst which multinucleated cells are evident, × 30.

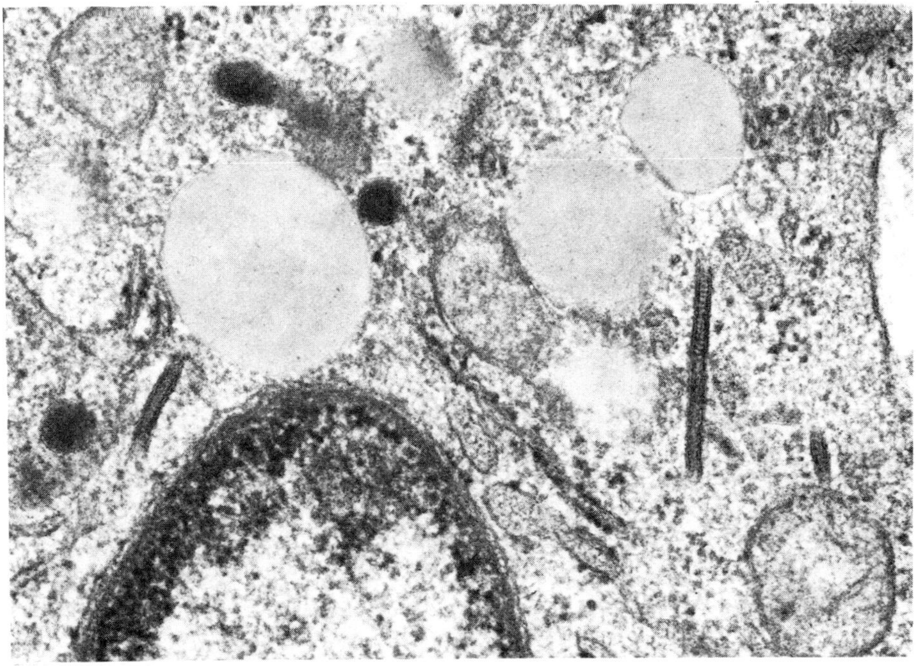

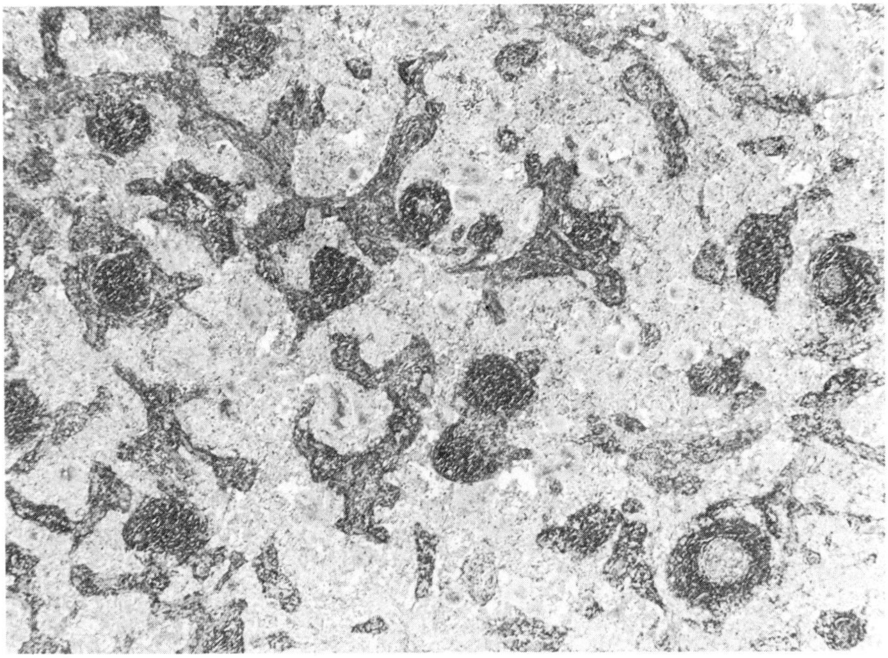

These cells have deeply infolded nuclei which are well seen in imprint preparations (Fig. 3.9). The chromatin is fine and dispersed and nucleoli small and inconspicuous (Fig. 3.10). In plastic sections the nuclear folds and the nucleoli are much more prominent (Fig. 3.11). These cells have abundant eosinophilic or slightly vacuolated cytoplasm. Giant cell forms with up to a dozen or more nuclei may be present. Mitotic figures are not usually seen and nuclear atypia is never a feature of these cells.

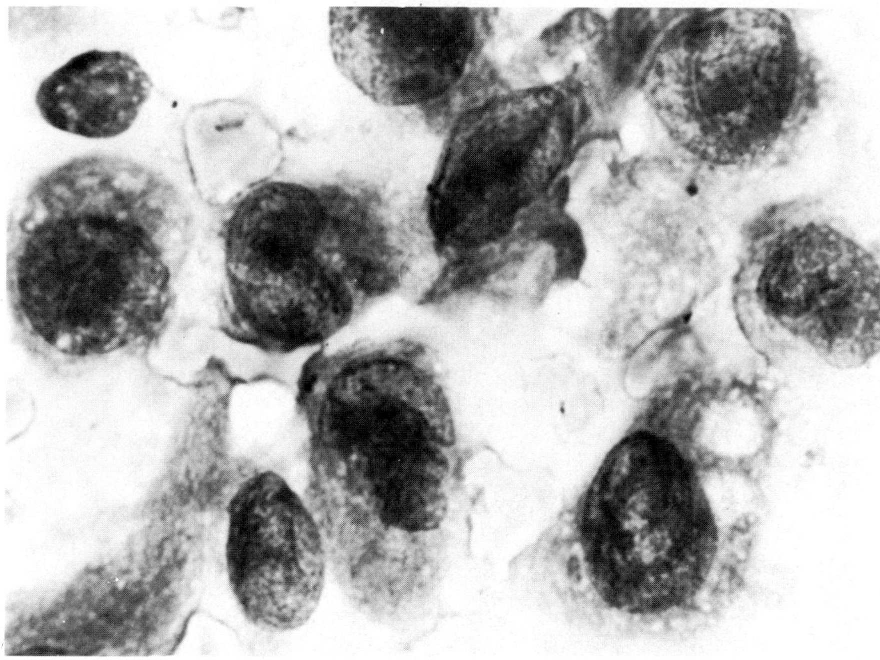

Fig. 3.9 Imprint preparation from a case of histiocytosis X. The characteristic nuclear folds are clearly evident. Giemsa, × 1200.

Phagocytosis including erythrophagocytosis is occasionally present. An infiltrate of eosinophils usually accompanies the histiocytes which may be scanty or constitute the predominant sinusoidal cell. In the latter cases eosinophil 'abscesses' may form. These occur in widely distended

---

Fig. 3.10 Characteristic intrasinusoidal infiltrate in histiocytosis X. The delicate folded nuclei have dispersed chromatin and small nucleoli, × 30.
Fig. 3.11 The infolding of the nuclei in histiocytosis X is well seen in plastic sections. The nucleoli are more prominent in this type of preparation. Toluidine blue, × 1200.

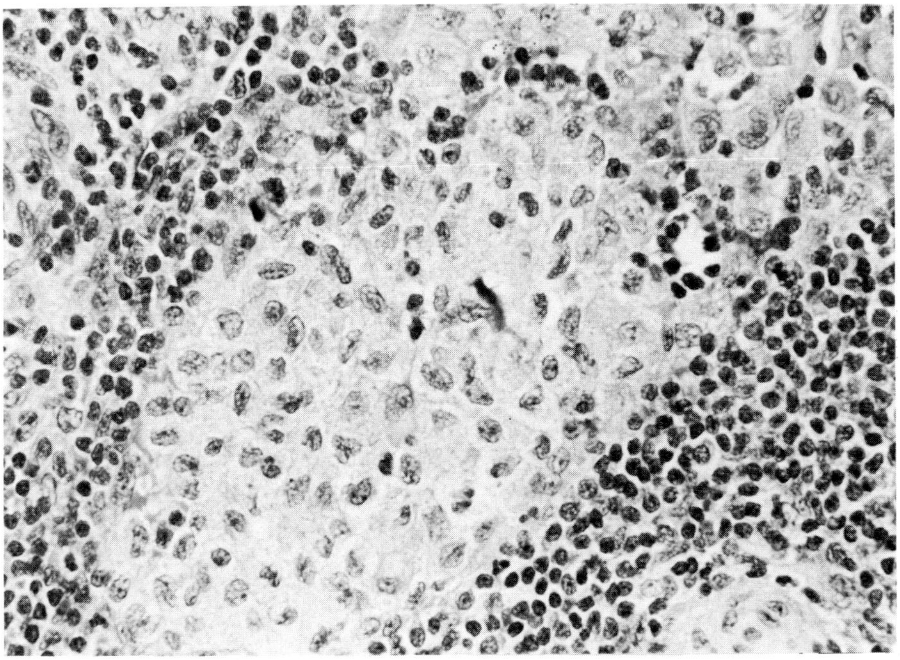

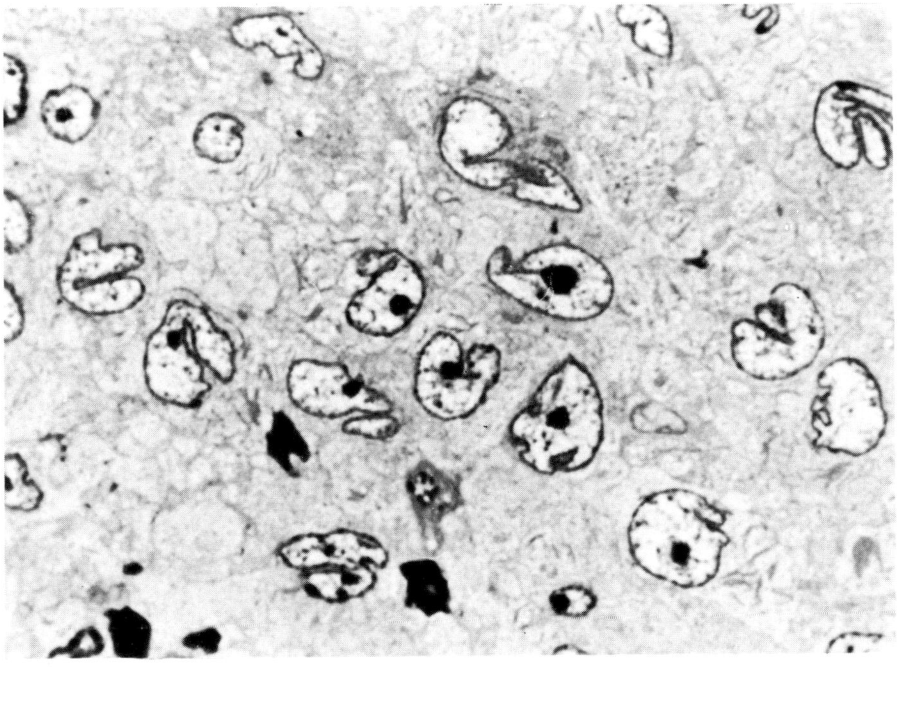

sinuses and consist of a central area of necrosis which appears to be composed of eosinophil debris surrounded by an intense infiltrate of intact eosinophils (Fig. 3.12).

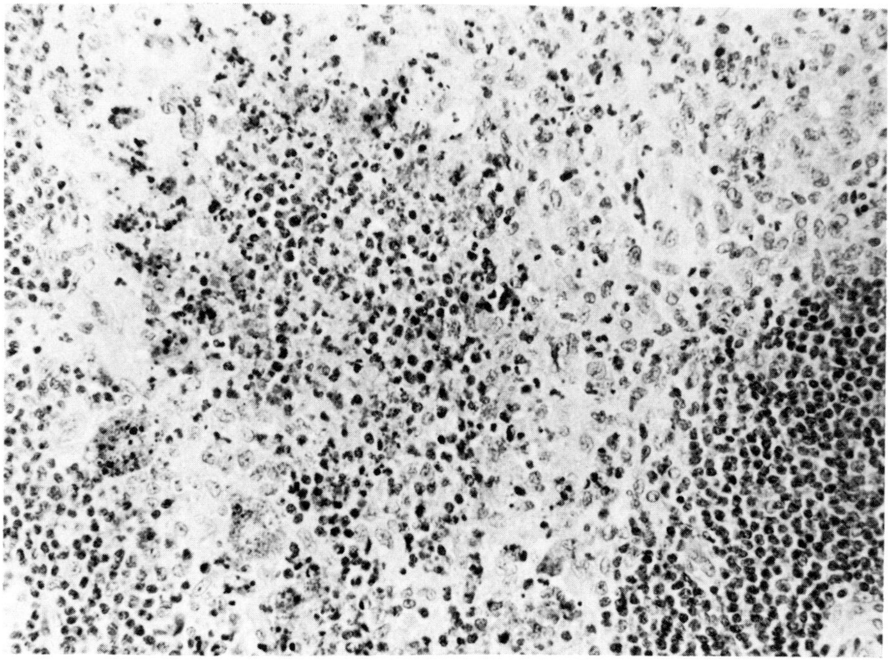

Fig. 3.12 An area of necrosis in a distended sinus from a case of histiocytosis X. Most of the necrotic cells are eosinophils forming a so-called 'eosinophilic abscess', × 250.

(b) *Differential diagnosis*

Histiocytosis X has to be distinguished from other sinus histiocyte proliferations. If attention is paid to the characteristic cytological features of the histiocytes in histiocytosis X this should rarely present difficulties. The accompanying cells may aid in the differential diagnosis; thus eosinophils, though not always present, are characteristic of histiocytosis X whereas plasma cell proliferation in the medullary cords is a distinctive feature of sinus histiocytosis with massive lymphadenopathy. Interdigitating reticulum cells and Langerhan's cells proliferate or accumulate in lymph nodes in dermatopathic lymphadenopathy. However, in this condition the cells are found predominantly in the paracortex and not in the sinusoids. When eosinophil 'abscesses' are a prominent feature of histiocytosis X the appearances may suggest an inflammatory lesion such as cat-scratch disease. In histiocytosis X the abscesses are always confined to the sinusoids and do not show the characteristic histiocyte pallisading of most non-pyogenic inflammatory lesions.

3.2.2 *Sinus histiocytosis with massive lymphadenopathy*

Synonyms: Rosai Dorfman disease
Lymphophagocytic histiocytosis

Sinus histiocytosis with massive lymphadenopathy (SHML) (Rosai and Dorfman, 1972) typically presents with massive bilateral painless cervical lymphadenopathy although other lymph node groups may be involved. Between a quarter and one-third of cases show involvement of extranodal sites including orbit and eyelid (Foucar *et al.*, 1979), upper respiratory tract and salivary glands (Foucar *et al.*, 1978), skin (Thawerani *et al.*, 1978), bone and testis (Azoury and Reed, 1966; Walker *et al.*, 1981), lung, kidney and retroperitoneum (Wright and Richards, 1981). The liver and spleen are usually of normal size. Weight loss, fever, leucocytosis with neutrophilia, an elevated ESR and polyclonal hypergammaglobulinaemia are common features. The disease occurs at all ages but predominates in the first two decades of life. It shows a male preponderance and occurs in Negroes more frequently than in other races. There is no consistent response to antibiotics, steroids, irradiation or chemotherapy, although local surgery may be of benefit. The disease usually follows a protracted indolent course with eventual spontaneous resolution of the lymphadenopathy.

The cause of SHML remains unknown, it may represent a specific infectious process (Lampert and Lennert, 1976) possibly occurring in patients with an underlying immunological deficit (Becroft *et al.*, 1973).

Imprint preparations show large histiocytes with abundant foamy cytoplasm exhibiting varying degrees of lymphophagocytosis. Associated with these cells are variable numbers of lymphocytes and plasma cells.

(a) *Histology*

Lymph node histology usually shows marked capsular and pericapsular fibrosis (Fig. 3.13). The lymph node sinuses are distended (Fig. 3.14) by a proliferation of histiocytes with abundant cytoplasm that is variably eosinophilic or vacuolated. The degree of sinusoidal distention varies possibly with the duration of the disease. Thus in some biopsies residual germinal follicles and prominent medullary cords are present whereas in others the proliferating sinusoidal histiocytes are almost confluent. The residual medullary cords contain large numbers of plasma cells that may contain prominent Russell bodies. Variable numbers of lymphocytes,

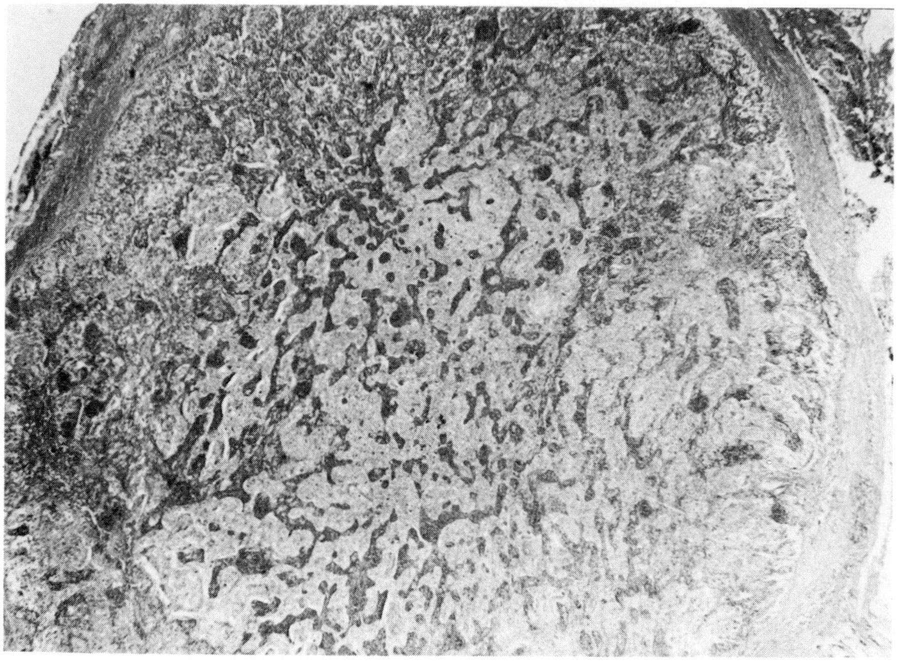

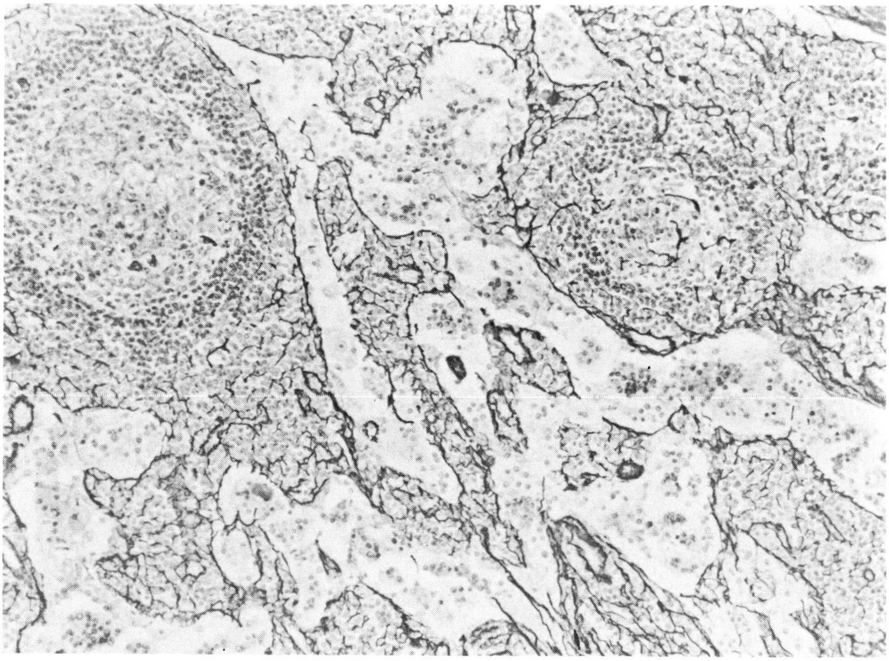

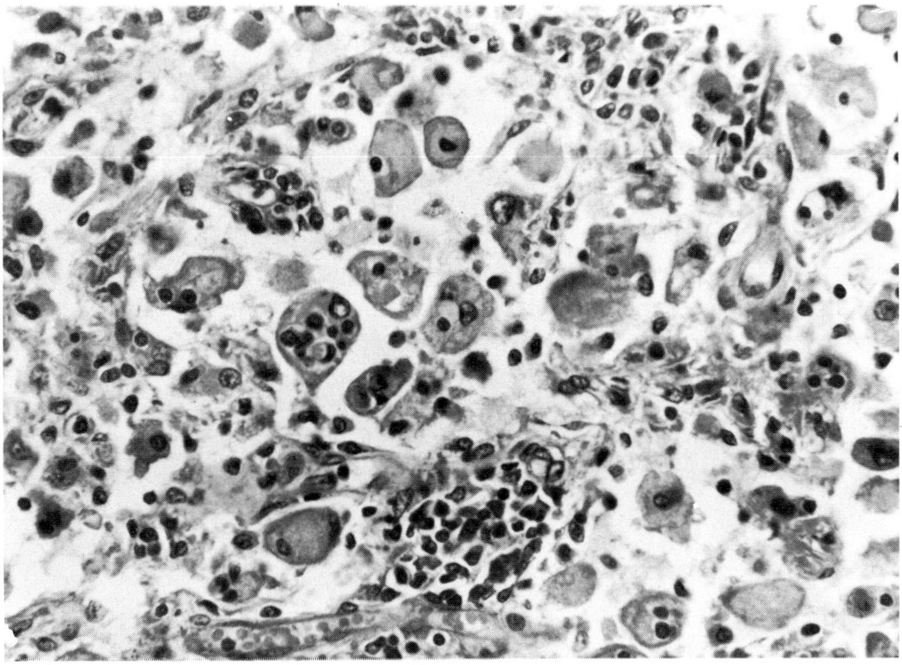

Fig. 3.15 SHML. Large intrasinusoidal macrophages can be seen to contain varying numbers of well-preserved lymphocytes and plasma cells, × 300.

polymorphs, haemosiderin-laden macrophages and histiocytes with abundant foamy cytoplasm may be present within the cords. The sinusoidal histiocytes are predominantly mononuclear with occasional multinucleate cells. Most cells have round or oval nuclei with one or two prominent eosinophilic nucleoli, nuclear atypia is present in occasional cells but is not prominent. The most characteristic feature of SHML is the presence of well-preserved lymphocytes and occasional plasma cells, polymorphs and erythrocytes in the cytoplasm of a variable number of the sinus histiocytes (Fig. 3.15). Several dozen cells may be seen within a single histiocyte.

Extranodal SHML may be less easily diagnosed because the characteristic sinusoidal distribution of the histiocytes is lacking and lymphophagocytosis is less pronounced than in nodal lesions. The histiocytes may

---

Fig. 3.13 Lymph node from cases of sinus histiocytosis with massive lymphadenopathy (SHML). There is marked capsular fibrosis and distention of the sinuses, × 12.

Fig. 3.14 Reticulin stain of a lymph node from a case of SHML showing residual follicles amidst distended sinuses, × 120.

nevertheless be found within spaces suggestive of lymph vessels and intervening infiltrates of lymphocytes, plasma cells and foamy macrophages are present.

(b) *Differential diagnosis*

SHML must be distinguished from other sinusoidal proliferative diseases. Reactive sinus histiocytosis is rarely massive enough to be confused with SHML and does not show lymphophagocytosis. Histiocytosis X primarily affecting lymph nodes may be confused with SHML (Williams and Dorfman, 1979). The cytological features of the histiocytes in histiocytosis X are characteristic and distinct from those in SHML. Lymphophagocytosis is not a feature of histiocytosis X nor is plasma cell proliferation in the medullary cords. Malignant histiocytosis (histiocytic medullary reticulosis) should not cause confusion clinically with SHML. The histiocytes in malignant histiocytosis exhibit greater atypia than those in SHML and do not show the same degree of lymphophagocytosis.

3.2.3 *Lymphangiogram effect*

Lymphangiography is now widely used as a method of staging a number of neoplasms and biopsy of the affect lymph nodes is frequently performed at subsequent staging laparotomies. The oily contrast medium used for lymphangiography is entrapped within the sinuses of the lymph nodes and induces a proliferation of histiocytes and giant cells. In the early stages large vacuoles corresponding to dissolved lipid globules are surrounded by histiocytes and giant cells (Figs 3.16 and 3.17). With time the globules break up into smaller droplets and finally disappear.

Lymphangiogram effects should cause little diagnostic difficulty since the distorted architecture of pathological nodes precludes the uptake of contrast medium. Thus in the search for lymphomatous involvement attention should be directed mainly to those areas within a node not showing lymphangiogram effect (Fig. 3.18).

3.2.4 *Kaposi's sarcoma*

Kaposi's sarcoma is an uncommon neoplasm in Europe and North America but accounts for up to 16% of all neoplasms in parts of tropical

---

Fig. 3.16 A paraaortic lymph node showing the effects of a lymphangiogram. The nodal architecture is distorted by large vacuoles caused by the lipid contrast medium, × 30.

Fig. 3.17 Lymphangiogram effect. Foreign body giant cells have accumulated around the collections of contrast medium, × 120.

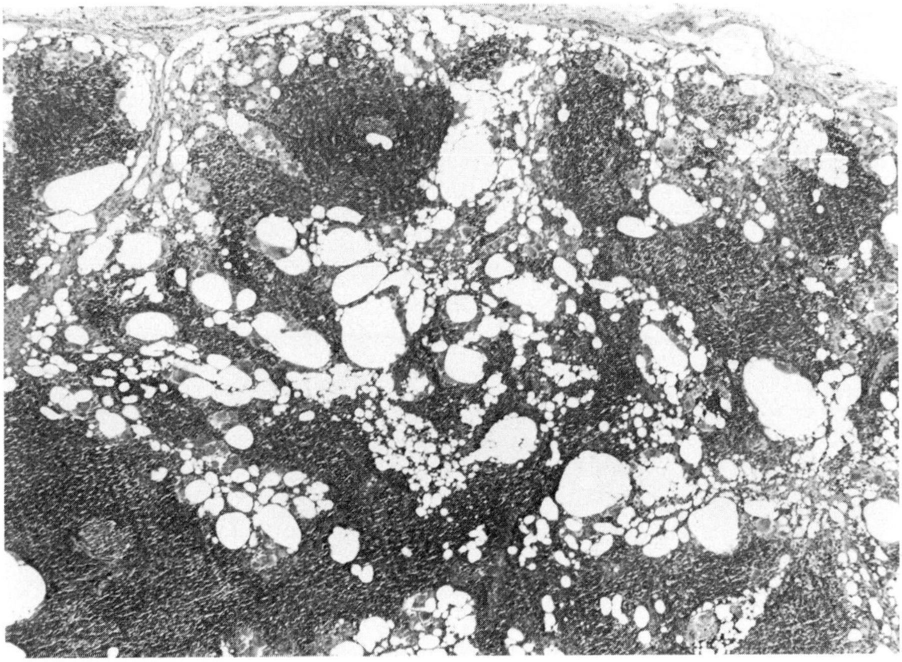

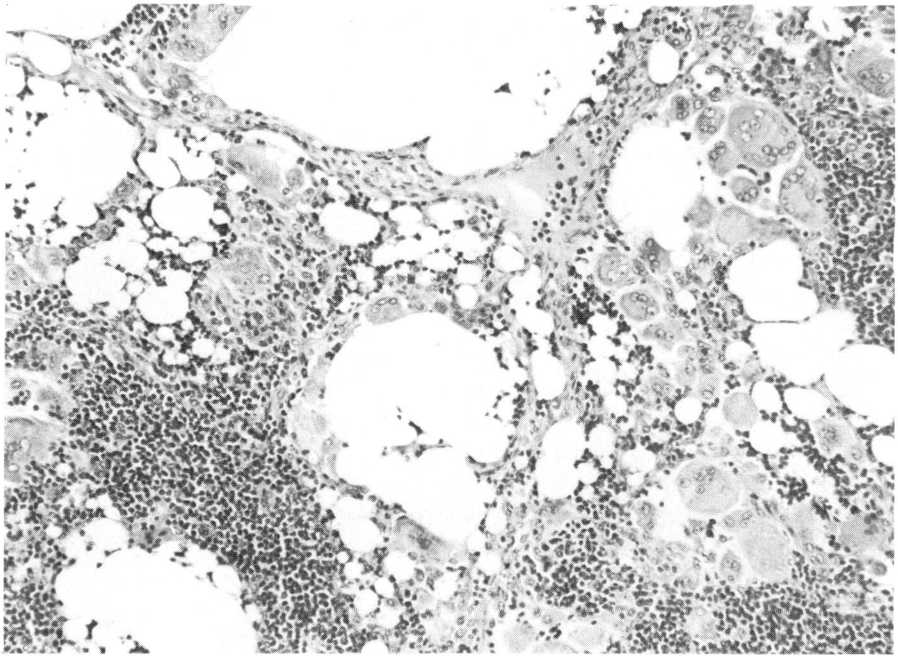

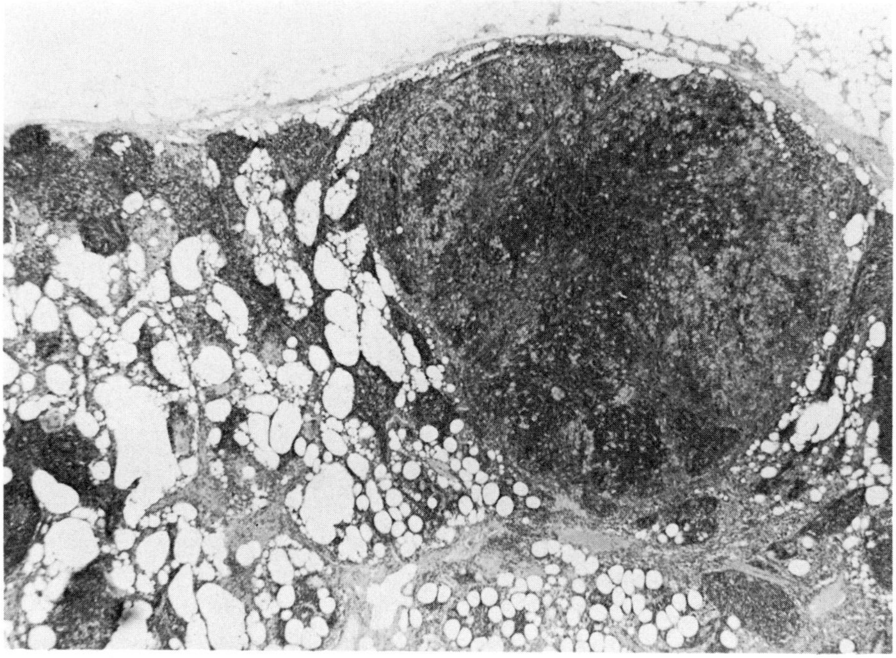

Fig. 3.18 Paraaortic lymph node from a staging laparotomy for Hodgkin's disease. The uninvolved part of the node shows lymphangiogram effect in contrast to the nodule of Hodgkin's tissue, × 20.

Africa. The usual presentation in adults is with nodular skin tumours, however, children and some adults may present with lymphadenopathy mimicking malignant lymphoma. Recently an aggressive form of the disease has been described in homosexual men, all of the eight cases reported had lymph node involvement (Hymes *et al.*, 1981). The histogenesis of Kaposi's sarcoma remains uncertain and it shows an intriguing association with malignant lymphomas and immunosuppression.

Kaposi's sarcoma is composed of plump spindle cells closely packed or forming a more open angiomatous pattern. Red blood cells lie between the spindle cells with no intervening endothelial cells. Large numbers of histiocytes are found throughout the tumour, which are more obvious when special staining techniques are used, and variable numbers of plasma cells are present. Within lymph nodes the tumour forms solid areas that partially or completely replace the node (Figs 3.19 and 3.20). The earliest changes in the lymph node involve the subcapsular and trabecular sinuses which show congestion and an angiomatous appearance (Dorfman and Warnke, 1974).

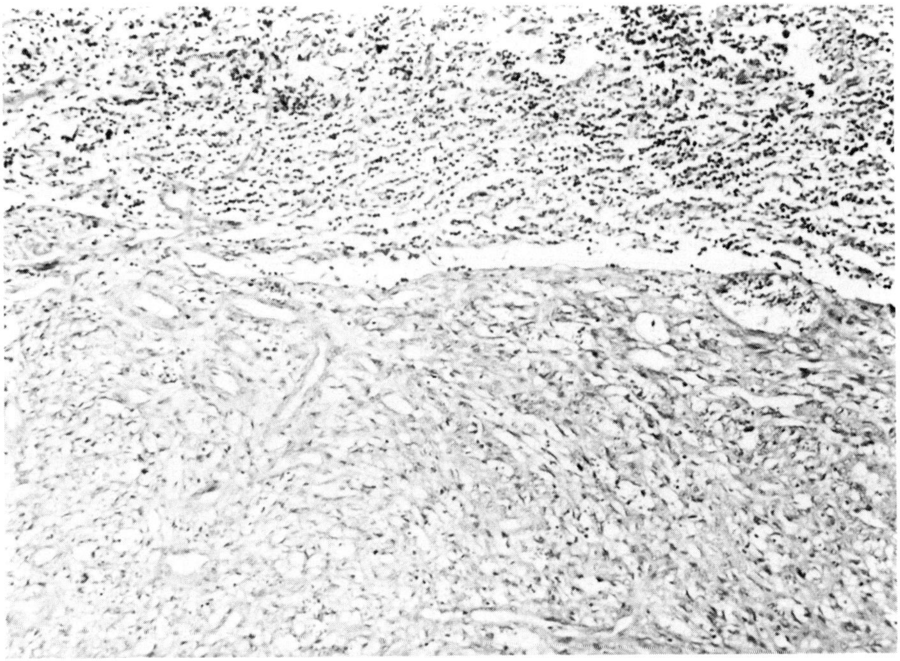

Fig. 3.19 A solid area of Kaposi's sarcoma within a lymph node, × 40.

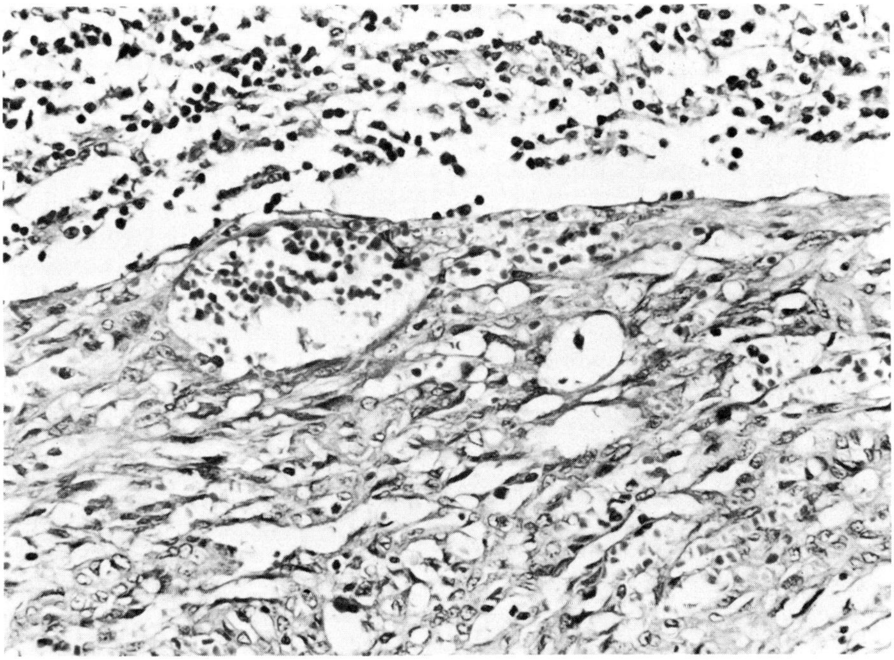

Fig. 3.20 Kaposi's sarcoma showing the characteristic non-endothelial lined vascular slits, × 200.

(a) *Differential diagnosis*

Passive venous congestion of lymph nodes may lead to the development of vascularized sinusoidal fibrosis (Haferkamp *et al.*, 1971; Dorfman and Warnke, 1974). This lesion can be distinguished from early Kaposi's sarcoma by the fact that the vascular spaces are lined by endothelial cells rather than spindle-shaped tumour cells.

3.3 Mixed and diffuse patterns

3.3.1 Angioimmunoblastic lymphadenopathy

Synonyms: Immunoblastic lymphadenopathy
Angioimmunoblastic lymphadenopathy with dysproteinaemia
Lymphogranulomatosis X

Angioimmunoblastic lymphadenopathy (AIL) mimicks malignant lymphoma in so far as it causes lymphadenopathy but it differs from most lymphomas in its rapidity of onset, fluctuant course and widespread distribution. The associated constitutional symptoms frequently raise suspicions of Hodgkin's disease although it is most unusual for Hodgkin's disease to present with generalized lymphadenopathy and hepatosplenomegaly. Skin rashes are frequent in AIL. The patients may have Coomb's positive haemolytic anaemia and polyclonal hypergammaglobulinaemia is common. There is often a history of exposure to drugs but no single drug or group of drugs appear to be implicated.

When Lukes and Tindle (1975) first described 32 cases with this condition they used the term immunoblastic lymphadenopathy. Frizzera *et al.* (1975) almost simultaneously, described 24 patients with a condition they called angioimmunoblastic lymphadenopathy with dysproteinaemia. It would appear that there is sufficient overlap between these two series of cases to categorize them as part of the same disease spectrum rather than as different entities. Dysproteinaemia is not a constant feature and we prefer the simpler title of angioimmunoblastic lymphadenopathy (AIL).

Three of the patients reported by Lukes and Tindle (1975) developed 'immunoblastic sarcomas' whereas Frizzera *et al.* (1975) stressed the distinction between AIL and lymphoma. Subsequently however, the same group (Nathwani *et al.*, 1978) reported 84 patients of whom 48 had AIL and 36 had features interpreted as a mixture of AIL and 'immunoblastic sarcoma'. The latter group had a substantially worse survival than the former. We have seen only one patient who developed malignant lymphoma following the diagnosis of AIL (Jones *et al.*, 1978); a high proportion of patients die with marrow failure and intercurrent infection within two years of diagnosis.

The nature of AIL remains a mystery. Lukes and Tindle (1975) proposed that it develops as a non-neoplastic hyperimmune proliferation of the B-cell system involving an exaggeration of lymphocyte transformation to lymphoblasts and plasma cells, triggered by an abnormal hypersensitivity response to therapeutic agents. Frizzera *et al.* (1975) suggested that the features of this condition are consistent with an autoimmune disorder in which a deficiency of the T-cell regulatory function predisposes to an abnormal proliferation of autoaggressive B-lymphocytes. AIL appears to be a hyperplastic process associated with disturbances of lymphocyte regulatory function which may predispose to the development of lymphoma. The vascular proliferation that is such a characteristic feature of this condition may be related to lymphocyte-induced angiogenesis (Sidky and Aurbach, 1975).

(a) *Histology*

The lymph nodes in AIL may be massively enlarged and have a homogeneous white or pale tan cut surface. Histologically the normal lymph node architecture may be effaced (Fig. 3.21) or there may be

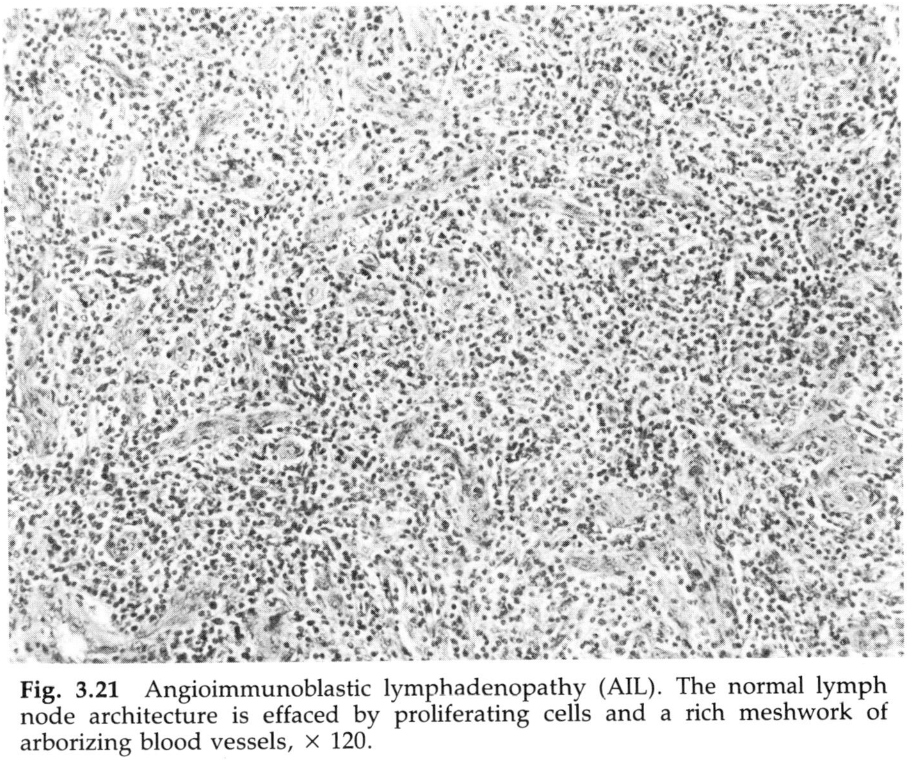

Fig. 3.21 Angioimmunoblastic lymphadenopathy (AIL). The normal lymph node architecture is effaced by proliferating cells and a rich meshwork of arborizing blood vessels, × 120.

residual atrophic lymphoid follicles. The proliferation sometimes extends through the lymph node capsule into the perinodal fat. AIL is characterized by a proliferation of arborizing small blood vessels (Fig. 3.22). These are lined by plump endothelial cells and may have

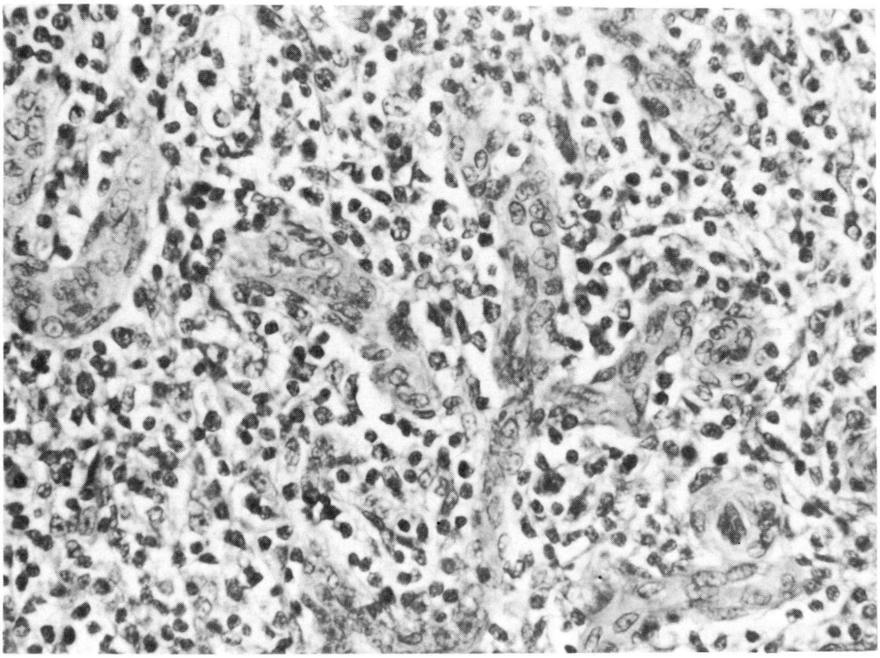

Fig. 3.22 Characteristic arborizing small blood vessels in AIL. Note the plump endothelial cells similar to those seen in postcapillary venules, × 300.

acidophilic, PAS-positive material in the wall. They are highlighted in sections stained for reticulin (Fig. 3.23) and by the PAS technique. The latter method will usually stain the plasma in the vessels darkly due to its high content of immunoglobulin. Between the blood vessels there is a variable infiltrate of small lymphocytes, blast cells and mature plasma cells (Figs 3.24 and 3.25). The blast cells may be either of the T-cell or B-cell series (Jones *et al.*, 1978) and are usually most prominent in sections stained by methyl green pyronin. Numerous mitotic figures are often

---

Fig. 3.23 The characteristic vascular pattern in AIL is well shown in this section stained for reticulin, × 30.

Fig. 3.24 The polymorphic cellular infiltrate in AIL consisting of a mixture of blast cells, plasma cells and small lymphocytes, × 400.

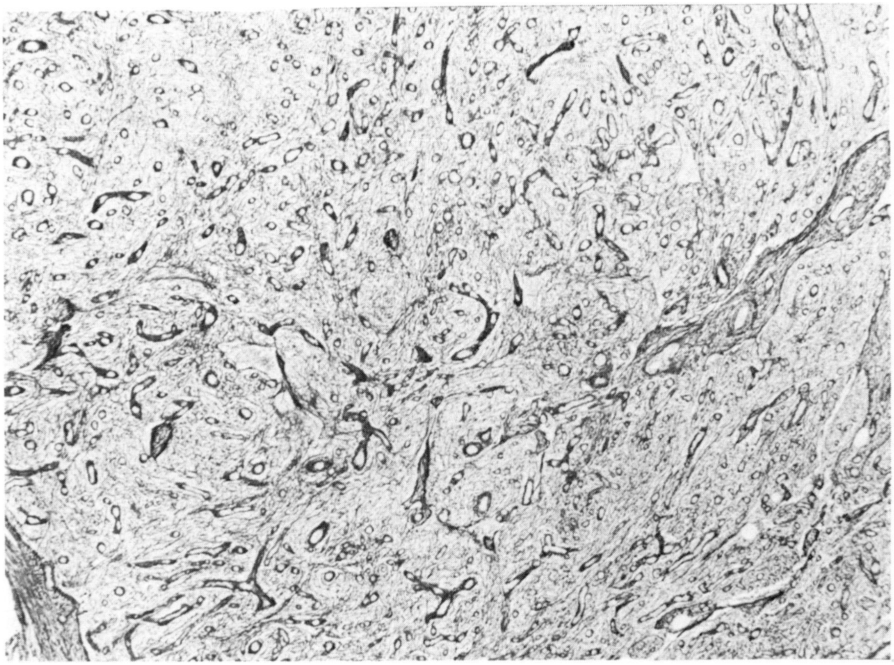

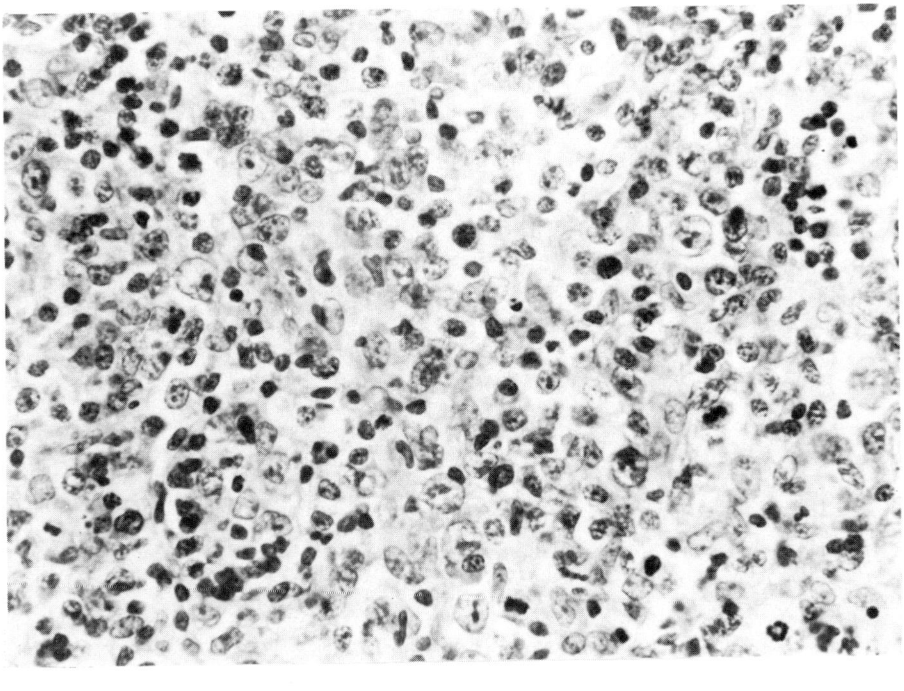

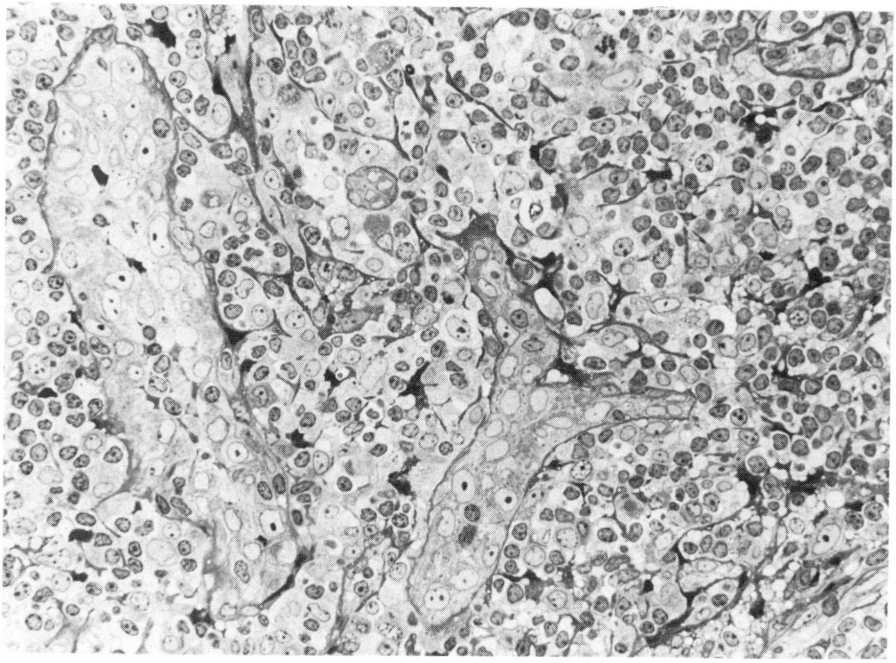

Fig. 3.25 The characteristic blood vessels in AIL are well shown in this plastic section as are the numerous nucleolated blast cells. Toluidine blue, × 300.

present. Immunoperoxidase stains for immunoglobulin show the plasmablasts and plasma cells to be polytypic while stains for lysozyme or other macrophage markers reveal many more histiocytes than are apparent in H and E stained sections. In some cases these histiocytes are seen in conventionally stained sections as epithelioid cell clusters. Some AIL biopsies contain large numbers of eosinophils; in others these cells are scanty or absent. Cellular atypia is not a prominent feature of AIL and should always raise suspicions of malignant lymphoma.

The tissue infiltrates of AIL in spleen, bone marrow, liver and skin are essentially similar to those seen in lymph nodes except that the proliferation of arborizing blood vessels is less easily identified. In our experience it could be difficult to make a definite diagnosis of AIL on biopsies of liver and skin without the knowledge that this disease has been diagnosed at some other site in the patient.

(b) *Differential diagnosis*

Blood vessel proliferation may be associated with a number of reactive diseases of the lymphoid system such as infectious mononucleosis and postvaccinial lymphadenitis. In these lesions, in contrast to AIL, the underlying nodal architecture is usually preserved and the blood vessels do not usually show the complex arborization seen in AIL. AIL may be confused with Hodgkin's disease particularly in those biopsies infiltrated by eosinophils. The absence of classic Reed–Sternberg cells in a lesion that otherwise resembles mixed cellularity Hodgkin's disease is against this diagnosis. In addition a proliferation of immunoblasts is not consistent with any type of Hodgkin's disease.

T-cell lymphomas are associated with a proliferation of blood vessels with plump endothelium and variable infiltrates of epithelioid cells and eosinophils. Watanabe *et al.* (1980) have described an adult T-cell lymphoma with hyperglobulinaemia that closely resembles AIL. In general the blood vessels in T-cell lymphomas do not show the arborizing pattern that is characteristic of AIL and plasma cells and their precursors are less frequent. A marked proliferation of blast cells should always raise suspicions of malignant lymphoma. In T-cell lymphomas these blast cells often exhibit considerable pleomorphism (see Chapter 9).

3.3.2 *Dermatopathic lymphadenopathy*

Synonyms: Lipomelanotic reticular hyperplasia
Lipomelanotic reticulosis

Regional or generalized lymph node enlargement may accompany chronic dermatoses, including the cutaneous T-cell lymphomas. The latter cases my present a difficult problem in the differentiation between dermatopathic lymphadenopathy alone and those cases in which there is infiltration of the lymph nodes by lymphoma cells (Scheffer *et al.*, 1980; Colby *et al.*, 1981).

(a) *Histology*

Enlargement of lymph nodes in dermatopathic lymphadenopathy is usually only moderate and is due mainly to expansion of the paracortex which often extends around the follicles to reach the capsular surface of the node (Figs 3.26 and 3.27). The expansion of the paracortex is due to proliferation or accumulation of interdigitating reticulum cells and Langerhan's cells together with lymphoid cells (Fig. 3.28). At light microscopy Langerhan's cells and interdigitating reticulum cells appear identical and can be differentiated only by the demonstration of Langerhan's granules by electron microscopy. The characteristic elongated irregular reniform nuclei and abundant pale-staining cytoplasm of Langerhan's cells and interdigitating reticulum cells are well seen in imprint preparations (Fig. 3.29), and with high magnification in paraffin sections (Fig. 3.30) and plastic embedded sections (Fig. 3.31). Phagocytozed melanin and haemosiderin may be seen in a proportion of the cells. The associated lymphoid cells include small lymphocytes and blast cells.

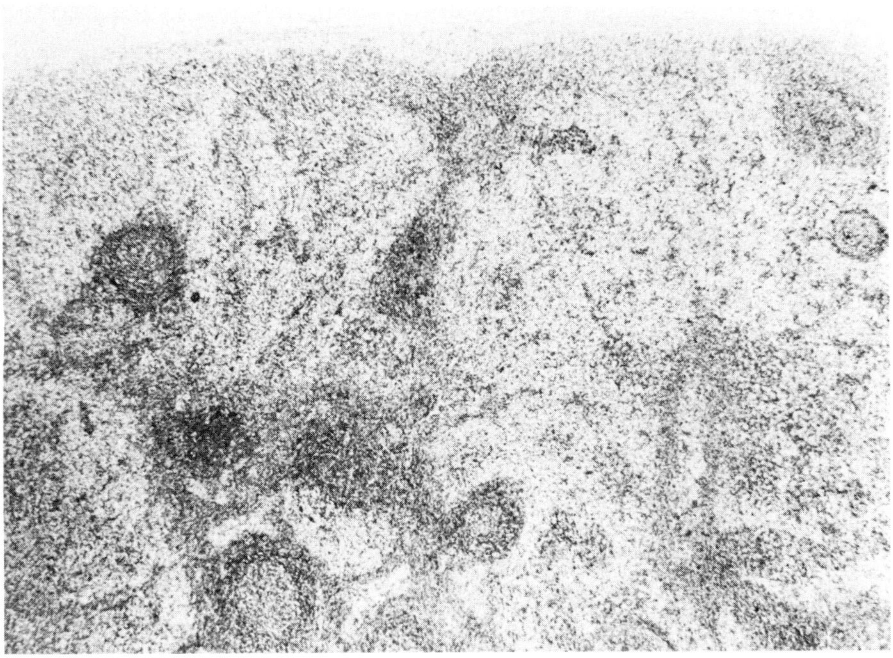

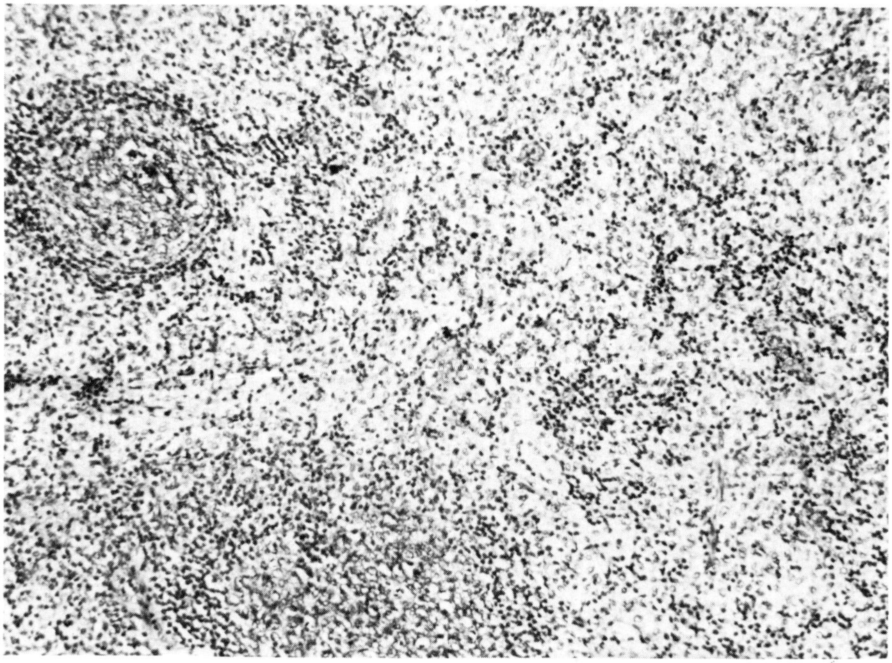

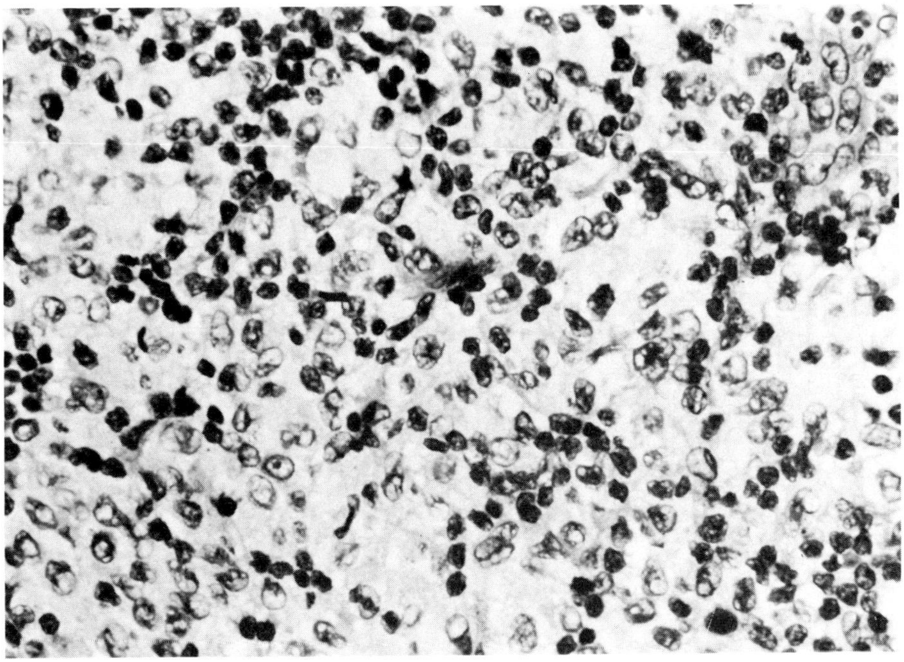

Fig. 3.28 High power view of the paracortical infiltrate in dermatopathic lymphadenopathy shows small lymphocytes and larger interdigitating reticulum and Langerhan's cells with pale-staining nuclei and abundant but indistinct cytoplasm, × 400.

Careful inspection of thin sections and in particular the use of plastic embedding techniques will reveal cerebriform cells amongst these lymphoid cells. This feature alone does not necessarily indicate involvement of the node by cutaneous T-cell lymphoma. Lymphomatous involvement can be recognized by the size of the cerebriform mononuclear cells, pleomorphism of these cells and the formation of large cellular aggregates that eventually obliterate the nodal structure (Scheffer *et al.*, 1980).

3.3.3 *Metastatic neoplasms simulating malignant lymphoma*

Metastatic neoplasms are probably the most frequent cause of lym-

---

Fig. 3.26 Dermatopathic lymphadenopathy. An infiltrate of pale-staining cells expands the paracortex and extends around the follicles to reach the marginal sinus, × 25.
Fig. 3.27 Dermatopathic lymphadenopathy. The infiltrate expanding the paracortex is seen to consist of a mixture of dark and light staining cells, × 100.

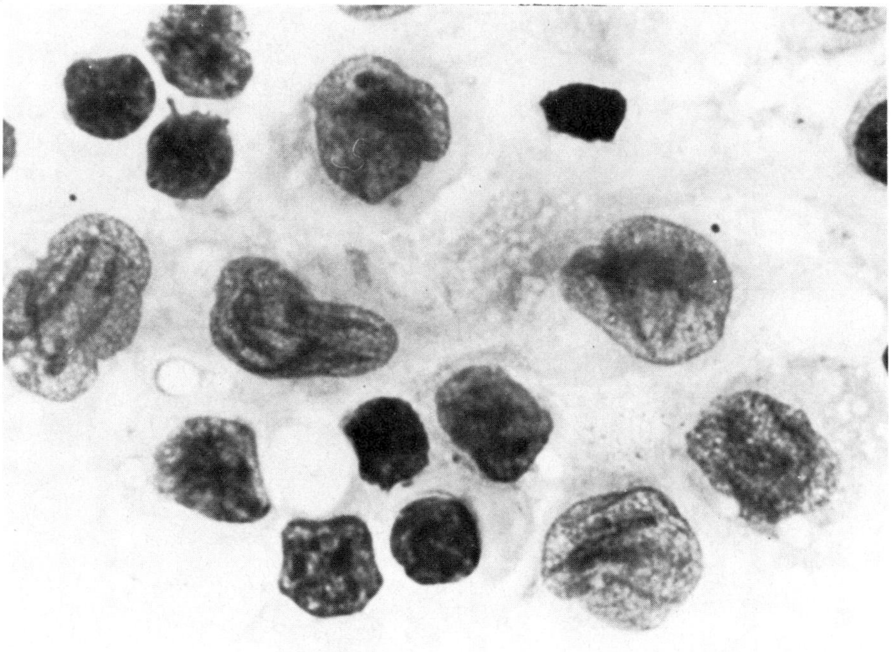

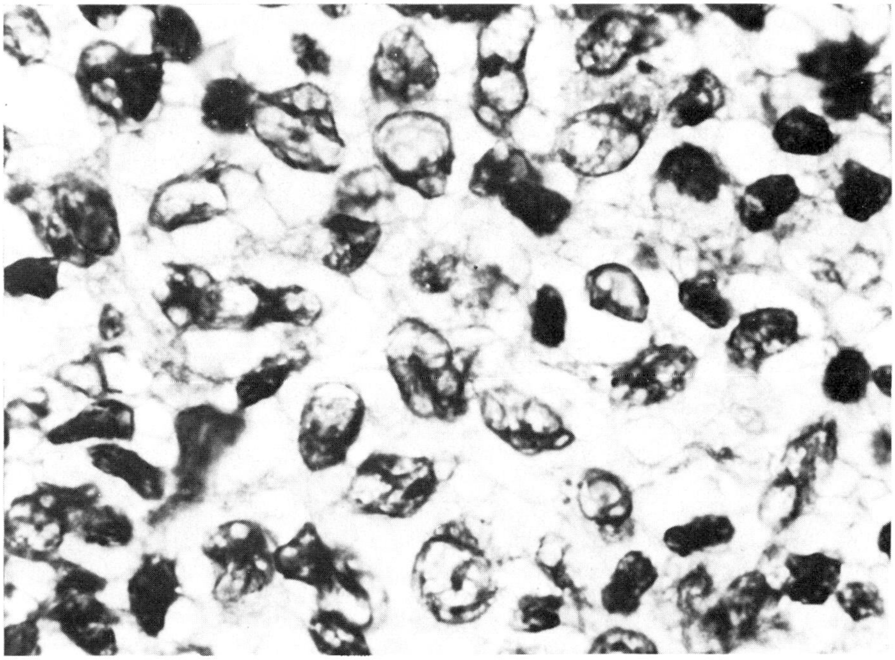

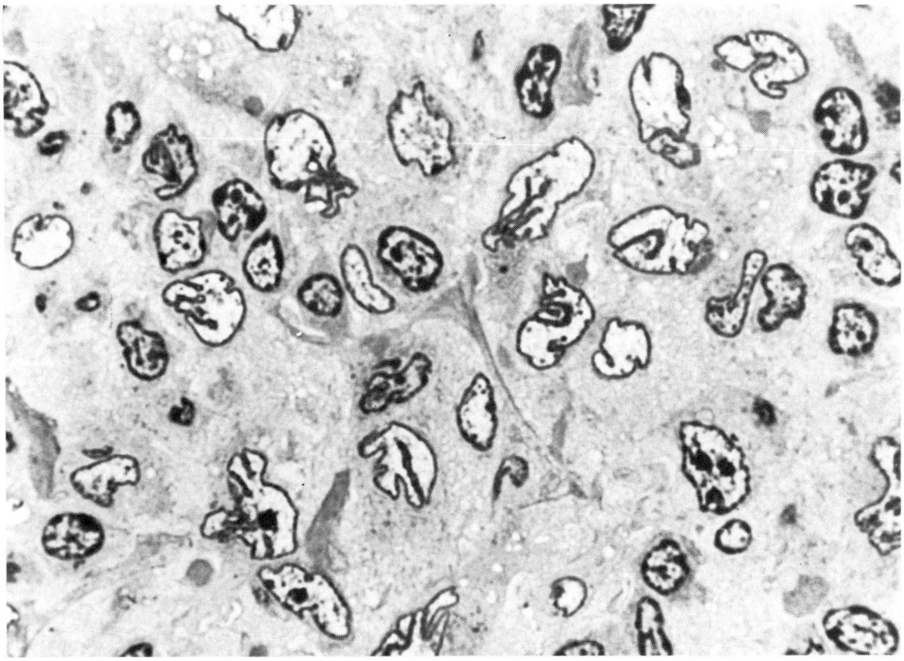

Fig. 3.31 Plastic embedded section of dermatopathic lymphadenopathy showing the characteristic nuclei of interdigitating reticulum cells. Toluidine blue, × 1200.

phadenopathy simulating malignant lymphoma. The distribution of the tumour within the node may give a clue to its nature. In general metastatic tumours spread to the subcapsular and trabecular sinuses first before spreading to the remainder of the node. Tumours may rarely mimic malignant histiocytosis at this stage. Cohesive cell masses and pushing rather than infiltrative margins (Figs 3.32 and 3.33) are usually present and are outlined by the reticulin stain (Fig. 3.34). Occasionally tumours are seen that have infiltrated most of the node resulting in an unusual mixture of tumour cells and lymphocytes (Figs 3.35 and 3.36). Lymphoid follicles may be preserved and the resulting histological appearance may thus simulate T-cell lymphoma. In this type of case the

---

Fig. 3.29 Imprint preparation from a case of dermatopathic lymphadenopathy. The large cells with abundant cytoplasm and delicately folded nuclei are interdigitating reticulum cells or Langerhan's cells. Giemsa, × 1200.
Fig. 3.30 High magnification of the paracortex in dermatopathic lymphadenopathy clearly distinguishes interdigitating reticulum cells and lymphocytes, × 1000.

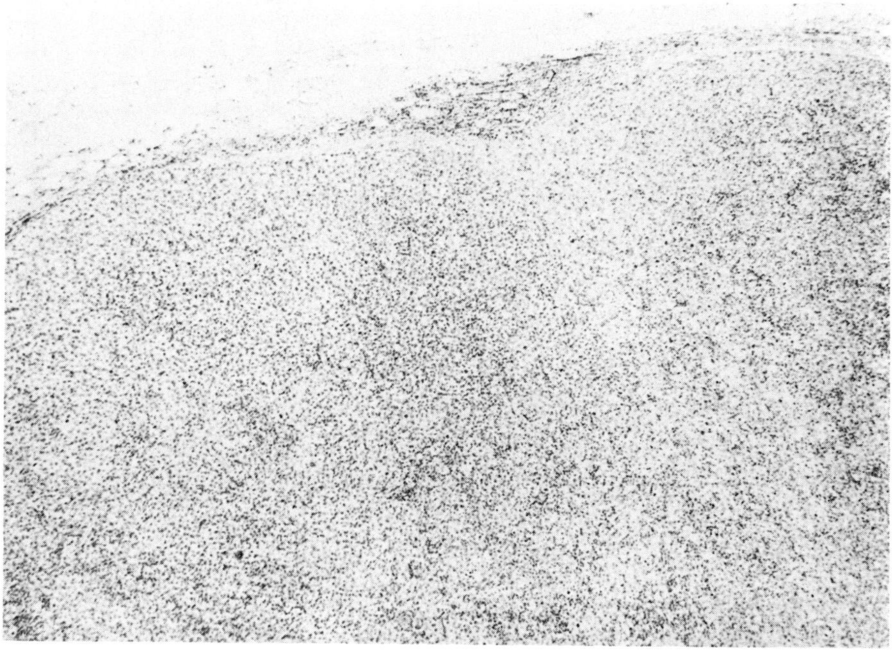

Fig. 3.32 Metastatic carcinoma of the breast replacing a lymph node and resembling malignant lymphoma. There is a narrow rim of compressed lymphoid tissue beneath the capsule, × 32.

separation of metastatic neoplasm from malignant lymphoma ultimately depends upon the cytology of the tumour cells. If strict attention is paid to the cytology of the tumour cells and an attempt is made to precisely identify the lymphoma type rather than making a generic diagnosis of malignant lymphoma non-lymphomatous neoplasms will often be recognized.

The two neoplasms that we have found to mimic malignant lymphoma most closely are postnasal space carcinoma and amelanotic melanoma. Both may have 'silent' primary sites. Although confluent sheets of tumour may be present in postnasal space carcinoma a degree of compartmentalization or packeting is usually evident in some areas and this is well shown with the reticulin stain (Figs 3.37 and 3.38). The tumour

---

Fig. 3.33 Higher power of the same section illustrated in Fig. 3.32, shows the pushing margin of metastatic tumour below a rim of lymphoid tissue above, × 250.

Fig. 3.34 Cohesive cell masses of metastatic carcinoma are outlined by the reticulin stain, × 32.

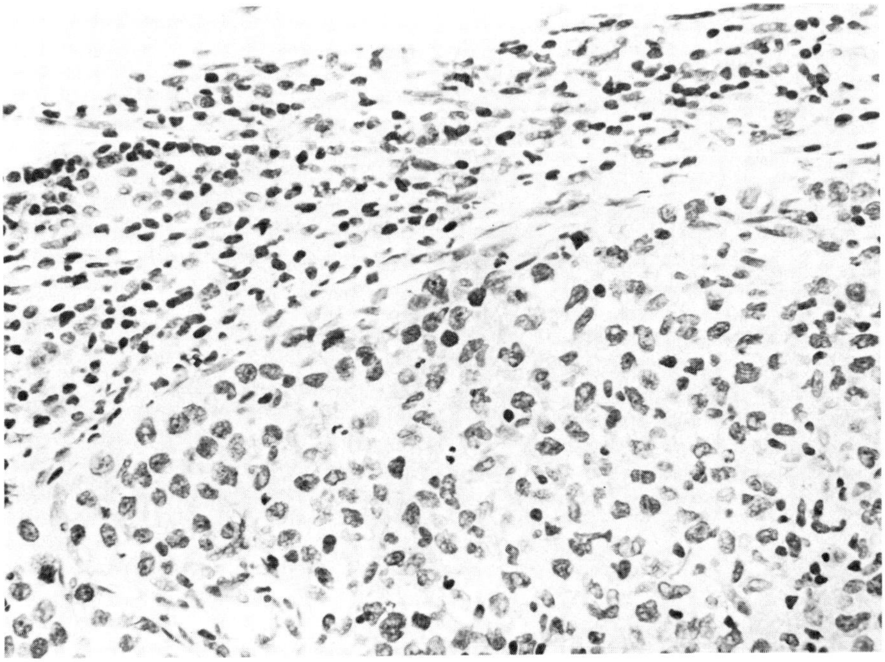

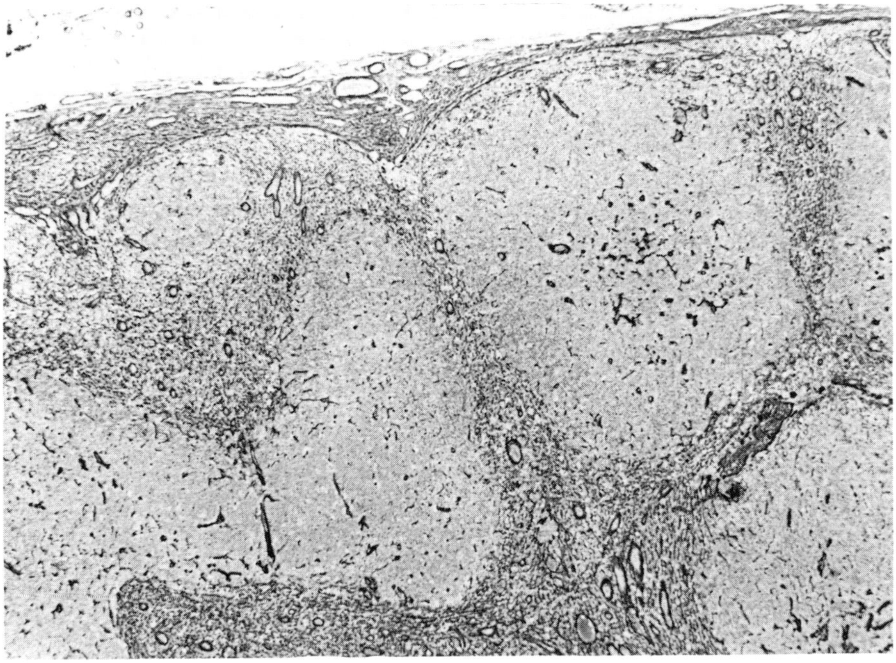

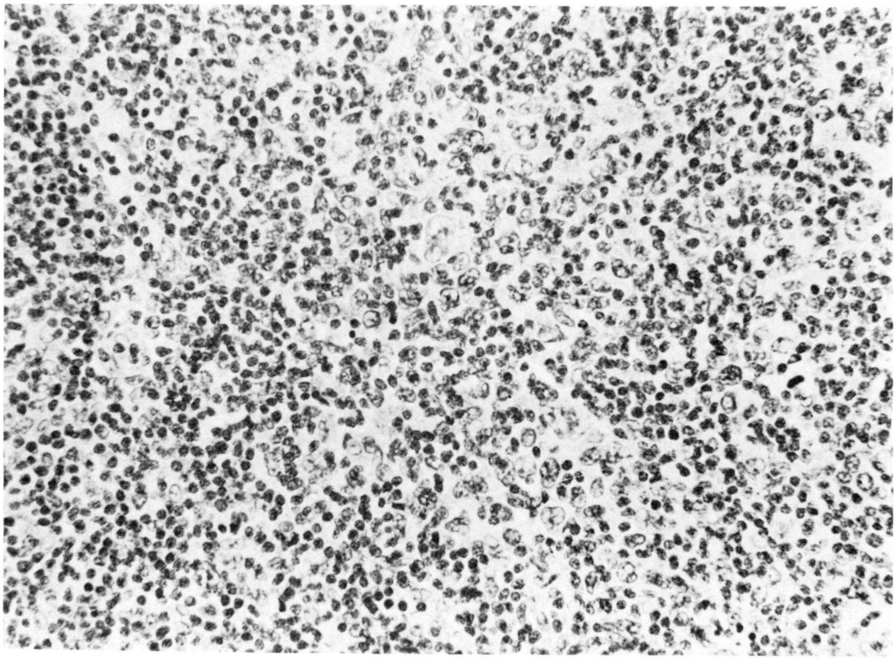

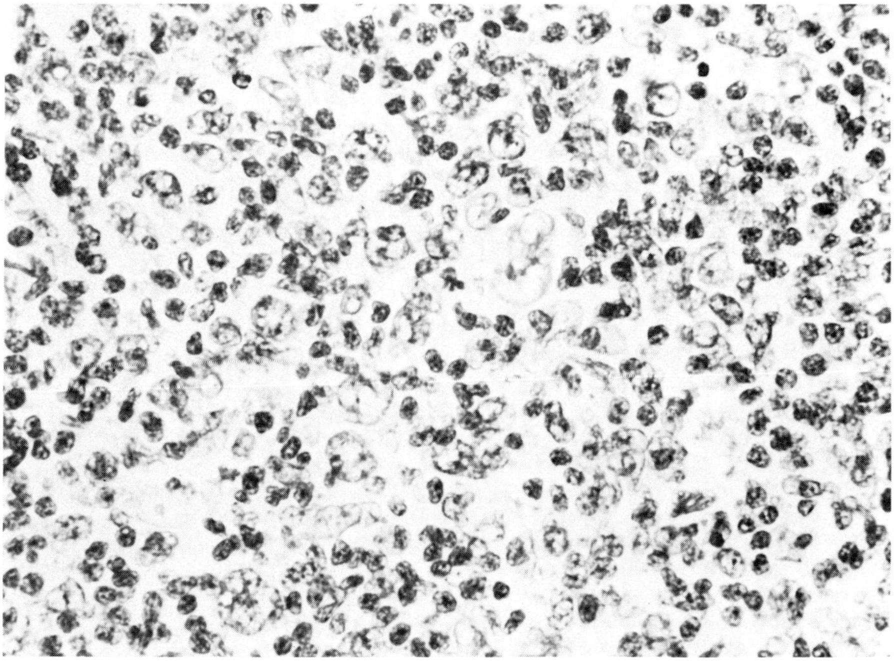

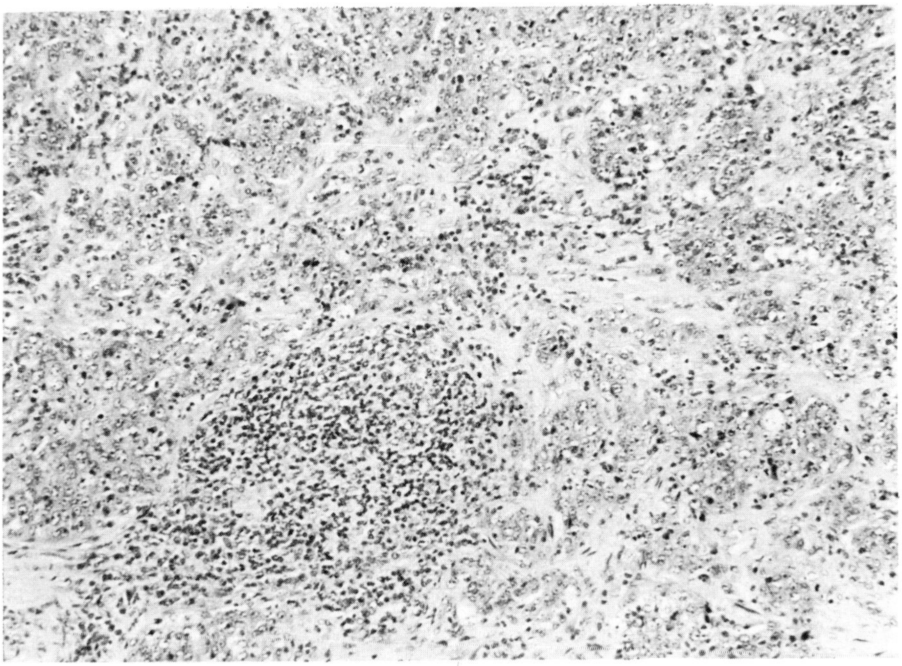

Fig. 3.37 Postnasal space carcinoma. There is packeting of the tumour cell infiltrate and an area of surviving lymphoid tissue, × 100.

cell nuclei may closely resemble centroblasts and interspersed macrophages can give the tumour a 'starry sky' appearance (Fig. 3.39). In replacing the entire node or filling out the sinuses and paracortex (Fig. 3.40) amelanotic melanoma may mimic malignant lymphoma. Again the reticulin stain can be helpful in demonstrating packeting of tumour cells (Fig. 3.41). Malignant melanocytes can bear a close resemblance to immunoblasts (Fig. 3.42) since their nuclei often contain large central nucleoli. A careful search will often reveal a few melanin-containing cells especially around islands of residual lymphoid tissue. Polymorph infiltration particularly around areas of tumour necrosis is more characteristic of carcinoma than lymphoma. Eosinophil infiltration is occasionally seen in carcinomas and should not in itself lead to a diagnosis of Hodgkin's disease. Binucleate cells superficially resembling Reed–Sternberg cells may be found in a number of anaplastic tumours but

---

Fig. 3.35 Metastatic carcinoma showing an unusual pattern of an intimate mixture of tumour cells and lymphoid cells, × 250.
Fig. 3.36 Higher power of Fig. 3.35 showing the cytology of large tumour cells which is not characteristic of any type of malignant lymphoma, × 400.

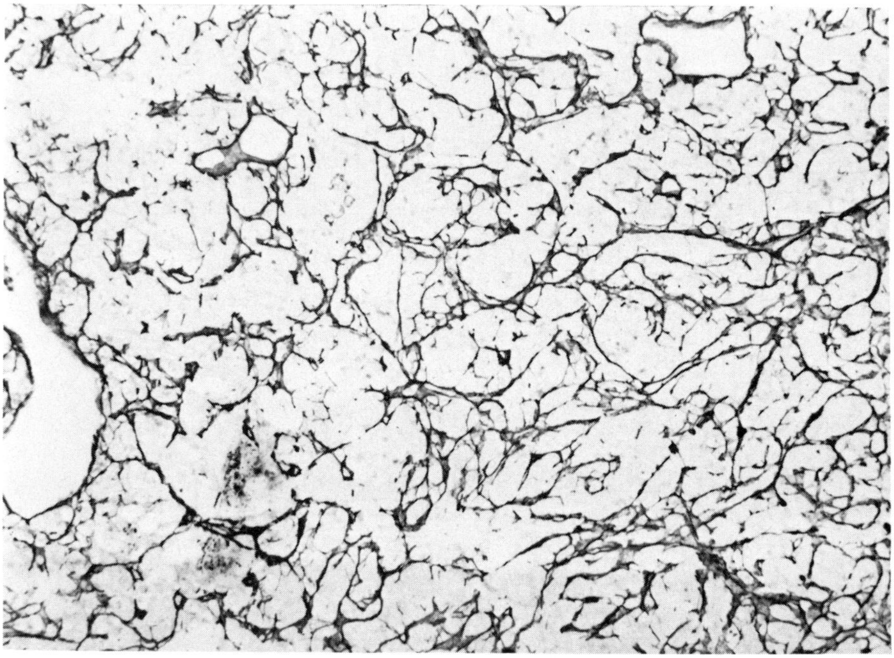

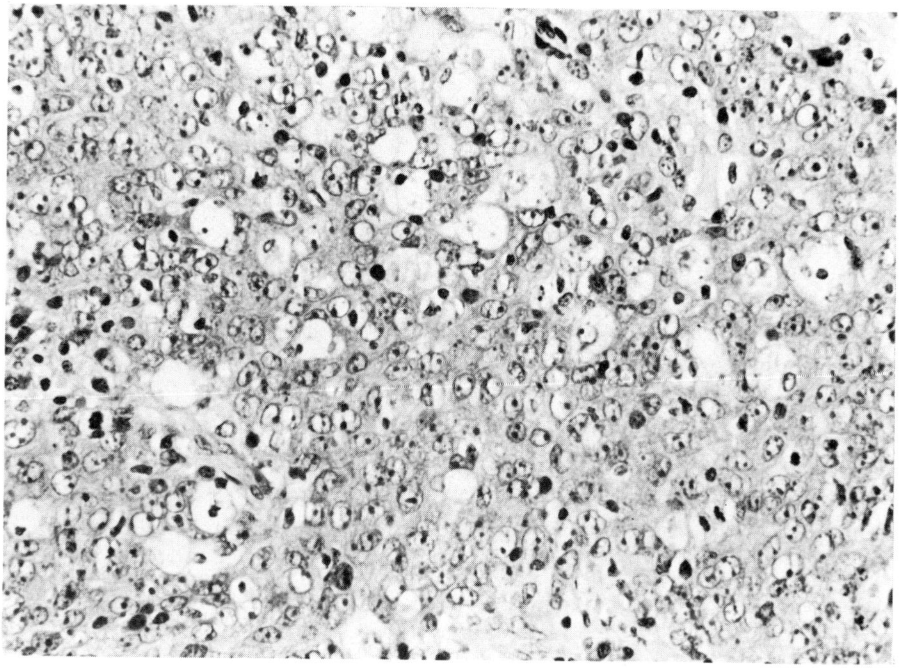

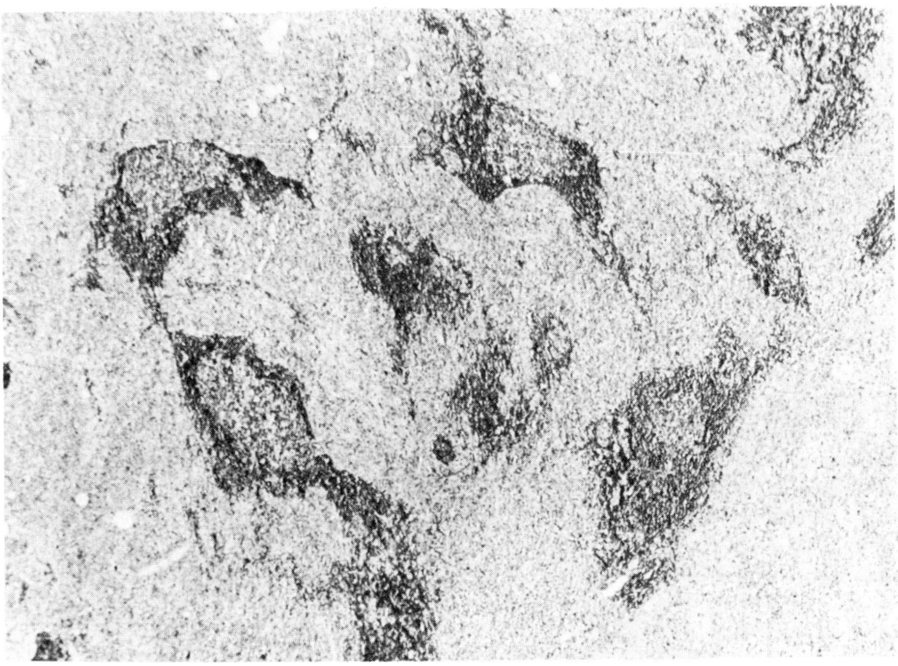

Fig. 3.40 Metastatic amelanotic melanoma filling out the sinuses and paracortex of a lymph node, × 400.

the background population of mononuclear tumour cells is usually inappropriate for any type of Hodgkin's disease.

3.3.4 *Silicone lymphadenopathy*

Silicone compounds have been used for many years in plastic surgery and in mammoplasty operations. In more recent years silicone elastomer prostheses have been employed to restore joint function in arthritic patients. Although relatively inert, silicone compounds can elicit a granulomatous reaction and when deposited in lymph nodes cause a significant lymphadenopathy (Kircher, 1980). In silicone lymphadenopathy the lymph node shows reactive changes and contains multinucleated giant cells in the paracortex and medullary cords (Fig. 3.43). Irregular granular fragments of silicone elastomer can be seen within the giant

---

Fig. 3.38 Postnasal space carcinoma. The packeting of the tumour cell infiltrate is emphasized by the reticulin stain, × 100.
Fig. 3.39 The cells of this postnasal space carcinoma resemble centroblasts. Interspersed macrophages give a 'starry sky' effect, × 400.

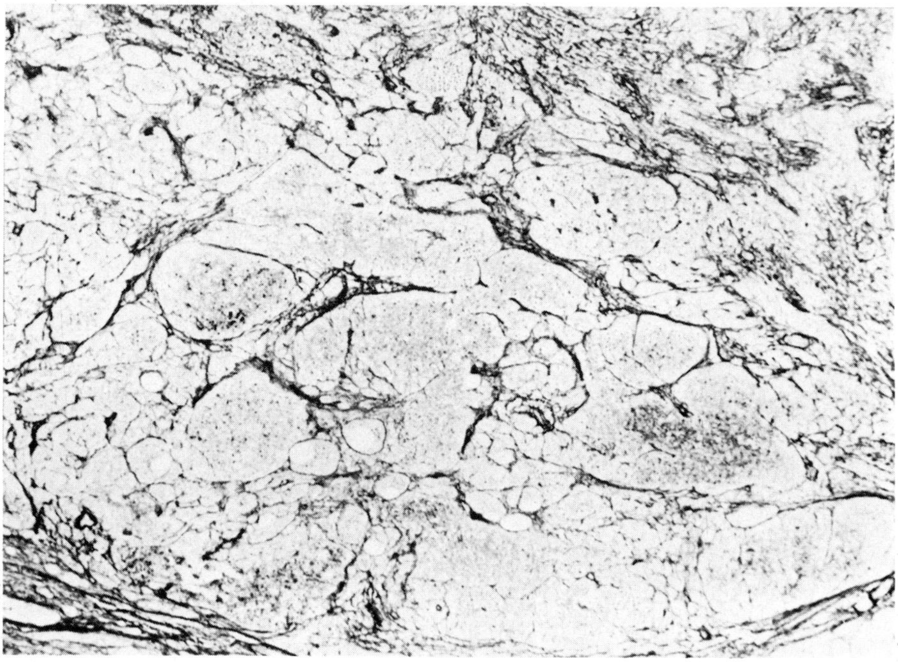

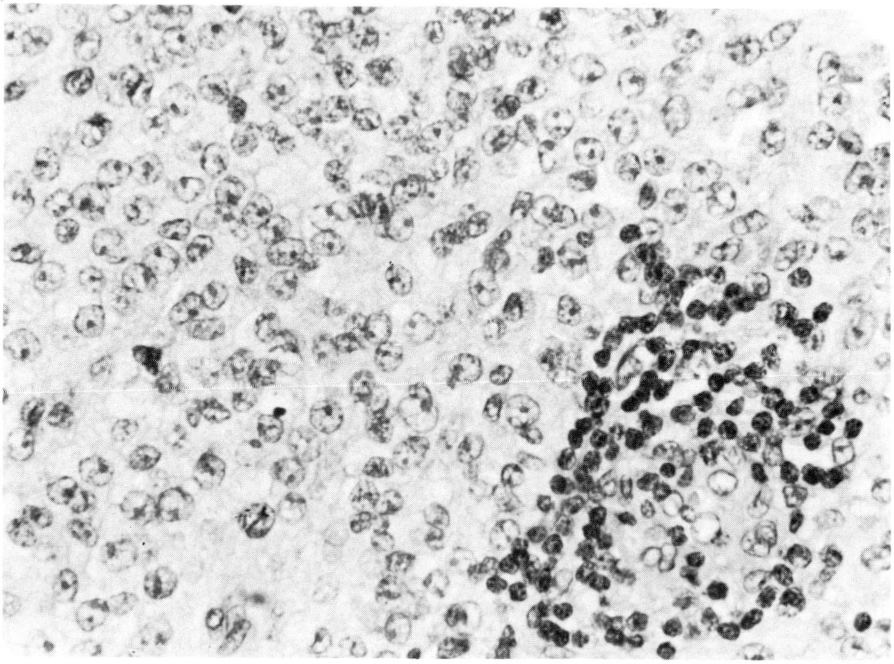

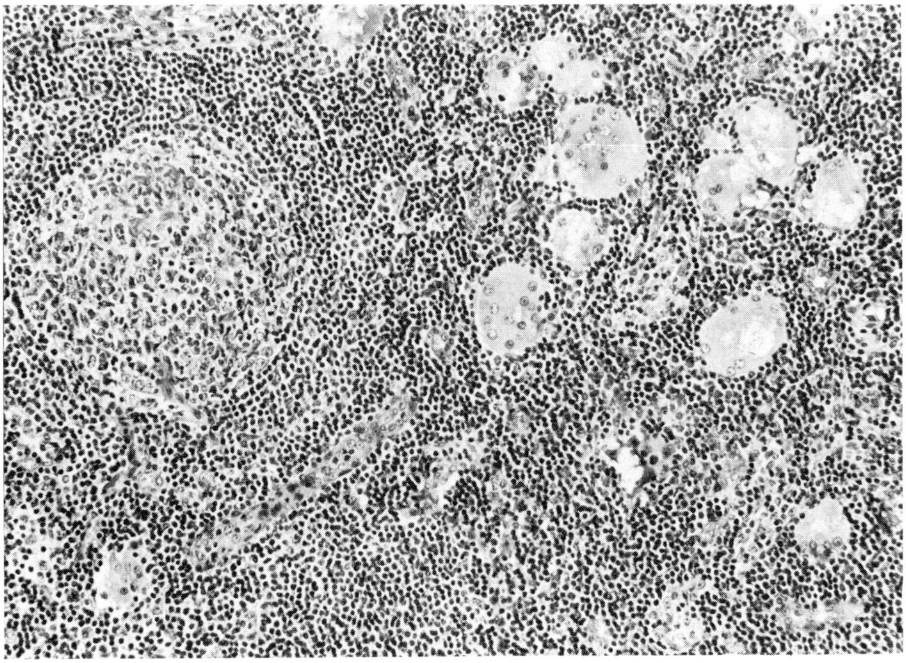

Fig. 3.43 Silicone lymphadenopathy showing multinucleated giant cells in the paracortex, × 120.

cells. This refractile material is not birefringent in polarized light. Asteroid bodies are seen in many of the giant cells (Fig. 3.44). Lymphadenopathy in patients with silicone elastomer prostheses is sometimes associated with malignant lymphoma (Digby and Wells, 1981) and in such cases silicone granulomas may be seen dispersed amongst the tumour cells (Fig. 3.45).

3.3.5 *Drug-induced lymphadenopathy*

Synonym: Diphenylhydantoin-induced lymphadenopathy
Dilantin hypersensitivity

Saltzstein and Ackerman (1959) described lymphadenopathy in patients receiving diphenylhydantoins in which there were prominent, some-

---

Fig. 3.41 Reticulin stain of metastatic amelanotic melanoma showing packeting of the tumour, × 40.
Fig. 3.42 The cells of metastatic amelanotic melanoma can, as shown here, bear a close resemblance to immunoblasts, × 400.

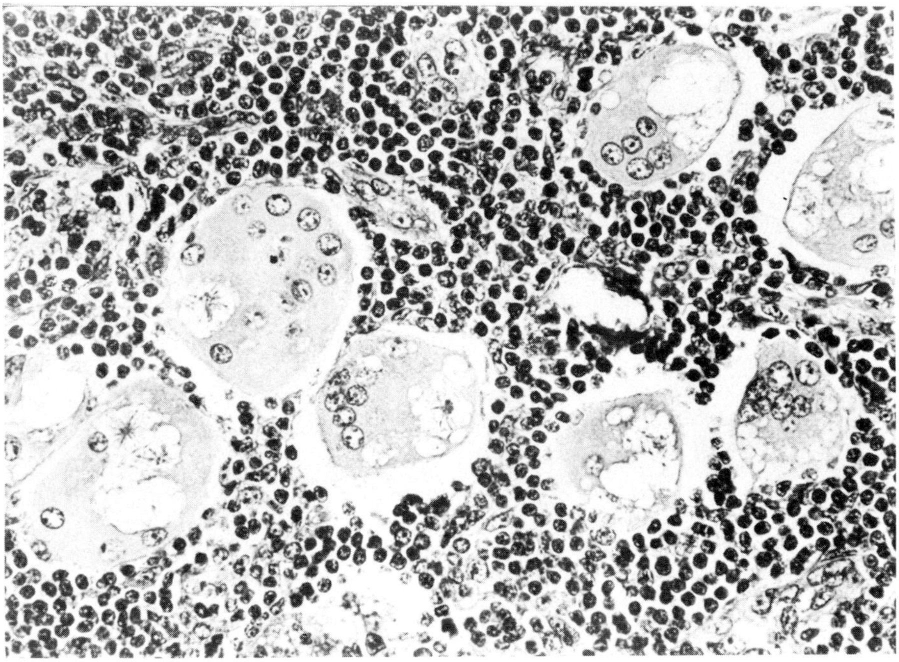

Fig. 3.44 Ateroid bodies and refractile material are characteristically present in the giant cells in silicone lymphadenopathy, × 300.

times pleomorphic, reticulum cells, eosinophils, neutrophils, plasma cells and areas of necrosis. In these patients lymphadenopathy regressed following cessation of treatment although some of them subsequently developed malignant lymphomas. Similar experiences have been reported by other authors (Hyman and Sommers, 1966; Dorfman and Warnke, 1974) suggesting that hydantoin-induced lymphadenopathy is either a preneoplastic state or occurs more frequently in patients at risk from lymphoma. Patients with angioimmunoblastic lymphadenopathy (AIL) frequently give a history of previous drug exposure and cases have been recorded following treatment with diphenylhydantoin (Lapes *et al.*, 1976). AIL and diphenylhydantoin-induced lymphadenopathy frequently present with fever, anaemia, lymphadenopathy and hepatosplenomegaly. In general patients with diphenylhydantoin-induced lymphadenopathy are younger than those with AIL, the lymphadenopathy regresses more consistently following drug withdrawal and is said to be most pronounced in the cervical region whereas in AIL it is frequently generalized.

Histologically diphenylhydantoin-induced lymphadenopathy shows distortion or partial effacement of nodal architecture. Vasculitis may be

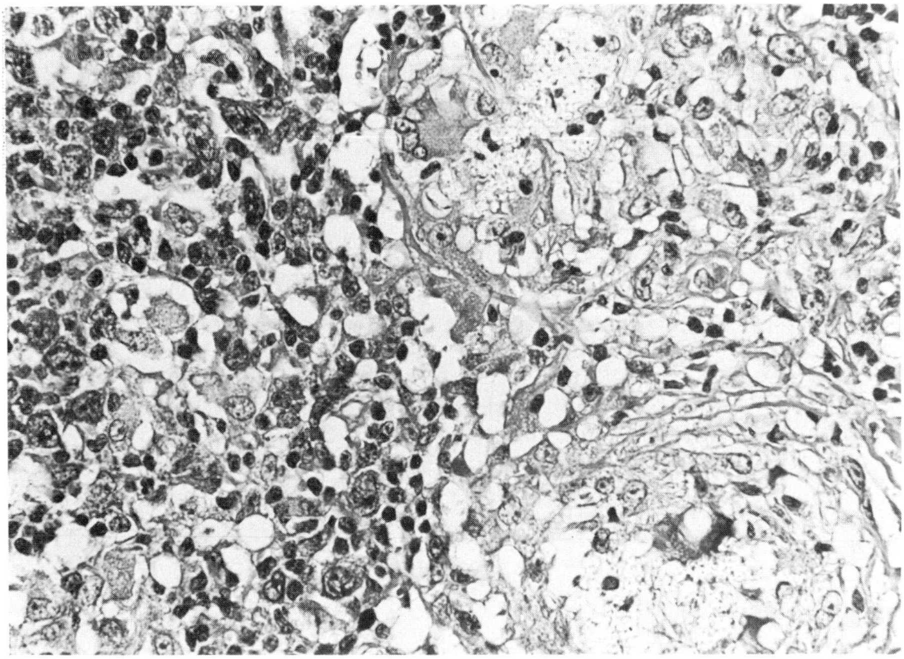

Fig. 3.45 Silicone lymphadenopathy occurring in association with a diffuse centroblastic/centrocytic lymphoma. Neoplastic centroblasts and centrocytes are seen to the left and histiocyte/giant cell granulomas surrounding refractile material to the right, × 300.

seen in the capsular vessels and there are associated areas of necrosis in the lymph node. Eosinophil infiltrates may be prominent. These appearances suggest a hypersensitivity reaction, possibly mediated by immune complexes whereas the changes in AIL suggest a more fundamental disorder of lymphocyte organization. Diphenylhydantoin-induced lymphadenopathy is an uncommon disorder in relation to the large numbers of patients receiving anticonvulsant therapy.

3.3.6 *Lupus erythematosus*

Lymphadenopathy is an unusual presenting feature of lupus erythmatosus and lymph node biopsy is rarely performed in this condition. Involved nodes may show varying degrees of follicular and parafollicular hyperplasia. More characteristic are small areas of necrosis often containing aggregates of nuclear debris (haematoxyphil bodies) probably within macrophages. Within these areas DNA may form a slightly granular haematoxyphilic deposit on collagen fibres and blood vessels.

Similar features are seen in malignant lymphomas and some metastatic neoplasms and care should be taken to exclude these.

3.3.7 Spontaneous infarction of lymph nodes

Lymph nodes have an abundant blood supply and infarction is rare. Davies and Stansfeld (1972) described five patients with spontaneous infarction of superficial lymph nodes, two of which were diagnosed clinically as fibroadenomas of the axillary tail of the breast and two as femoral hernias. They observed thrombosed and partially recanalized veins within the substance and the hila of the affected nodes and attributed the infarction to venous thrombosis. In practice infarction of lymph nodes is most frequently associated with metastatic neoplasms or lymphomas. The infarction in such cases can be almost total. A search should be made for residual tumour cells around blood vessels and within or just beneath the capsule. The character of the cell ghosts may aid the identification of pre-existing neoplasm and the reticulin stain is often of value in determining the underlying structure of the node.

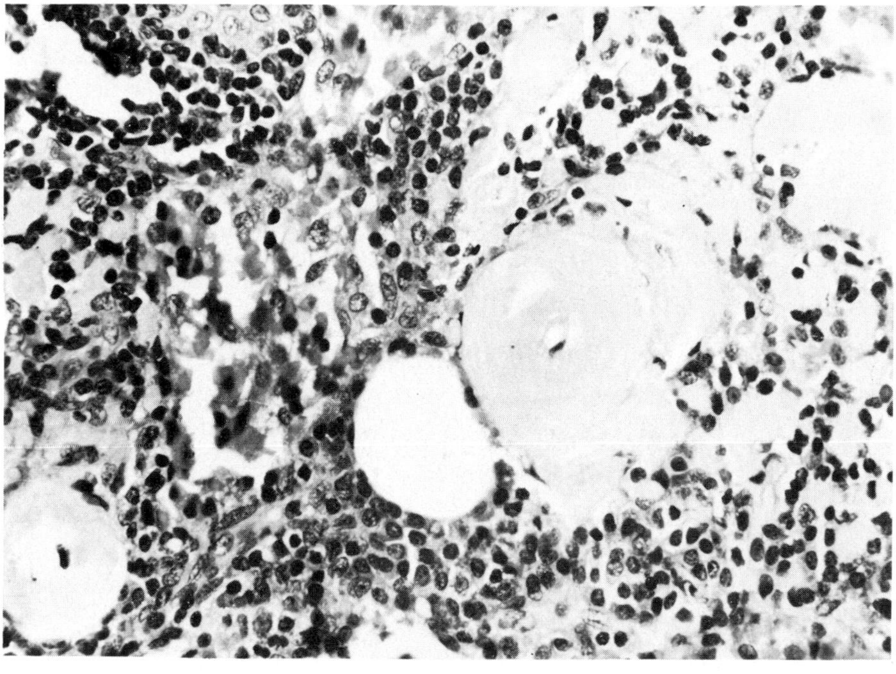

Fig. 3.46 Amyloidosis inolving a lymph node showing concentric perivascular deposition of amyloid, × 300.

3.3.8 *Amyloidosis*

Lymph nodes may be affected by amyloidosis, and show moderate enlargement. The amyloid is often deposited in concentric perivascular rings (Fig. 3.46) and gradually displaces the cells from the node. It may be associated with lymphoplasmacytic and plasmacytic neoplasms although the acidophilic hyaline material found in such cases is usually hyalinized collagen or inspissated protein. Infiltration of the lymphoid follicles or medullary cords of the spleen is well recognized in systemic amyloidosis.

References

Azoury, F. J. and Reed, R. J. (1966), Histiocytosis: report of an unusual case. *New Engl. J. Med.*, **274**, 928–30.

Bartoli, E., Massarelli, G., Soggia, G. and Tanda, F. (1980), Multicentric giant lymph node hyperplasia. A hyperimmune syndrome with a rapidly progressive course. *Am. J. Clin. Pathol.*, **73**, 423–6.

Becroft, D. M. O., Dix, M. R., Gillman, J. C. *et al.* (1973), Benign sinus histiocytosis with massive lymphadenopathy: transient immunological defects in a child with mediastinal involvement. *J. Clin. Path.*, **26**, 463–9.

Butler, J. J. (1969), Non-neoplastic lesions of lymph nodes of man to be differentiated from lymphomas. *Natl Cancer Inst. Monogr.*, **32**, 233–55.

Castleman, B., Iverson, L. and Menendez, V. P. (1956), Localized mediastinal lymph node hyperplasia resembling thymoma. *Cancer*, **9**, 822–30.

Colby, T. V., Burke, J. S. and Hoppe, R. T. (1981), Lymph node biopsy in mycosis fungoides. *Cancer*, **47**, 351–9.

Davies, J. D. and Stansfeld, A. G. (1972), Spontaneous infarction of superficial lymph nodes. *J. Clin. Pathol.*, **25**, 689–96.

Diamond, L. W. and Braylan, R. C. (1980), Immunological markers and DNA content in a case of giant lymph node hyperplasia (Castleman's disease). *Cancer*, **46**, 730–5.

Digby, J. and Wells, A. L. (1981), Malignant lymphoma with intranodal refractile particles after insertion of silicone prosthesis. *Lancet*, **ii**, 580.

Dorfman, R. F. and Warnke, R. (1974), Lymphadenopathy simulating the malignant lymphomas. *Human Pathol.*, **5**, 519–50.

Foucar, E., Rosai, J. and Dorfman, R. F. (1978), Sinus histiocytosis with massive lymphadenopathy. Ear, nose and throat manifestations. *Arch. Otolaryngol.*, **104**, 687–93.

Foucar, E., Rosai, J. and Dorfman, R. F. (1979), The ophthalmologic manifestations of sinus histiocytosis with massive lymphadenopathy. *Am. J. Ophthamol.*, **87**, 354–67.

Frizzera, G., Moran, E. M. and Rappaport, H. (1975), Angioimmunoblastic lymphadenopathy: diagnosis and clinical course. *Am. J. Med.*, **59**, 803–18.

Gaba, A. R., Stein, R. S., Sweet, D. L. and Variakojis, D. (1978), Multicentric giant lymph node hyperplasia. *Am. J. Clin. Pathol.*, **69**, 86–90.

Haferkamp, O., Roseneau, W. and Lennert, K. (1971), Vascular transformation of lymph node sinuses due to venous obstruction. *Arch. Pathol.*, **92**, 81–3.

Hyman, G. A. and Sommers, C. (1966), The development of Hodgkin's disease and lymphoma during anticonvulsant therapy. *Blood*, **28**, 416–27.

Hymes, K. B., Cheung, T., Greene, J. B. *et al.* (1981), Kaposi's sarcoma in homosexual men – A report of eight cases. *Lancet*, **ii**, 598–600.

Jones, D. B., Castleden, M., Smith, J. L. *et al.* (1978), Immunopathology of angioimmunoblastic lymphadenopathy. *Br. J. Cancer*, **37**, 1053–62.

Keller, A. R., Hochholzer, L. and Castleman, B. (1972), Hyaline-vascular and plasma cell types of giant lymph node hyperplasia of the mediastinum and other locations. *Cancer*, **29**, 670–83.

Kircher, T. (1980), Silicone lymphadenopathy. A complication of silicone elastomer finger joint prostheses. *Human Pathol.*, **11**, 240–4.

Lampert, F. and Lennert, K. (1976), Sinus histiocytosis with massive lymphadenopathy. Fifteen new cases. *Cancer*, **37**, 783–9.

Lapes, M. J., Vivacqua, R. J. and Antoniades, K. (1976), Immunoblastic lymphadenopathy associated with phenytoin. (Diphenylhydantoin.) *Lancet*, **i**, 198.

Lattes, R. and Pachter, M. R. (1962), Benign lymphoid masses of probable hamartomatous nature. *Cancer*, **15**, 197–214.

Lukes, R. J. and Tindle, B. H. (1975), Immunoblastic lymphadenopathy. A hyperimmune entity resembling Hodgkin's disease. *New Engl. J. Med.*, **292**, 1–8.

Nathwani, B. N., Rappaport, H., Moran, E. M. *et al.* (1978), Malignant lymphoma arising in angioimmunoblastic lymphadenopathy. *Cancer*, **41**, 578–606.

Robb-Smith, A. H. T. (1947), The lymph node biopsy. In *Recent Advances in Clinical Pathology* (ed. S. C. Dyke), Churchill Livingstone, London, pp. 350–77.

Rosai, J. and Dorfman, R. F. (1972), Sinus histiocytosis with massive lymphadenopathy: a pseudolymphomatous benign disorder. Analysis of 34 cases. *Cancer*, **30**, 1174–88.

Saltzstein, S. L. and Ackerman, L. V. (1959), Lymphadenopathy induced by anticonvulsant drugs and mimicking clinically and pathologically malignant lymphoma. *Cancer*, **12**, 164–82.

Scheffer, E., Meijer, C. J. L. M. and Vanvloten, W. A. (1980), Dermatopathic lymphadenopathy and lymph node involvement in mycosis fungoides. *Cancer*, **45**, 137–48.

Schroer, K. R. and Franssila, K. O. (1979), Atypical hyperplasia of lymph nodes: A follow-up study. *Cancer*, **44**, 1155–63.

Sidky, Y. A. and Aurbach, R. (1975), Lymphocyte induced angiogenesis; a quantitative and sensitive assay of the graft vs. host reaction. *J. Exp. Med.*, **141**, 1084–100.

Thawerani, H., Sanchez, R. L., Rosai, J. and Dorfman, R. F. (1978), The cutaneous manifestations of sinus histiocytosis with massive lymphadenopathy. *Arch. Dermatol.*, **114**, 191–7.

Walker, P., Rosai, J. and Dorfman, R. F. (1981), The osseous manifestations of sinus histiocytosis with massive lymphadenopathy. *Am. J. Clin. Pathol.*, **75**, 131–9.

Watanabe, S., Shinosato, Y., Shimoyama, M. *et al.* (1980), Adult T-cell lymphoma with hypergammaglobulinaemia. *Cancer*, **46**, 2472–83.

Williams, J. and Dorfman, R. F. (1979), Lymphadenopathy as the initial manifestation of histiocytosis X. *Am. J. Surg. Pathol.*, **3**, 405–21.

Wright, D. H. and Richards, D. B. (1981), Sinus histiocytosis with massive lymphadenopathy (Rosai–Dorfman disease): Report of a case with widespread nodal and extranodal dissemination. *Histopathology*, **5**, 697–709.

4 Hodgkin's disease

The debate as to whether Hodgkin's disease is an inflammatory or neoplastic disease appears to have been settled in favour of the latter. The main evidence supporting a neoplastic proliferation is the relentless progression of the disease when untreated, the morphological atypia of some of the component cells and the finding of aneuploidy in cytogenetic preparations made from Hodgkin's tissue (Kaplan, 1980). The Reed–Sternberg (RS) cell and its mononuclear counterpart (often referred to as the Hodgkin cell) are regarded as the neoplastic cells whereas the other components of Hodgkin's disease tissue are thought to be reactive. The presence of RS cells is mandatory for a diagnosis of Hodgkin's disease, but since morphologically identical or closely similar cells may be seen in other lymphoproliferative or neoplastic diseases the diagnosis of Hodgkin's disease should be made only when RS cells are seen in a cellular setting appropriate for one of the morphological subtypes of that disease. The composition of the reactive cells forming that setting, the numerical relationship of those cells to the RS cells and variations in the morphology of the RS cells are used to define the histological subtypes of Hodgkin's disease (Table 4.1) (Lukes and Butler, 1966).

Partial involvement of lymph nodes may occur in Hodgkin's disease. In the early stages this may be focal involving the parafollicular areas of the node (Fig. 4.1). In lymph nodes removed from patients with suspected Hodgkin's disease or removed at staging laparotomy that appear on low power examination to show follicular hyperplasia only, it is worthwhile critically examining the parafollicular areas for evidence of Hodgkin's disease (Strum and Rappaport, 1970). Progression of the disease gradually obliterates the interfollicular structures so that atrophic follicles are isolated in a sea of Hodgkin's tissue before the node is eventually totally replaced.

The histogenesis of RS cells remains a subject of speculation and controversy (Kaplan, 1980). Morphological similarities between these cells and transformed lymphocytes, together with the demonstration of

Table 4.1 Classification of Hodgkin's disease

Type of Hodgkin's disease	Classic RS cells	RS cell variants	Lymphocytes	Epithelioid histiocytes	Eosinophils	Other features/comments
Lymphocyte predominant:						
Nodular	±	Polylobated type	+++	+ → +++	±	Nodular structure
Diffuse	±	Polylobated type	+++	+ → +++	±	Classic Hodgkin's paragranuloma
Mixed cellularity	+ → ++	–	+ → ++	+ → ++	± → ++	Classic Hodgkin's granuloma
Nodular sclerosing	± → +	Lacunar type	+ → ++	+ → ++	± → ++	Divided into nodules by bands of collagen
Nodular sclerosing cellular phase	± → +	Lacunar type	+ → ++	+ → ++	± → ++	Lacunar RS cells but no fibrosis
Lymphocyte depleted:						
Reticular	+ → +++	–	± → +	± → +	+ → ++	Classic Hodgkin's sarcoma
Diffuse	± → +	–	± → +	± → +	± → +	Hypocellular tissue with eosinophilic PAS-positive interstitial material

± Very scanty
\+
++ ↓
+++ Plentiful

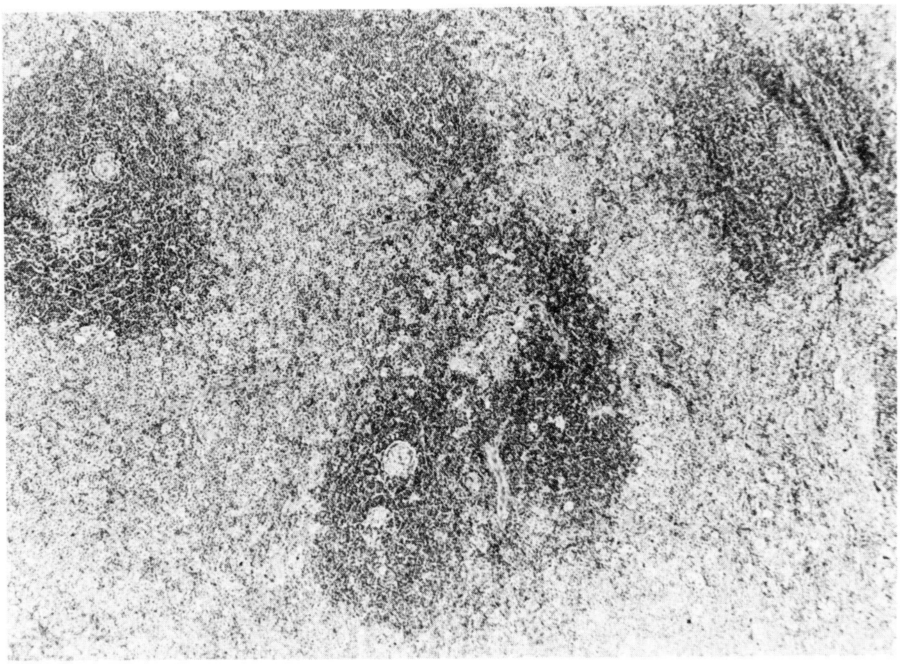

Fig. 4.1 Lymph node showing early involvement by Hodgkin's disease. The tumour infiltrates the paracortex of the node leaving residual atrophic follicles, × 40.

immunoglobulin in their cytoplasm (Garvin *et al.*, 1974; Taylor, 1976) was thought to favour an origin from B-lymphocytes. Subsequent studies showed that the immunoglobulin is polytypic (includes both light chains) and frequently associated with other serum proteins (Poppema, 1978; Payne *et al.*, 1982). These observations suggest that the RS cell takes up protein from its environment. Elegant tissue culture studies of RS cells by Kadin *et al.* (1978) have confirmed this suggestion. This observation together with the finding that some RS cells contain granular alpha-1-antitrypsin (Payne *et al.*, 1982) and fibronectin (Resnick and Nachman, 1981) could be interpreted as favouring a monocyte/macrophage-derived cell. The studies of cultured RS cells by Kaplan and his colleagues support this interpretation (Kaplan, 1980).

Kaplan and Smithers (1959) noted similarities between Hodgkin's disease tissue and tissues from animals with graft versus host disease, and suggested that Hodgkin's disease might represent a lymphocyte war. With this concept in mind the reactive cells in Hodgkin's tissue might represent at least in part, a 'host' reaction against the tumour cells. The high ratio of lymphocytes to RS cells in the prognostically favourable subtypes of Hodgkin's disease could be regarded as indicating good host immune response to the neoplastic cells. This, however, is probably a naive concept since the lymphocytes do not appear to exert a cytotoxic action against the RS cells (Payne *et al.*, 1980). There appears to be a profound disturbance of lymphoreticular physiology in Hodgkin's tissue that is frequently associated with generalized disturbances of immune reactivity, particularly of T-lymphocyte function. This may be related to the aetiology of the disease but the substantial restoration of immune function that follows successful therapy suggests that the disease causes the immunological perturbation (Kaplan, 1980).

Hodgkin's disease shows a number of clinical features that set it apart from other malignant lymphomas. It has a bimodal age distribution with a peak incidence in adolescence and early adult life and a second peak after the age of 50. It shows a predilection for the central (axial) lymph node groups and tends to spare peripheral and mesenteric lymph nodes. Involvement of the extranodal lymphoid tissues of the nasopharynx and gastrointestinal tract is very uncommon. The disease usually spreads in a predictable fashion to contiguous lymph node groups presumably via lymphatics. Haematogenous spread to the liver and bone marrow may follow splenic involvement but almost never occurs in the absence of splenic tumour. This pattern of spread provides a rational basis for the staging and treatment of Hodgkin's disease.

4.1 Classification of Hodgkin's disease (Table 4.1)

Jackson and Parker (1947) divided Hodgkin's disease into paragranuloma, granuloma and sarcoma. Although Hodgkin's paragranuloma has a good prognosis and sarcoma has a bad prognosis the majority of patients fall into the granuloma group and this classification does not provide an adequate subdivision of cases for the analysis of treatment trials. Lukes and his coworkers proposed six histological categories of Hodgkin's disease (Lukes and Butler, 1966; Lukes *et al.*, 1966a) that were reduced to four groupings in the Rye classification (Lukes *et al.*, 1966b). This reduction was undertaken for the ease of clinical comparisons but since this book is directed principally to the diagnostic histopathologist, and the six subgroups are histologically distinct, we have reverted to the original Lukes classification.

Although the presence of RS cells is essential for the diagnosis of any subtype of Hodgkin's disease it should be noted that the morphology of these cells differs in the three main subtypes (Fig. 4.2 (a), (b) and (c)). The 'classic' RS cell should be sought in all subtypes but is found most easily in mixed cellularity Hodgkin's disease. This cell has darkly-staining amphophilic cytoplasm and usually appears multinucleated although in

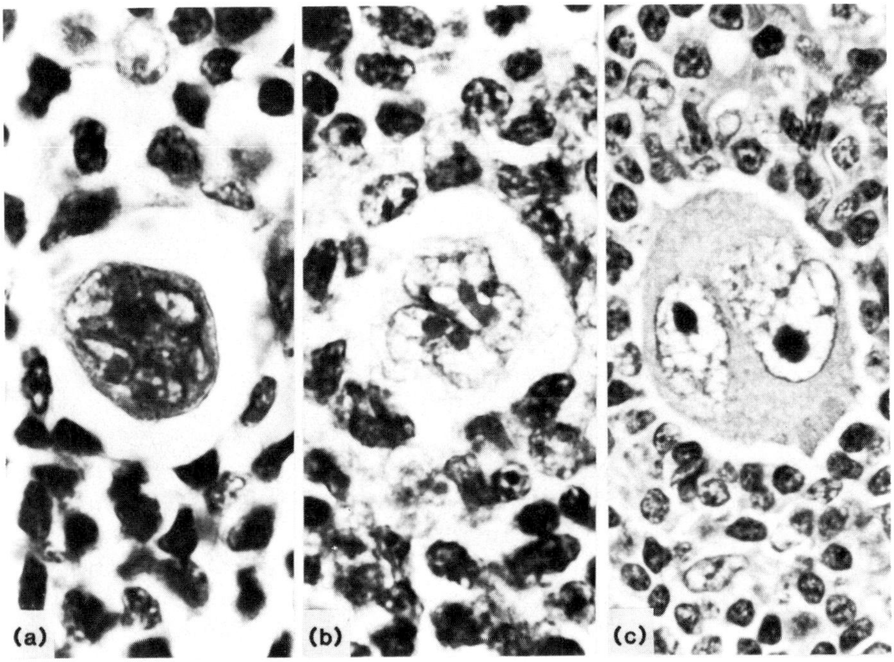

Fig. 4.2 (a) Polylobated Reed–Sternberg cell in lymphocyte/histiocyte predominant Hodgkin's disease, × 800.
(b) Lacunar Reed–Sternberg cell in nodular sclerosing Hodgkin's disease, × 800.
(c) Classic Reed–Sternberg cell in mixed cellularity Hodgkin's disease, × 800.

some instances ultrastructural studies have shown connected nuclear lobes rather than separate nuclei. Characteristically these cells have prominent large eosinophilic nucleoli attached to condensed heterochromatin at the nuclear membrane by delicate strands of chromatin.

The lacunar RS cell characterizes the nodular sclerosing variant of Hodgkin's disease. This cell has relatively abundant pale-staining or finely vacuolated cytoplasm which often shrinks away from the surrounding structures in formalin-fixed tissues leaving the cell in a clear lacuna. The nucleus of the lacunar RS cell is often markedly polylobated; it usually has finer nuclear chromatin and smaller nucleoli than classic RS cells (Fig. 4.3). The RS cell of lymphocyte-histiocyte predominant Hodgkin's disease is also often multilobated. This cell usually has granular nuclear chromatin and smaller and less conspicuous nucleoli than the other variants of RS cells. It does not show the clear cytoplasm and cytoplasmic shrinkage of the lacunar RS cell. The term 'Hodgkin's cell' is often applied to the mononuclear form of the classic RS cell (Fig. 4.4). Cells with a similar morphology may be found in other types of

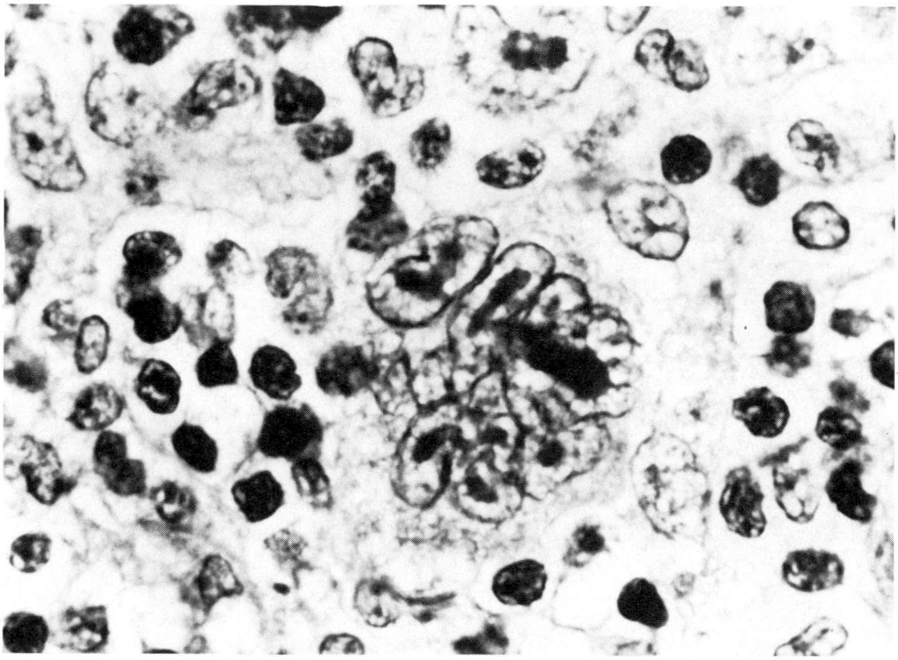

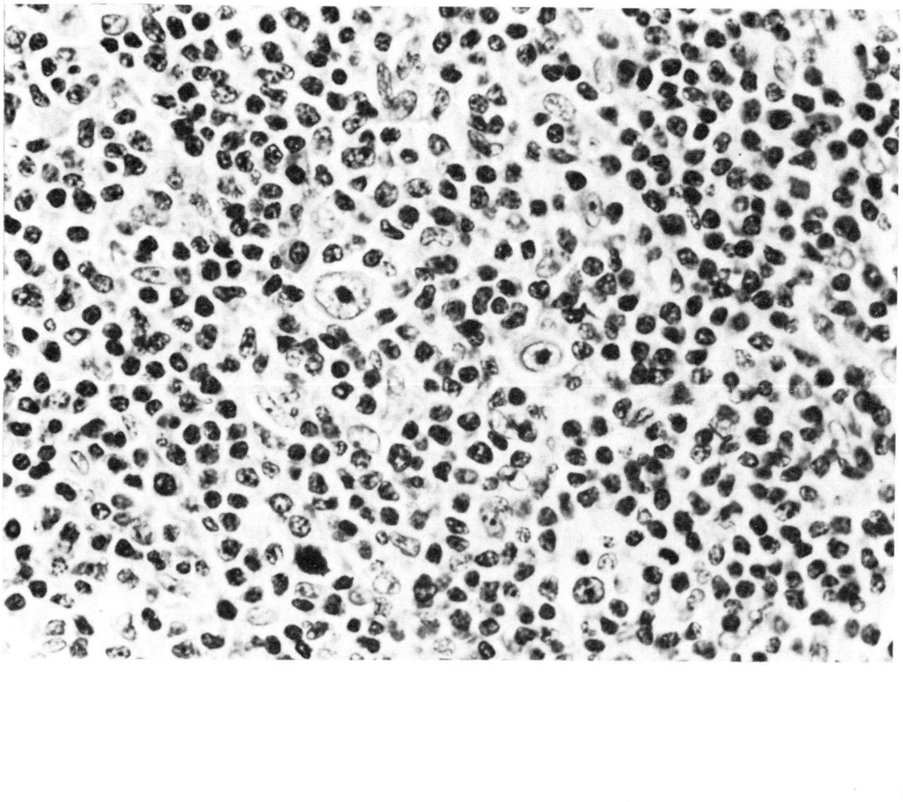

lymphadenopathy and a diagnosis of Hodgkin's disease should not be based on the finding of Hodgkin's cells in the absence of RS cells.

4.1.1 *Lymphocyte and/or histiocyte (L and H) predominant Hodgkin's disease*

(a) *Nodular*

Low power scanning shows this tumour to have a nodular or nodular and diffuse structure (Figs 4.5 and 4.6). Partial involvement of nodes is

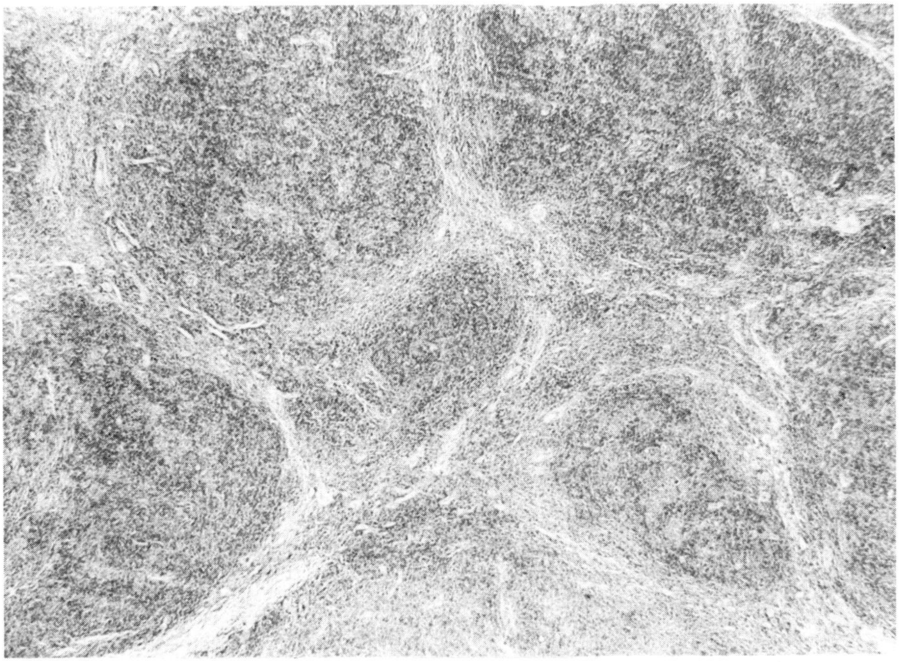

Fig. 4.5 Lymphocyte/histiocyte predominant Hodgkin's disease nodular. Large nodules of darkly staining lymphoid tissue outlined by paler zones containing large numbers of blood vessels, × 32.

uncommon although atrophic reactive follicles may be seen at the periphery of the node. The Hodgkin's tissue is composed predominantly of small lymphocytes arranged in ill-defined nodules outlined by areas of less dense cellularity containing scattered blood vessels. Variable numbers

---

Fig. 4.3 Lacunar Reed–Sternberg cell showing extreme nuclear pleomorphism, × 1000.
Fig. 4.4 Mononuclear 'Hodgkin's cells' with a single nucleus and prominent central nucleolus, × 250.

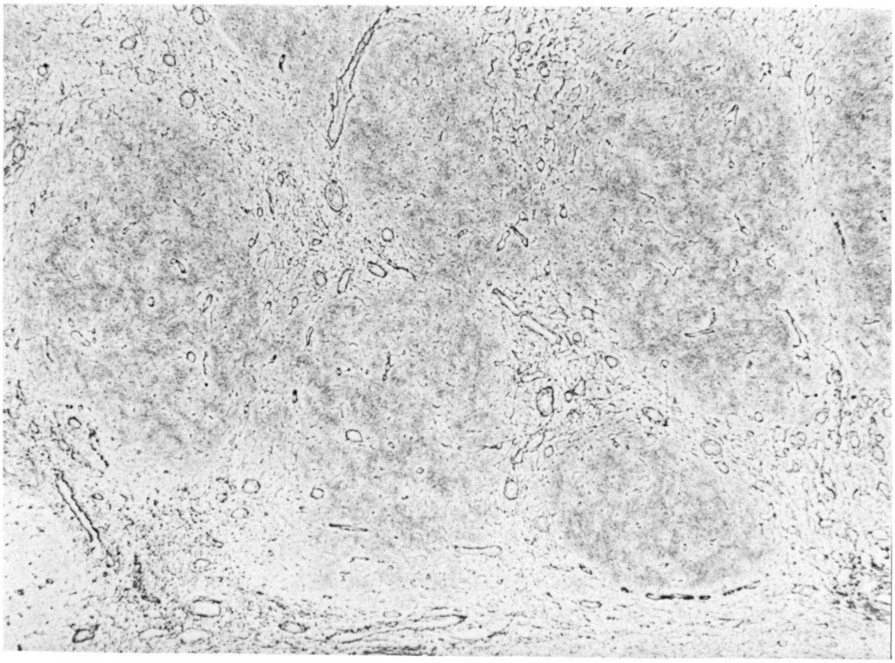

Fig. 4.6 Reticulin stain of tumour shown in Fig. 4.5. Condensed reticulin and blood vessels are seen around the lymphoid nodules, × 32.

of epithelioid histiocytes distributed either singly or in small groups are characteristic of this variant of Hodgkin's disease although they are not usually as abundant as in the diffuse L and H predominant form. Classic RS cells are very scanty and several blocks or levels may have to be scanned before one is found. Cells corresponding to the polylobated variant of the RS cell may, however, account for up to 10% of the cells in this tumour (Lukes *et al.*, 1966a). These cells have complex polylobated nuclei, fine nuclear chromatin and small nucleoli. Their cytoplasm is well defined, basophilic in Giemsa-stained imprints and sections and markedly pyroninophilic. The methyl green pyronin stain is a useful technique for highlighting these cells. In the nodular form of L and H predominant Hodgkin's disease they are frequently aggregated towards the centre of the nodules (Fig. 4.7)

(b) *Diffuse*

The cellular composition of this variant of Hodgkin's disease is similar to that of the nodular subtype except that epithelioid histiocytes tend to be more frequent. The tumour has a diffuse structure (Figs 4.8 and 4.9).

(c) *Differential diagnosis*

The nodular variant of L and H predominant Hodgkin's disease differs

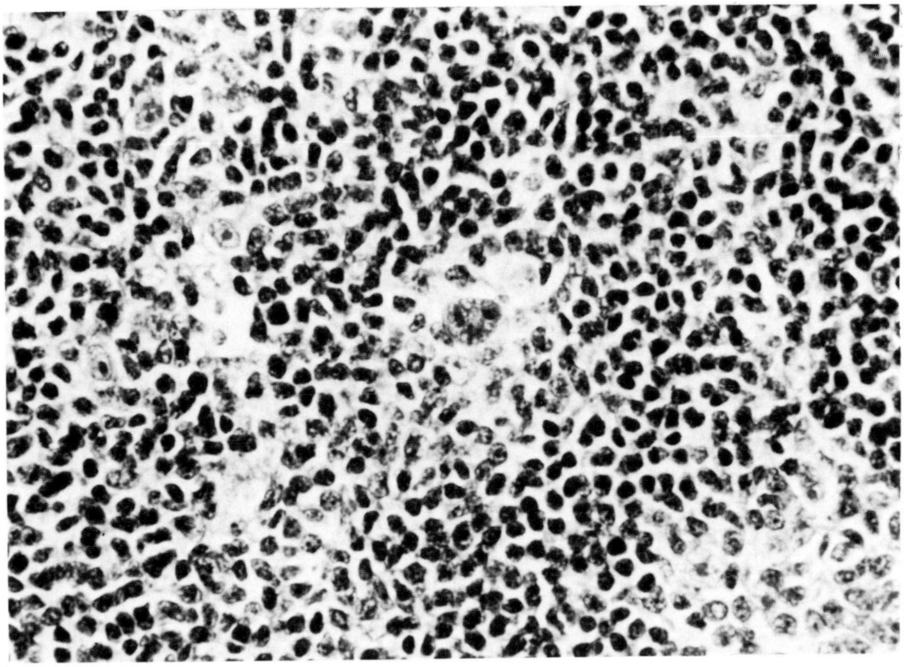

Fig. 4.7 Lymphocyte/histiocyte predominant Hodgkin's disease. Polylobated Reed–Sternberg cells and Hodgkin's cells aggregated towards the centre of the lymphoid nodules, × 250.

from follicular lymphoma in that the follicles are larger, usually less well defined and are composed of small lymphocytes and histiocytes rather than follicle centre cells.

L and H predominant cases of Hodgkin's disease composed mainly of small lymphocytes may be confused with small lymphocytic lymphoma. Since small lymphocytic lymphoma is essentially a disease of later life this type of Hodgkin's disease should always be considered in a young patient with a lymphoma consisting mainly of small lymphocytes. The presence of RS cells and their polylobated variants will distinguish the two lesions.

RS-like cells may be seen in the T-cell lymphoma of pleomorphic type which also frequently contains large numbers of epithelioid histiocytes. It is not surprising therefore that this tumour is sometimes confused with L and H predominant Hodgkin's disease. The main feature that differentiates the two is that the lymphoid cells in the pleomorphic T-cell lymphoma show all gradations from small lymphocytes to large T-blasts, many of them with convoluted nuclei, whereas in Hodgkin's disease the lymphoid cells are all small lymphocytes. The presence of high

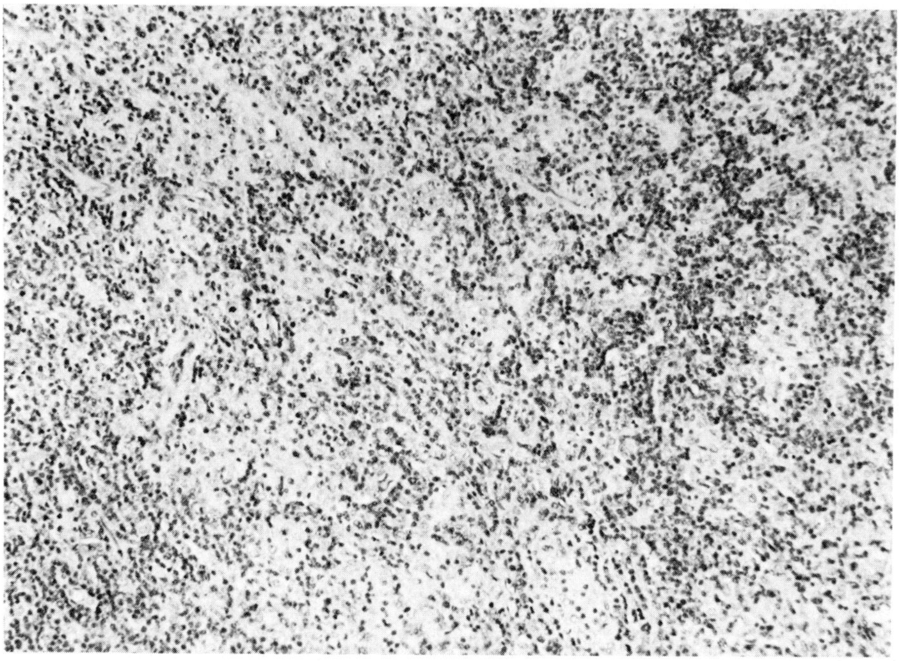

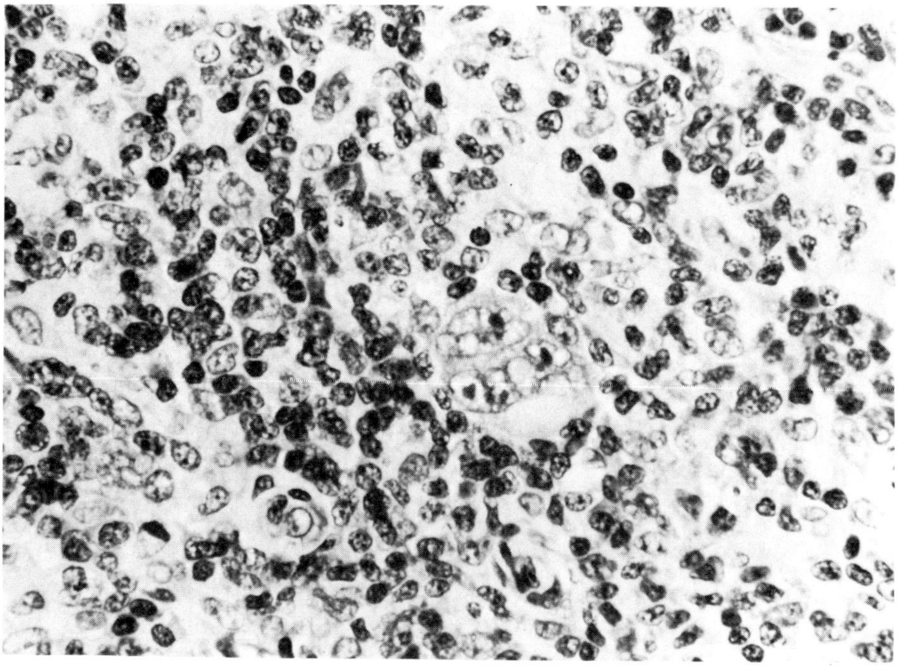

endothelial vessels and compartmentalizing PAS-positive reticulin bands in the T-cell lymphoma may assist this differentiation.

Large numbers of epithelioid histiocytes may be found in non-Hodgkin's lymphomas of differing histogenesis. One of these appears to be of T-cell origin and is often designated Lennert's lymphoma (Lennert, 1981). The differentiation between L and H predominant Hodgkin's disease and Lennert's lymphoma may be difficult. The diagnosis of Hodgkin's disease depends upon the finding of RS cells which will be accompanied by variable numbers of small lymphocytes. The lymphoid cells in Lennert's lymphoma are often irregular with squiggly nuclei and show transitions to blast cells.

4.1.2 Hodgkin's disease mixed cellularity

The cellular composition of this variant of Hodgkin's disease covers a spectrum from lymphocyte-histiocyte predominance through to lymphocyte depletion, the dividing line between these subtypes being to some extent arbitrary. The presence of more than very occasional RS cells would place a case in the mixed cellularity rather than the lymphocyte predominance group (Figs 4.10, 4.11 and 4.12). When RS cells and their variants equal or exceed other cells in the biopsy the case should be categorized as reticular Hodgkin's disease. Problems may rarely arise with nodes that show variations in their cellular composition in different areas. These should be categorized according to the predominant pattern.

In addition to a variable content of small lymphocytes epithelioid histiocytes may be present singly or in clusters. Immunoperoxidase staining for lysozyme always reveals many more histiocytes than are apparent in H and E stained sections. Eosinophils and neutrophils may be present in variable numbers and frequently accumulate around areas of necrosis. Plasma cells may be seen scattered throughout the Hodgkin's tissue, particularly in methyl green pyronin stained sections, but they are usually most abundant at the periphery of the node and in areas of partial involvement. Silver staining reveals a dense reticulin network but mature collagen is usually only seen in residual nodal structures.

Fig. 4.8 Lymphocyte/histiocyte predominant Hodgkin's disease diffuse. The tissue is composed predominantly of epithelioid histiocytes and small lymphocytes, × 100.

Fig. 4.9 The same section as illustrated in Fig. 4.8 showing a polylobated Reed–Sternberg cell surrounded by large numbers of lymphocytes and epithelioid histiocytes, × 400.

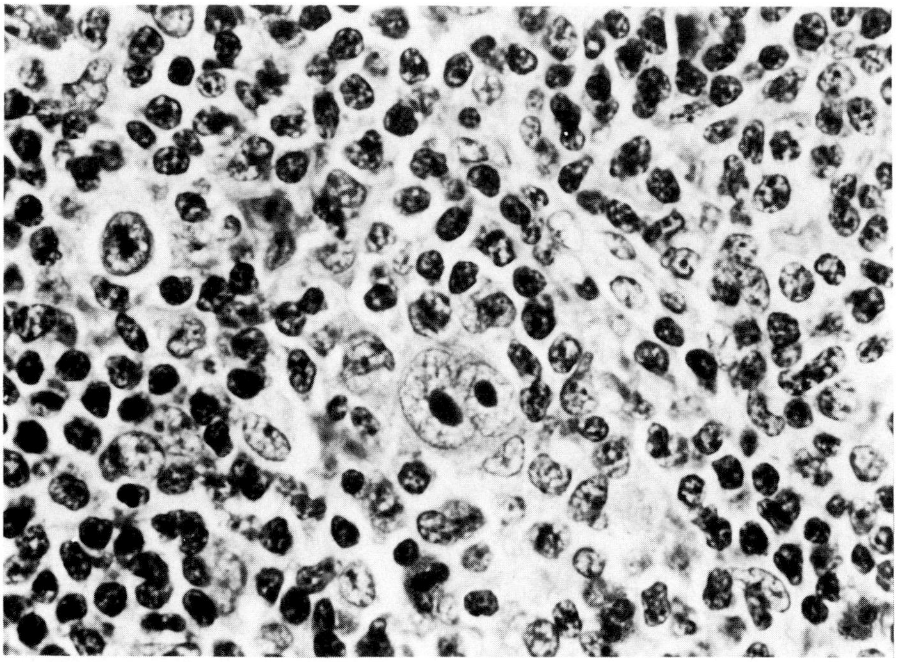

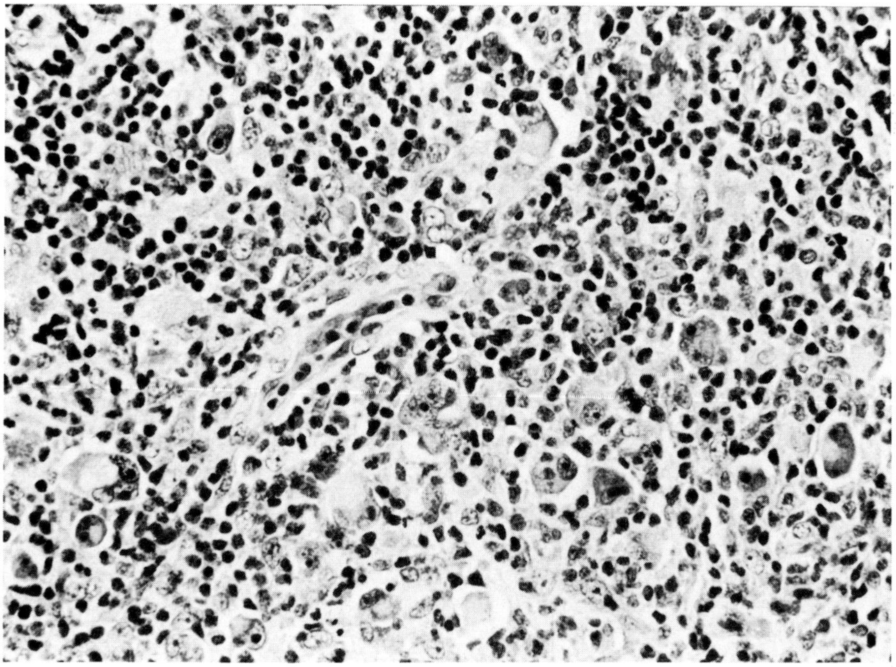

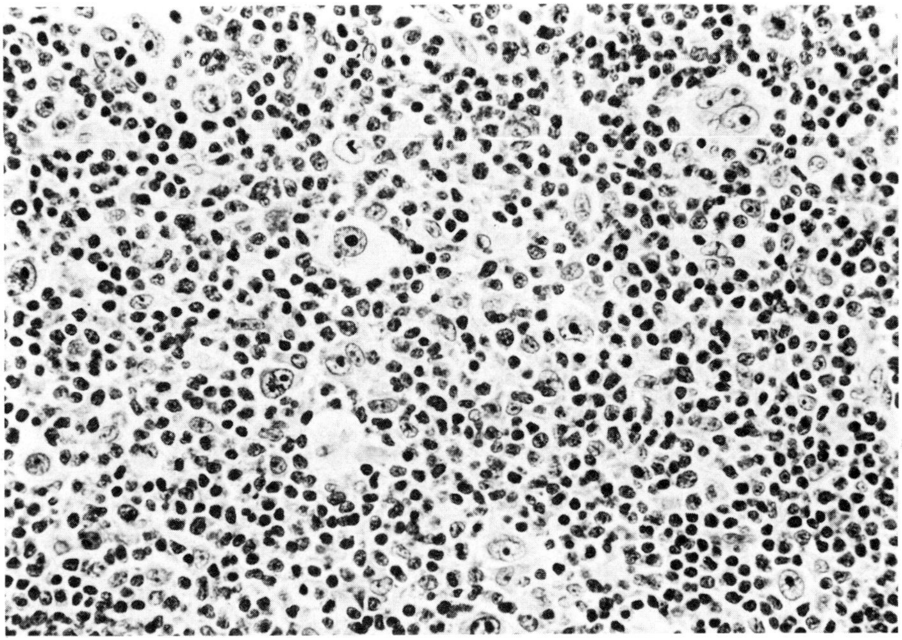

Fig. 4.12 Mixed cellularity Hodgkin's disease showing large numbers of Reed–Sternberg cells and mononuclear Hodgkin's cells, × 250.

(a) *Differential diagnosis*

Various reactive proliferations including drug-induced lymphadenopathy and angioimmunoblastic lymphadenopathy may simulate mixed cellularity Hodgkin's disease. Neoplastic lesions that are frequently confused with this disease are large cell lymphomas, particularly the polymorphic type of T-cell lymphoma, and anaplastic carcinomas that contain multinucleate forms and that are infiltrated by inflammatory cells. The presence of eosinophils in particular appears to influence pathologists into making the diagnosis of Hodgkin's disease. If the basic rule – *that Reed–Sternberg cells must be identified in a cellular environment appropriate for one of the subtypes of Hodgkin's disease* – is applied this error will not be committed.

Fig. 4.10 Mixed cellularity Hodgkin's disease. A Reed–Sternberg cell is seen in a setting composed predominantly of lymphocytes. Scattered atypical cells with prominent nucleoli are also seen. There are too many atypical cells for this to be categorized as lymphocyte predominant Hodgkin's disease, × 480.

Fig. 4.11 Mixed cellularity Hodgkin's disease showing large numbers of Reed–Sternberg cells in a setting of lymphocytes and histiocytes. Numerous eosinophils are also present but do not show up well in this photograph, × 250.

4.1.3 Nodular sclerosing Hodgkin's disease

Nodular sclerosing Hodgkin's disease, previously included with the mixed cellularity type as Hodgkin's granuloma is the most common subtype seen in Europe and North America. It has a higher female-to-male ratio than other types of Hodgkin's disease and shows a predilection for the mediastinum. This variant of Hodgkin's disease is characterized by the presence of lacunar-type RS cells and bands of fibrous tissue that extend into the lymph node from a thickened capsule and divide the tumour into nodules (Figs 4.13, 4.14 and 4.15).

The lacunar RS cell has abundant pale-staining cytoplasm that frequently retracts in formalin-fixed paraffin-embedded tissues leaving

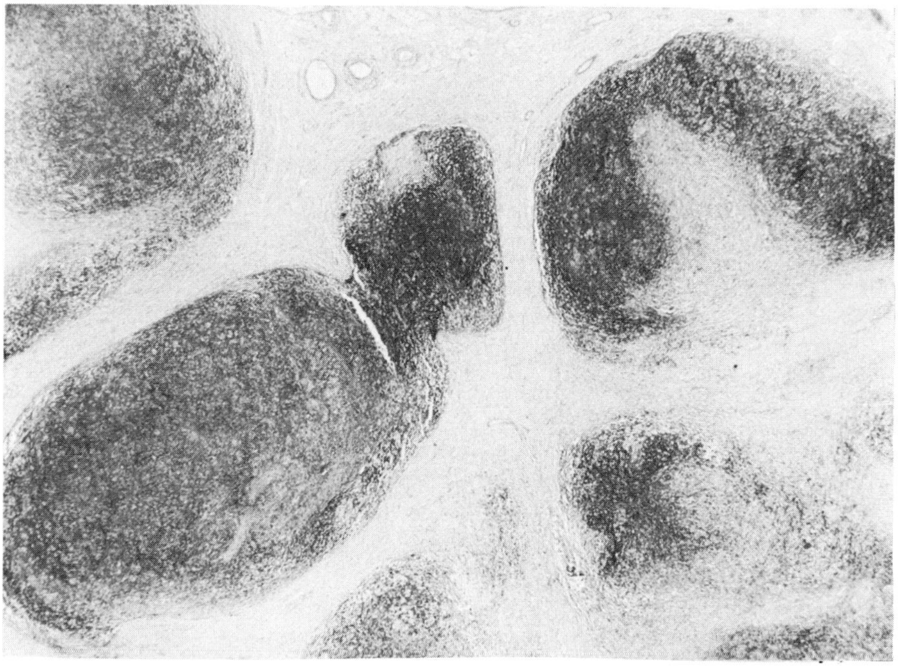

Fig. 4.13 Nodular sclerosing Hodgkin's disease. Nodules of lymphoid tissue are surrounded by dense bands of fibrous tissue. This extends into some of the nodules partially obliterating them, × 12.

Fig. 4.14 Nodular sclerosing Hodgkin's disease. The Hodgkin's tissue has a 'salt and pepper' appearance due to the presence of large numbers of lacunar Reed–Sternberg cells, × 30.

Fig. 4.15 Nodular sclerosing Hodgkin's disease showing large numbers of lacunar cells surrounded predominantly by small lymphocytes, × 120.

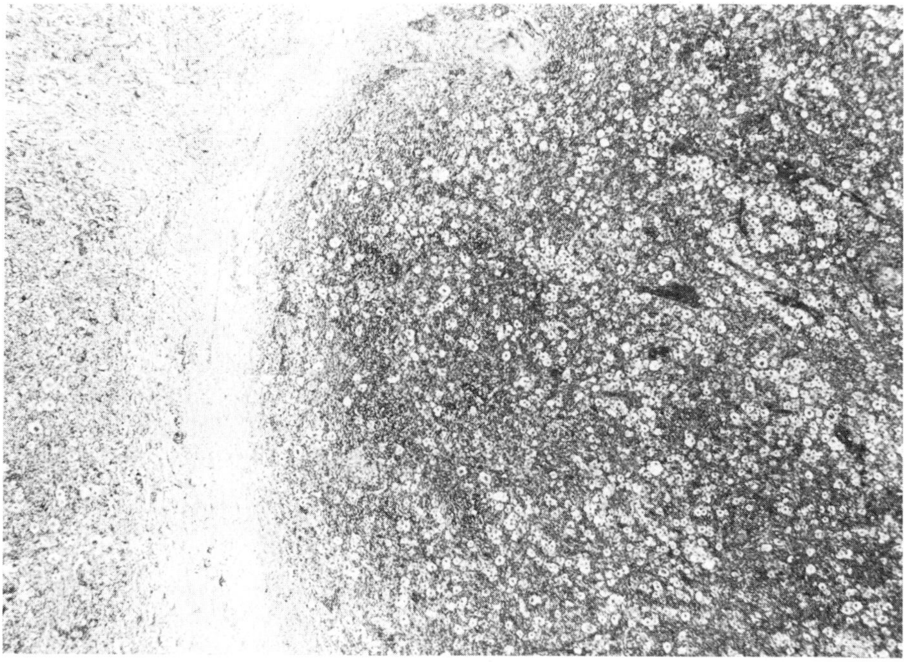

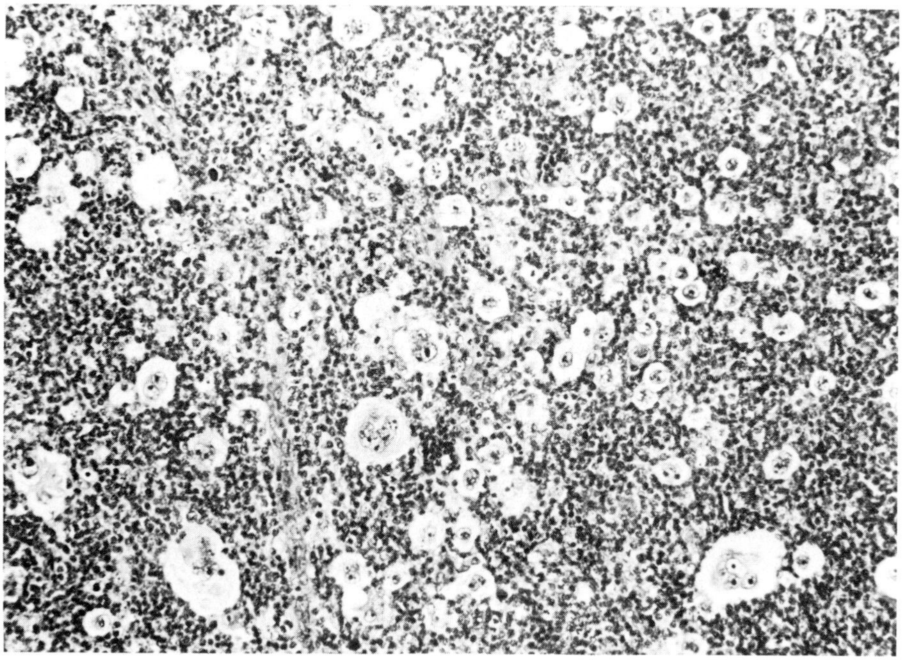

the cell in the centre of a clear space or lacuna. In imprint preparations (Fig. 4.16) they have multiple nuclei or a single complex polylobated nucleus with fine nuclear chromatin and prominent nucleoli. The cytoplasm is abundant and pale staining. Although lacunar cells are often present in large numbers classic RS cells may be difficult to find in nodular sclerosing Hodgkin's disease.

The cellular composition of the nodules in nodular sclerosing Hodgkin's disease varies from lymphocyte predominance to lymphocyte depletion in which the majority of the cells are lacunar cells, or mononuclear cells with similar cytological qualities. These latter tumours are frequently heavily infiltrated by polymorphs and show areas of necrosis. Plasma cells are most abundant in residual lymph node adjacent to tumour and in the fibrous bands. Fibrosis appears to increase with duration of the disease. In the early stages of sclerosis the fibrous bands may be highlighted by reticulin and connective tissue stains or by their birefringence in polarized light. As the disease progresses the fibrous tissue may extend into the nodules and obliterate the Hodgkin's tissue leaving only scattered lymphocytes and histiocytes.

In some cases of nodular sclerosing Hodgkin's disease very little

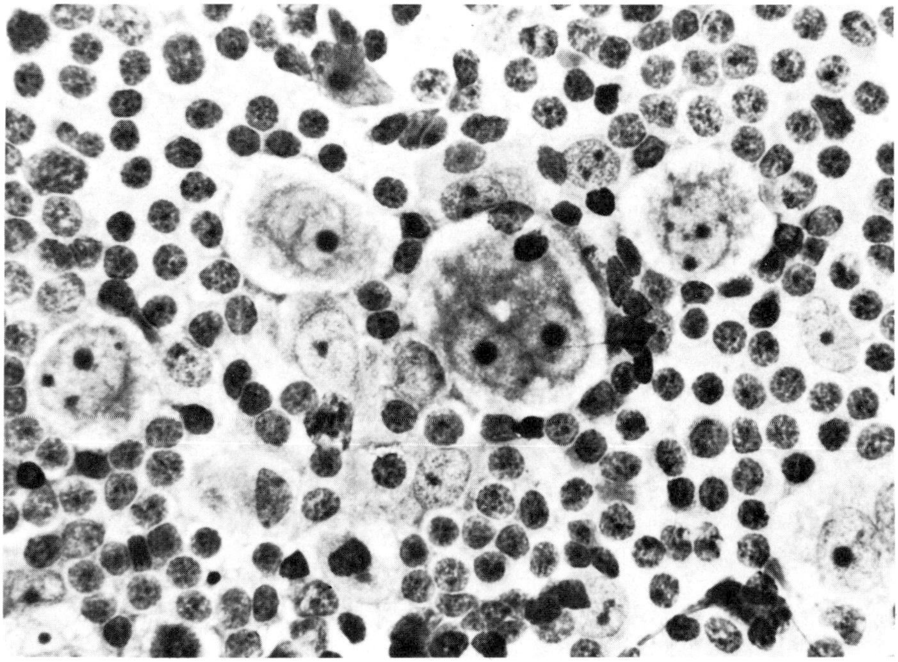

Fig. 4.16 Nodular sclerosing Hodgkin's disease. Imprint preparation showing bilobed and mononuclear lacunar cells. Giemsa, × 480.

sclerosis is evident although there may be numerous lacunar cells (Figs 4.17 and 4.18). These cases are categorized as nodular sclerosis, cellular phase on the grounds that the classical appearances of nodular sclerosis may be found at other sites or appear in subsequent biopsies.

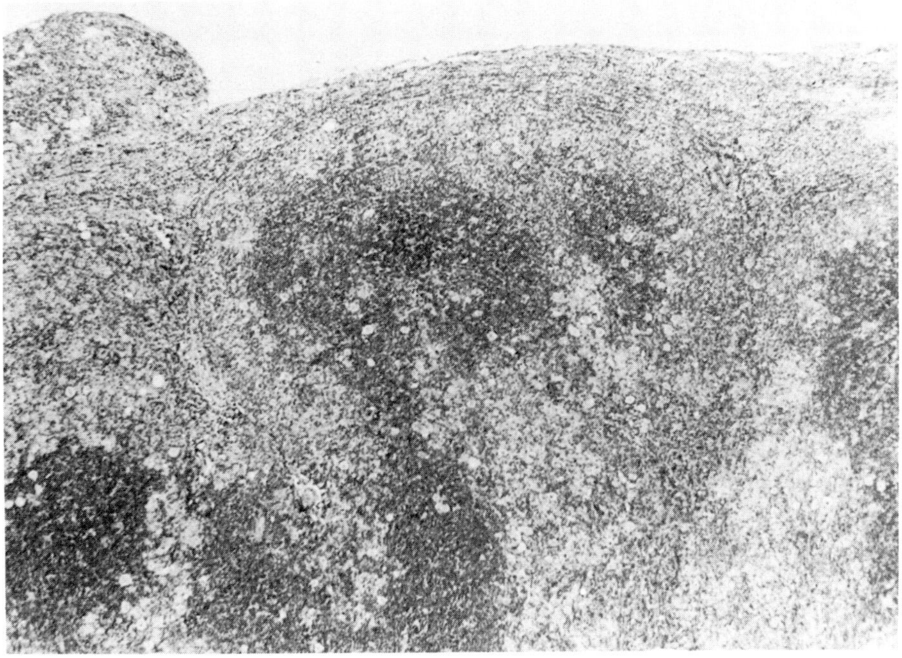

Fig. 4.17 Nodular sclerosing Hodgkin's disease, cellular phase. Numerous lacunar cells are just apparent at this magnification but there is no apparent fibrosis, × 32.

(a) *Differential diagnosis*

Very rarely inflammatory and reactive lesions and lymphomas other than Hodgkin's disease are associated with degrees of fibrosis similar to that seen in nodular sclerosing Hodgkin's disease. The cellular phase of nodular sclerosing and lymphocyte-histiocyte predominant Hodgkin's disease can be distinguished by the presence of lacunar cells in the former. Lymphocyte-depleted variants of nodular sclerosing Hodgkin's disease may show a florid proliferation of lacunar cells and atypical histiocytes with areas of necrosis and polymorph infiltration but very few lymphocytes. Pathologists may incline towards diagnosing these as lymphocyte-depleted Hodgkin's disease. However, although within the nodular sclerosing subtype they may have a worse prognosis than the

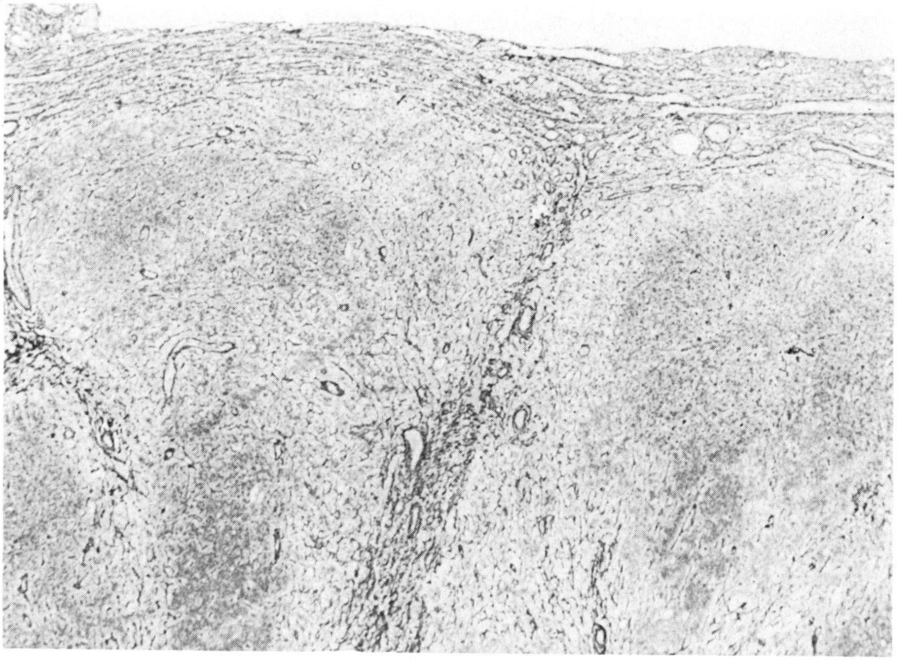

Fig. 4.18 Reticulin stain of the same section shown in Fig. 4.17. This shows condensation of reticulin in the capsule with extension into the node giving a nodular appearance, × 32.

lymphocyte-predominant forms (Bennett *et al.*, 1981) they have a better prognosis than lymphocyte-depleted Hodgkin's disease.

4.1.4 Lymphocyte depleted – reticular type

Reticular Hodgkin's disease, previously called Hodgkin's sarcoma, accounts for less than 5% of most reported series of this disease. The predominant cells in the tumour are RS cells, mononuclear Hodgkin's cells and pleomorphic variants of these (Figs 4.19 and 4.20). Moderate numbers of lymphocytes, histiocytes and plasma cells may be present. Polymorph leucocytes, particularly eosinophils may be abundant and are

---

Fig. 4.19 Lymphocyte-depleted Hodgkin's disease, reticular type. Reed–Sternberg cells, Hodgkin's cells and atypical cells in a setting composed predominantly of histiocytes and polymorphs, × 250.

Fig. 4.20 Hodgkin's disease, lymphocyte depleted, reticular type. Numerous multinucleated cells, some of which resemble Reed–Sternberg cells in a setting composed predominantly of histiocytes and polymorphs, × 250.

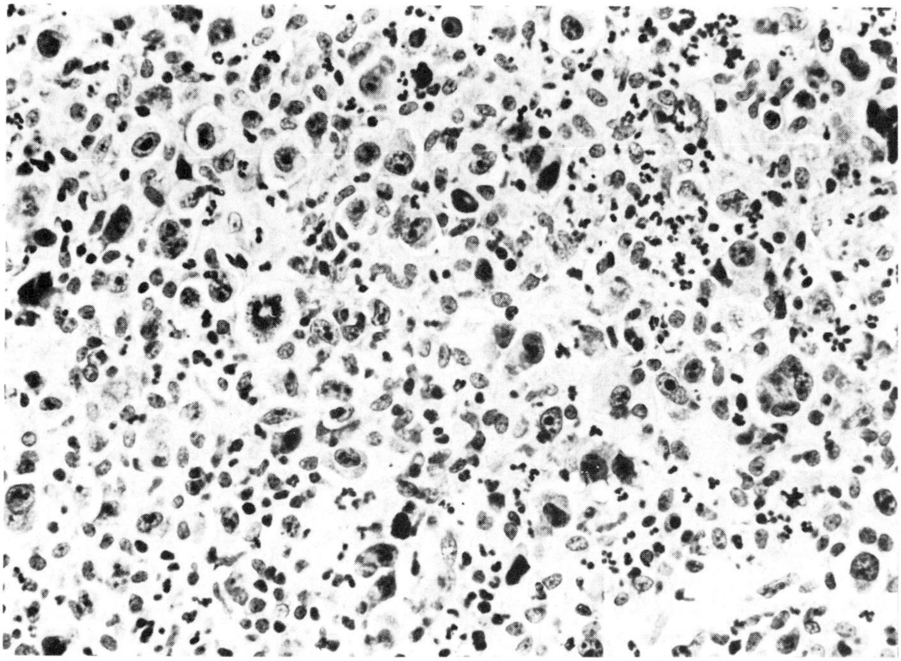

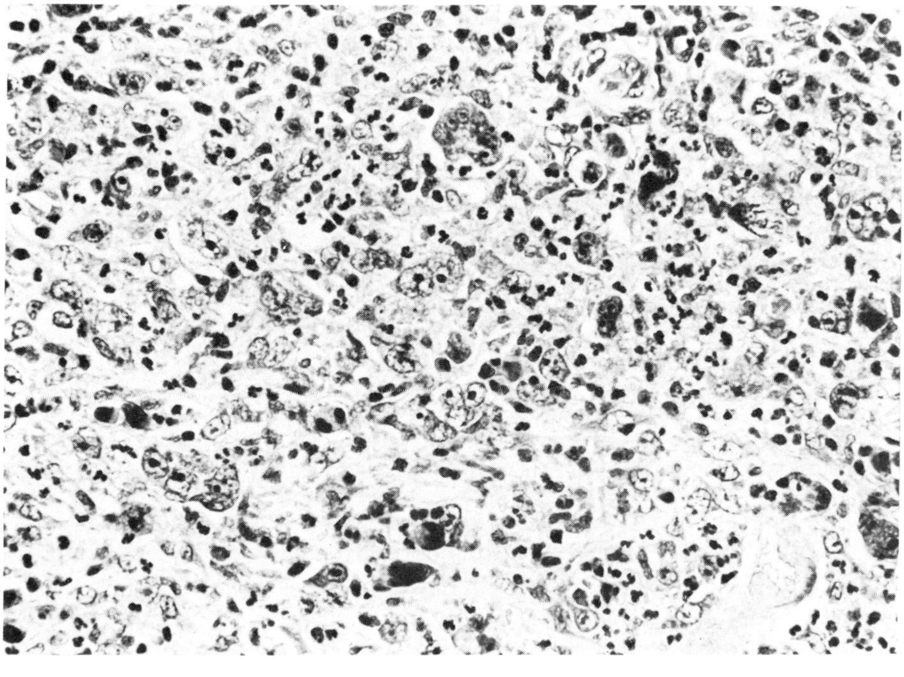

usually most marked around areas of necrosis that may be extensive. Silver stains show a moderately dense reticulin pattern within the tumour.

(a) *Differential diagnosis*

As stated above the dividing line between the lymphocyte-depleted end of mixed cellularity and reticular Hodgkin's disease is not well defined. Reticular Hodgkin's disease is probably the most frequently misdiagnosed variant of Hodgkin's disease. Anaplastic carcinomas and pleomorphic variants of large cell lymphomas, particularly when they contain multinucleated cells and are infiltrated by eosinophils, are frequently misdiagnosed as Hodgkin's disease. The pleomorphic variants of centroblastic lymphomas and immunoblastic sarcomas can be identified by the presence of a large population of monomorphic tumour cells as well as the multinucleate cells that may resemble Reed–Sternberg cells. Immunohistochemical studies and surface markers will usually confirm the B-cell nature of these tumours.

Many examples of malignant histiocytosis of the intestine have been labelled as Hodgkin's disease because of the presence of multinucleated tumour cells associated with eosinophils and other inflammatory or reactive cells. Histiocytic lymphomas are frequently infiltrated by eosinophils and plasma cells. They can be differentiated from Hodgkin's by the relative monomorphism of the tumour cells and the paucity or absence of cells that fulfil the criteria for classic RS cells.

We have seen several anaplastic carcinomas, particularly of the thyroid and gastrointestinal tract, that have been diagnosed as Hodgkin's disease on the basis of the presence of multinucleated cells and an intense infiltrate of inflammatory cells including eosinophils. Examination of further tissue blocks will often reveal areas of cellular cohesion or of glandular differentiation in these tumours, PAS staining may reveal secretory products and electron microscopy frequently permits the identification of epithelial cell characteristics. Primary Hodgkin's disease is very uncommon at extra nodal sites and it is probably wisest to assume that all tumours resembling Hodgkin's disease at these sites are anaplastic carcinomas or lymphomas other than Hodgkin's disease until critical examination has excluded these possibilities.

4.1.5 *Lymphocyte depleted – diffuse fibrosis*

Neiman *et al.* (1973) reported this as a distinct variant of Hodgkin's disease affecting an elderly population with a marked male preponderance and very poor prognosis. Patients usually present with malaise fever and weight loss, often manifest anaemia and have hepatosplenomegaly without marked peripheral adenopathy. Needle biopsies of the liver and bone marrow trephine specimens may be the only tissues available for making the ante-mortem diagnosis. In a subsequent study Bearman *et al.* (1978) found no clinical or survival differences between the reticular and diffuse fibrosis subtypes of Hodgkin's disease and were able to establish the diagnosis on a peripheral lymph node biopsy in 81% of their cases. They concluded that lymphocyte-depleted Hodgkin's disease is not a distinct clinicopathological entity.

If Hodgkin's disease is thought of as a lymphocyte war, diffuse fibrosis must represent a situation in which the combatants have annihilated each other. The tissue is markedly hypocellular (Fig. 4.21) and consists

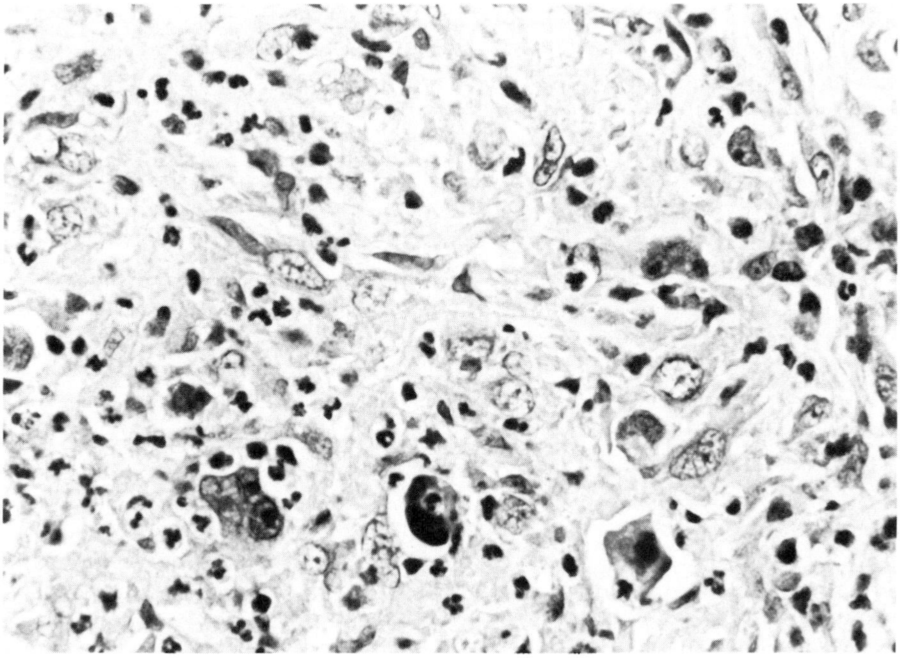

Fig. 4.21 Hodgkin's disease, lymphocyte depleted, diffuse fibrosis. The tissue is markedly hypocellular containing scattered atypical cells with occasional Reed–Sternberg cells. Some of the atypical cells appear degenerate and are surrounded by polymorphs, × 400.

predominantly of amorphous eosinophilic PAS-positive material containing a meshwork of reticulin fibres but no mature collagen. The term diffuse fibrosis is therefore a misnomer. Necrosis may be prominent and pyknotic cells and cell debris is usually seen throughout the tissue. The few residual cells usually include granulocytes and histiocytes, atypical hyperchromatic cells and scanty to moderate numbers of RS cells.

(a) *Differential diagnosis*
Areas of diffuse fibrosis may be seen in mixed cellularity or reticular subtypes of Hodgkin's disease. In these cases the tumour should be categorized according to the predominant histological pattern. Tissues from patients with end stage angioimmunoblastic lymphadenopathy and lymphomas other than Hodgkin's disease that have been intensively treated by chemotherapy may show a hypocellular pattern suggestive of diffuse fibrosis, but will not contain RS cells.

4.2 Staging laparotomy

The rational treatment of Hodgkin's disease depends upon accurate staging of the tumour. Clinical and radiological examinations can identify involvements of most lymph node groups except those in the upper abdomen. Involvement of the spleen cannot be accurately determined except by direct examination since normal sized organs may contain Hodgkin's tissue and moderate enlargement may occur without tumour infiltration (Farrer-Brown *et al.*, 1971; Kadin *et al.*, 1971). For these reasons many centres perform a laparotomy with splenectomy for the staging of Hodgkin's disease. In addition to removal of the spleen it is usual to sample upper abdominal lymph nodes and any other nodes that are enlarged and to mark the residual nodes with radiopaque clips to monitor tumour progression. Any suspicious lesions in the liver are biopsied. If the organ appears normal it is usual to perform a random wedge biopsy and one or more needle biopsies from each lobe. In young females surgeons usually take the opportunity provided by the staging laparotomy to move the ovaries towards the midline, out of the field of radiation encompassed by a lower mantle.

Examination of the bone marrow should be included with the staging procedures for Hodgkin's disease. Marrow smears are not satisfactory for the identification of Hodgkin's tissue and either the marrow fragments should be filtered and sectioned or a marrow trephine should be performed (Lukes, 1971).

4.2.1 Spleen

Infiltration by Hodgkin's tissue may be present in a spleen of normal size, conversely enlarged spleens do not necessarily contain tumour although those over 600 g usually do. The tumour may be visible on the capsular surface as elevated and sometimes bossilated nodules. On the cut surface macroscopic tumour nodules vary from little larger than normal Malpighian corpuscles to lobulated masses that may occupy much of the spleen. The tumour usually has a variegated cut surface often with areas of necrosis and fibrosis and lacks the more homogeneous 'fish-flesh' appearance of many lymphomas other than Hodgkin's disease. When obvious tumour tissue is not visible macroscopically at least five blocks of spleen should be taken including any Malpighian corpuscles that appear slightly enlarged.

The microscopic features of Hodgkin's disease in the spleen are essentially the same as those seen in lymph nodes and in any one patient the subtype seen in the spleen usually corresponds to that seen in the original diagnostic lymph node biopsy (Dorfman, 1971). In nodular sclerosing Hodgkin's disease haemosiderin deposits around the tumour are usually more prominent in the spleen than in lymph nodes. When the spleen does not appear to be involved macroscopically the search for microscopic foci should be concentrated on the periarteriolar lymphoid sheath (Figs 4.22 and 4.23). Occasionally large numbers of granulocytes including eosinophils may be found in the red pulp, these are not indicative of splenic involvement. The importance of determining whether the spleen is involved by Hodgkin's tissue arises from the fact that it appears to act as the centre for haematogenous spread. In the

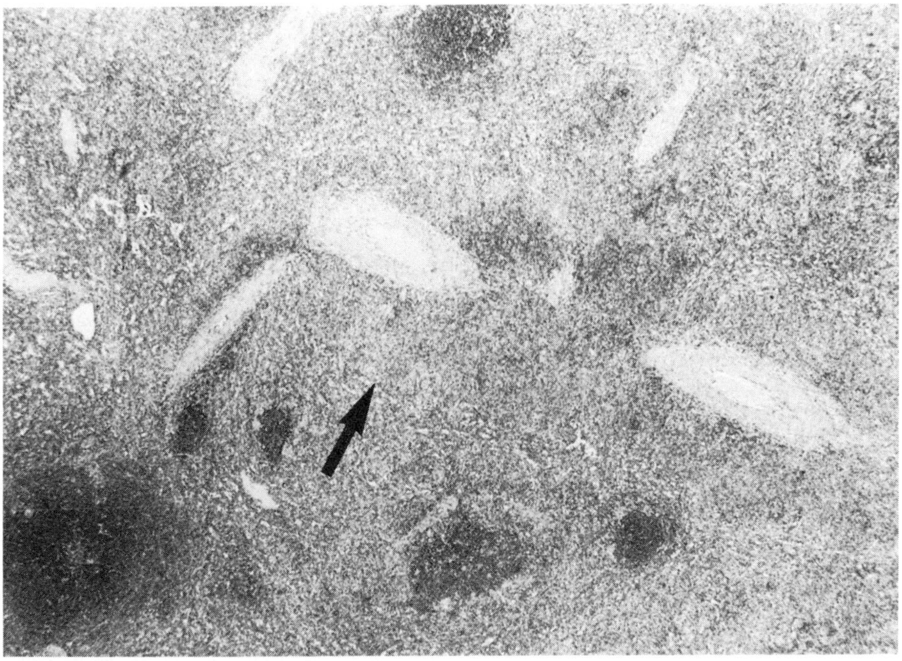

Fig. 4.22 Early involvement of the spleen by mixed cellularity Hodgkin's disease. The tumour involves the periarteriolar sheath running diagonally across the photograph (arrow), × 40.

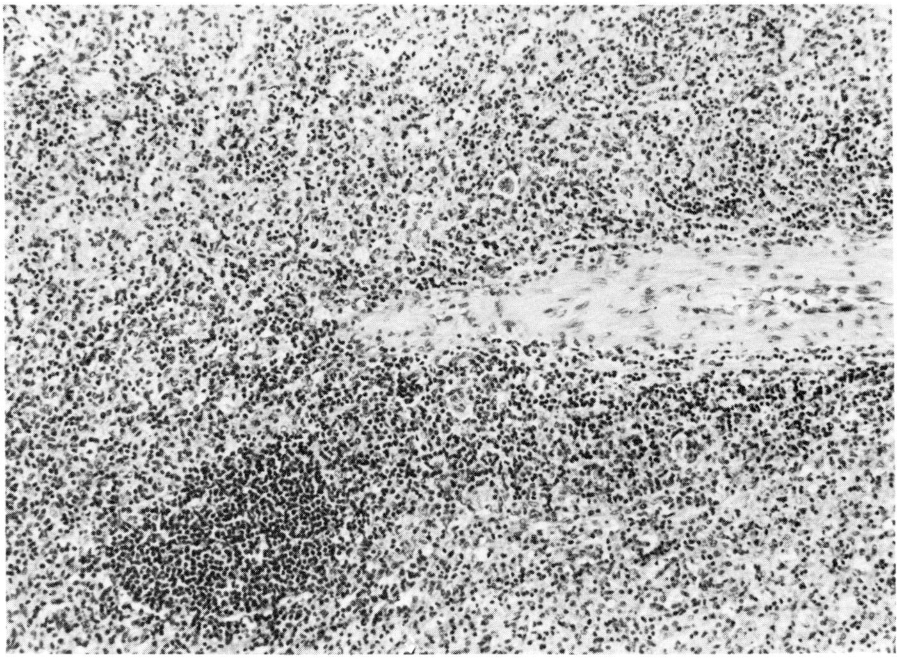

Fig. 4.23 Higher power of Fig. 4.22 showing the Hodgkin's tissue in periarteriolar sheath, × 100.

absence of splenic tumour involvement of the liver and bone marrow almost never occurs.

Collections of epithelioid histiocytes and giant cells forming loose non-caseous granulomas are found in the periarteriolar sheath of about 10% of splenectomies from patients with Hodgkin's disease (Figs 4.24 and 4.25). Similar granulomas may be seen in the paracortex of lymph nodes (Fig. 4.26) and in liver biopsies (Fig. 4.27) from patients with Hodgkin's disease (Abt *et al.*, 1974; Kadin *et al.*, 1970; Sacks *et al.*, 1978). Their presence should not be interpreted as evidence for Hodgkin's disease at that site. The finding of granulomas does not adversely influence the prognosis of Hodgkin's disease (O'Connell *et al.*, 1975).

Fig. 4.24 Section of spleen from a patient with Hodgkin's disease showing large epithelioid cell giant cell granulomas surrounding the arterioles but not extending into the follicles, × 40.

Fig. 4.25 Higher power of Fig. 4.24 showing epithelioid giant cell granulomas in the periarteriolar sheath, × 100.

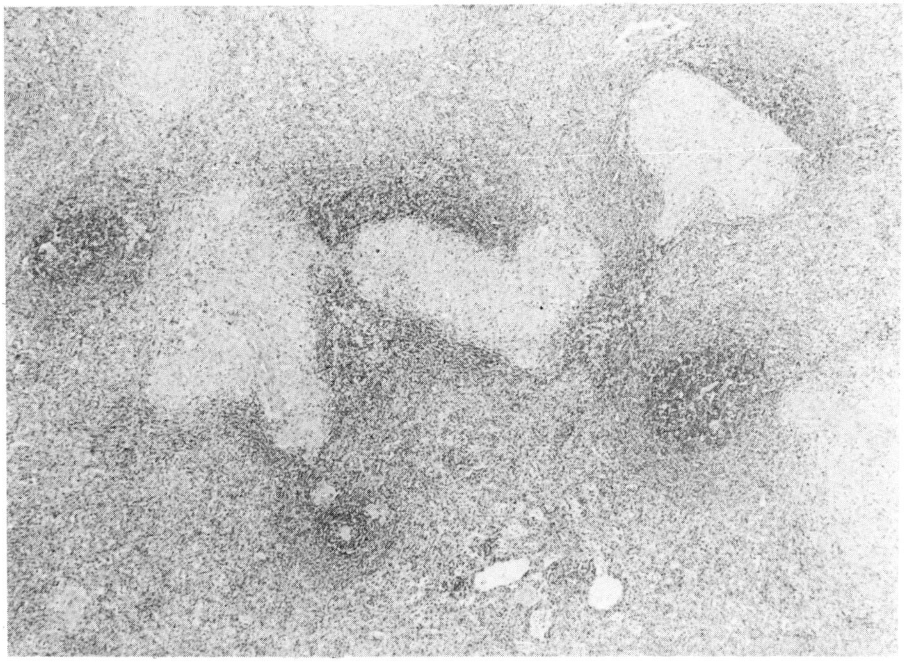

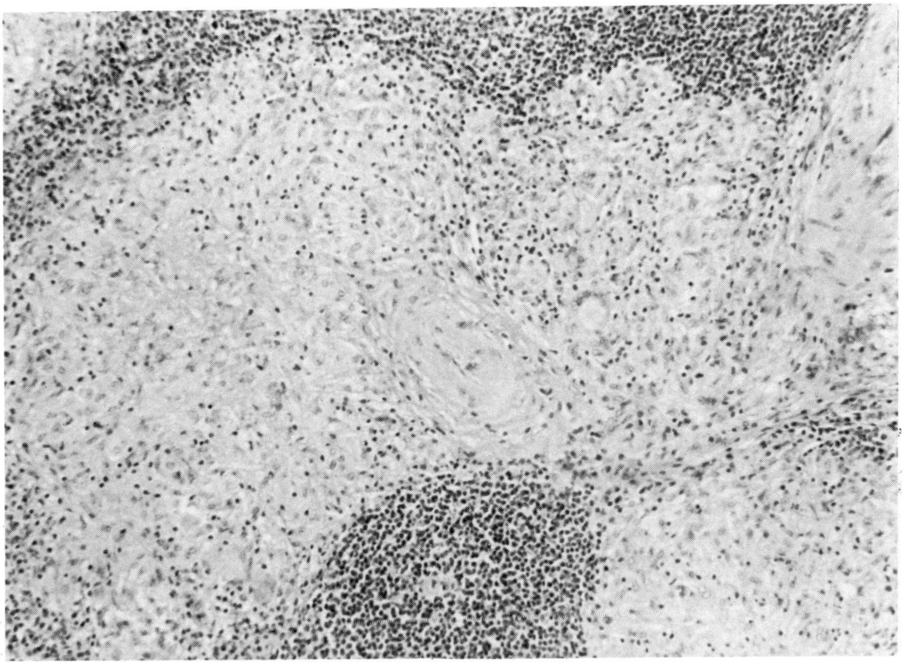

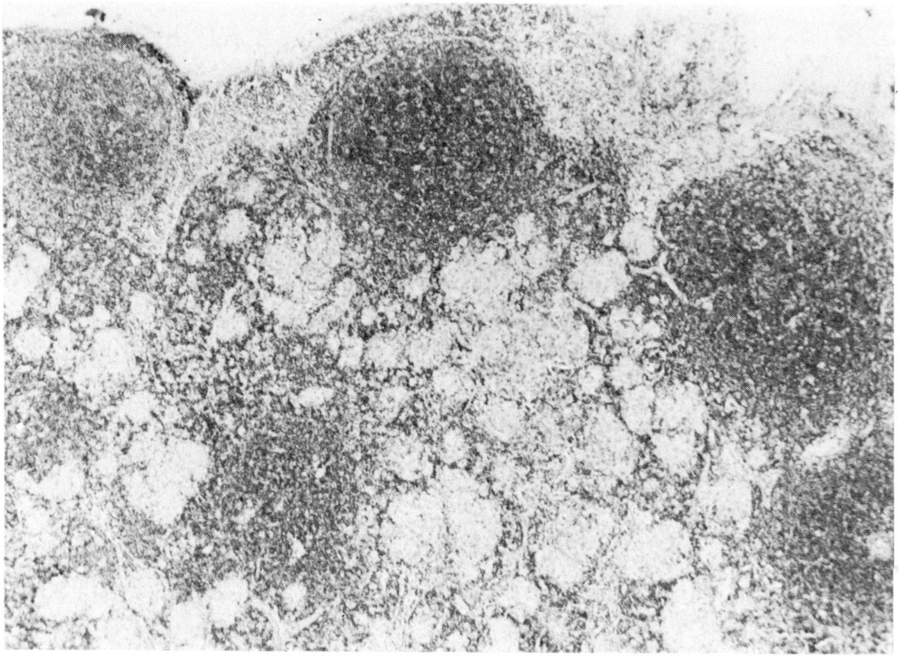

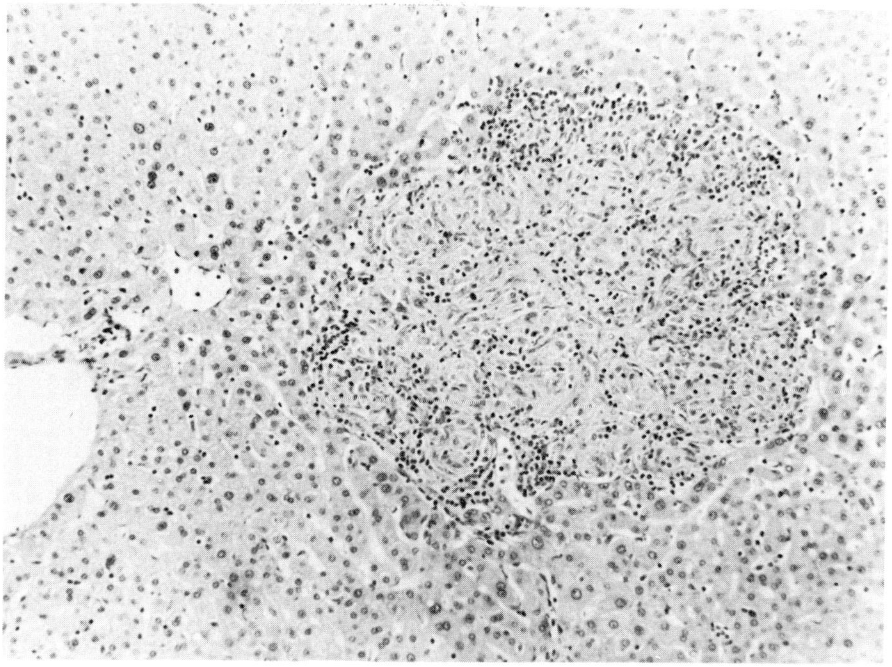

4.2.2 Liver

The pathologist's approach to a liver biopsy should be slightly different if the biopsy is part of a staging laparotomy in a patient already diagnosed as having Hodgkin's disease than if it is a percutaneous biopsy in an undiagnosed patient. In the latter case a confident diagnosis of Hodgkin's disease can be made only if Reed–Sternberg cells are seen in an appropriate setting. In specimens removed at staging laparotomy less critical criteria are acceptable for the recognition of Hodgkin's tissue in view of the small amount of liver that is usually sampled (Figs 4.28 and 4.29). The finding of mononuclear Hodgkin's cells in an appropriate

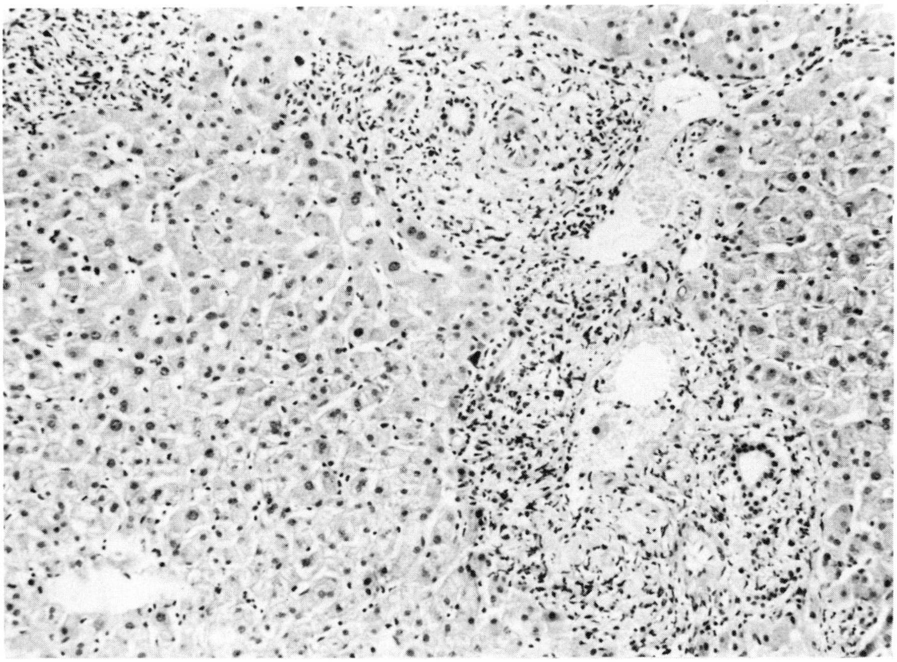

Fig. 4.28 Liver biopsy from a patient with mixed cellularity Hodgkin's disease showing an increased cellularity of the portal areas, × 100.

Fig. 4.26 Lymph node removed at staging laparotomy from a patient with Hodgkin's disease. Hodgkin's tissue is not present in this node but there are large numbers of epithelioid giant cell granulomas in the paracortical areas, × 40.
Fig. 4.27 Liver biopsy removed at staging laparotomy from a patient with Hodgkin's disease. The section shows a large epithelioid cell granuloma in the portal tract. Similar granulomas were seen in the spleen of this patient but there was no evidence of Hodgkin's tissue in either organ, × 100.

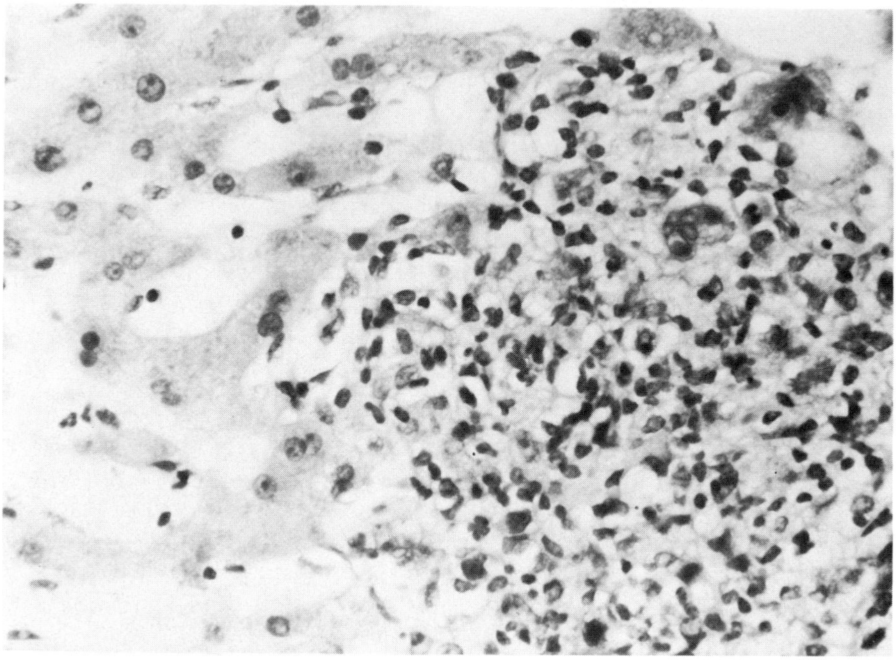

Fig. 4.29 Higher power of Fig. 4.28 showing large numbers of lymphocytes and histiocytes in the portal tract. A single Reed–Sternberg cell is present, × 300.

cellular background is sufficient for a diagnosis of Hodgkin's disease in these circumstances (Rappaport *et al.*, 1971). If cells showing cytological atypia are seen in the portal tracts the biopsy should be serially sectioned and a search made for Hodgkin's or Reed–Sternberg cells.

4.3 Thymus

Hodgkin's disease, particularly the nodular sclerosing subtype, may involve the thymus. It is not appropriate to use the term granulomatous thymoma for this condition.

References

Abt, A. B., Kirschner, R. H., Belliveau, R. E. *et al.* (1974), Hepatic pathology associated with Hodgkin's disease. *Cancer*, **33**, 1564–71.

Bearman, R. M., Pangalis, G. A. and Rappaport, H. (1978), Hodgkin's disease, lymphocyte depletion type: a clinicopathologic study of 39 patients. *Cancer*, **41**, 293–302.

Bennett, M. H., Tu, A. and Vaughan Hudson, B. (1981), Analysis of Grade I

Hodgkin's disease (Report No. 6) Part 2. Nodular sclerotic Hodgkin's disease. Cellular subtypes related to prognosis. *Clin. Radiol.*, **32**, 491–8.
Dorfman, R. F. (1971), Relationship of histology to site in Hodgkin's disease. *Cancer Res.*, **31**, 1786–93.
Farrer-Brown, G., Bennett, M. H., Harrison, C. V. *et al.* (1971), The pathological findings following laparotomy in Hodgkin's disease. *Br. J. Cancer*, **25**, 449–57.
Garvin, A. J., Spicer, S. S., Parmley, R. T. and Munster, A. M. (1974), Immunohistochemical demonstration of IgG in Reed–Sternberg and other cells in Hodgkin's disease. *J. Exp. Med.*, **139**, 1077–83.
Jackson, H. Jr. and Parker, F. Jr. (1947), *Hodgkin's Disease and Allied Disorders*, Oxford University Press, Oxford, New York.
Kadin, M. E., Donaldson, S. S. and Dorfman, R. F. (1970), Isolated granulomas in Hodgkin's disease. *New Engl. J. Med.*, **283**, 859–61.
Kadin, M. E., Glatstein, E. and Dorfman, R. F. (1971), Clinical-pathological studies of 117 untreated patients subjected to laparotomy for the staging of Hodgkin's disease. *Cancer*, **27**, 1277–94.
Kadin, M. E., Stites, D. P., Levy, R. and Warnke, R. (1978), Exogenous origin of immunoglobulin in Reed–Sternberg cells of Hodgkin's disease. *New Engl. J. Med.*, **299**, 1208–14.
Kaplan, H. D. (1980), *Hodgkin's Disease*, Harvard University Press, Cambridge, Massachusetts; London, England.
Kaplan, H. S. and Smithers, D. W. (1959), Autoimmunity in man and homologous disease in mice in relation to the malignant lymphomas. *Lancet*, **ii**, 1–4.
Lennert, K. (1981), *Histopathology of Non-Hodgkin's Lymphomas (Based on the Kiel Classification)*, Springer-Verlag, Berlin.
Lukes, R. J. (1971), Criteria for involvement of lymph node, bone marrow, spleen and liver in Hodgkin's disease. *Cancer Res.*, **31**, 1755–67.
Lukes, R. J. and Butler, J. J. (1966), The pathology and nomenclature of Hodgkin's disease. *Cancer Res.*, **26**, 1063–81.
Lukes, R. J., Butler, J. J. and Hicks, E. B. (1966a), Natural history of Hodgkin's disease as related to its pathological picture. *Cancer*, **19**, 317–44.
Lukes, R. J., Craver, L. F., Hall, T. C. *et al.* (1966b), Report of the nomenclature committee. *Cancer Res.*, **26**, 1311.
Neiman, R. S., Rosen, P. J. and Lukes, R. J. (1973), Lymphocyte depletion Hodgkin's disease. A clinicopathologic entity. *New Engl. J. Med.*, **288**, 751–5.
O'Connell, M. J., Schimpff, S. F., Kirschner, R. H. *et al.* (1975), Epithelioid granulomas in Hodgkin's disease – a favorable prognostic sign? *JAMA*, **233**, 886–9.
Payne, S. V., Newell, D. G., Jones, D. B. and Wright, D. H. (1980), The Reed–Sternberg cell/lymphocyte interaction. Ultrastructure and characteristics of binding. *Am. J. Pathol.*, **100**, 7–24.
Payne, S. V., Wright, D. H., Jones, K. J. M. and Judd, M. A. (1982), The macrophage origin of Reed–Sternberg cells. An immunohistochemical study. *J. Clin. Pathol.*, **35**, 159–66.
Poppema, S., Elema, J. D. and Halie, M. R. (1978), The significance of intracytoplasmic proteins in Reed–Sternberg cells. *Cancer*, **42**, 1793–1803.
Rappaport, H., Berard, C. W., Butler, J. J. *et al.* (1971), Report of the committee on histopathological criteria contributing to staging of Hodgkin's disease. *Cancer Res.*, **31**, 1864–5.

Resnick, G. D. and Nachman, R. L. (1981), Reed–Sternberg cells in Hodgkin's disease contain fibronectin. *Blood*, **57**, 339–42.
Sacks, E. L., Donaldson, S. S., Gordon, J. and Dorfman, R. F. (1978), Epithelioid granulomas associated with Hodgkin's disease. Clinical correlations in 55 previously untreated patients. *Cancer*, **41**, 562–7.
Strum, S. B. and Rappaport, H. (1970), Significance of focal involvement of lymph nodes for the diagnosis and staging of Hodgkin's disease. *Cancer*, **25**, 1314–19.
Taylor, C. R. (1976), An immunohistochemical study of follicular lymphoma, reticulum cell sarcoma and Hodgkin's disease. *Eur. J. Cancer*, **12**, 61–75.

5 The classification and terminology of malignant lymphomas other than Hodgkin's disease (non-Hodgkin's lymphomas – NHL)

The semantic and conceptual confusion that has surrounded the classification of malignant lymphomas in recent years has caused bewilderment and despair amongst diagnostic histopathologists. The introduction of the Rappaport classification in 1966 (Table 5.1) and its wide acceptance at least in the English-speaking world promoted a considerable advance in the study, comparison and therapy of NHL. The Rappaport classification made two particularly important contributions.

Table 5.1 Classification of non-Hodgkin's lymphomas (Rappaport, 1966)

Nodular		Diffuse
	Lymphocytic well differentiated	
	Lymphocytic poorly differentiated	
	Mixed (lymphocytic-histiocytic)	
	Histiocytic	
	Undifferentiated	

The first was the recognition that many lymphomas of similar cytology occurred in both diffuse and nodular forms and the second was to relate histology to prognosis. The impact of this classification was so great that despite its undisputed deficiencies it is still used in a modified form (Table 5.2) by many pathologists and oncologists today. The deficiencies of the Rappaport classification are its failure to clearly identify tumours of follicle centre cell origin and the use of the term 'histiocytic' for large cell lymphomas of variable histogenesis, most of which are not derived from histiocytes.

A major recent advance in lymphoma classification has been the realization that the majority of NHL are derived from cells that constitute the follicle centre. This concept put forward almost simultaneously by Lennert and his colleagues in Kiel, Germany and Lukes and Collins in

Table 5.2 Modified Rappaport classification (Nathwani, 1979)

Nodular and/or diffuse
Poorly differentiated lymphocytic
Mixed (lymphocytic-histiocytic)
'Histiocytic'
Burkitt's lymphoma
Undifferentiated non-Burkitt's
Diffuse
Well-differentiated lymphocytic (WDL)
WDL with plasmacytoid differentiation
Intermediate lymphocytic
Immunoblastic
Lymphoblastic
NHL of 'Lennert's' type
Mycosis fungoides
Plasmacytoma
Unclassifiable
Composite
Malignant histiocytosis

America was originally founded on morphological analysis alone but has had its validity established by the use of immunologic and immunohistochemical techniques. The Kiel classification and the Lukes and Collins classification are shown in Tables 5.3 and 5.4. While these two classifications disagree in some detail and use different terminologies they are conceptually very similar and it is possible to equate most entities diagnosed using the one classification with an equivalent in the other. It is important to realize that neither of these classifications is entirely satisfactory nor static and that they will continue to change as our understanding of lymphoreticular malignancy develops. Several other classifications of NHL have been proposed. We recognize that these may have contributed to individual therapeutic trials but it is our opinion that they are all inferior to the Kiel or Lukes and Collins classification and it serves no purpose to enumerate a host of different terms for the same entity.

In this book we have, with a few exceptions, used the terminology of the Kiel classification which we consider to be more elegant and precise than the terminology of the Lukes and Collins classification; for example the centrocyte is categorized as a cleaved cell in the Lukes and Collins classification yet nuclear cleavage is not particularly characteristic of these cells in histological sections whereas it is a much more prominent feature of many T-cell lymphomas. We cannot sufficiently stress the importance of attempting precisely to classify each case of NHL. It is only by

Table 5.3 Modified Kiel classification (Lennert, 1978)

I *Low grade malignancy*
- ML Lymphocytic
  - B-CLL
  - T-CLL
  - Hairy cell leukaemia
  - Mycosis fungoides and Sezary's syndrome
  - T-zone lymphoma
- ML Lymphoplasmacytic/lymphoplasmacytoid (LP immunocytoma)
- ML Plasmacytic
- ML Centrocytic
- ML Centroblastic/centrocytic
  - Follicular
  - Follicular and diffuse
  - Diffuse
  - With or without sclerosis

II *High grade malignancy*
- ML Centroblastic
  - Primary
  - Secondary
- ML Lymphoblastic
  - B-lymphoblastic, Burkitt type and others
  - T-lymphoblastic, convoluted cell type and others
  - Unclassified
- ML Immunoblastic
  - With plasmablastic/plasmacytic differentiation (B)
  - Without plasmablastic/plasmacytic differentiation (B or T)

exercising this discipline that common errors, such as mistaking metastatic carcinoma for lymphoma can be avoided. Standard light microscopy alone, if of high quality, is sufficient to identify the majority of cases of NHL as we hope to show in the following chapters. However, in a small proportion of cases the use of special techniques such as immunological markers, immunohistochemistry, cytochemistry and electron microscopy are necessary for precise identification.

The Kiel classification, along with most other classifications, lays great stress on the prognostic implication of its different categories. While broadly agreeing with these at present we do not feel that prognosis should govern the order and lay-out of classification since with new treatments prognoses can change. It is more important that a classification should have a structured histogenetic basis in which related entities are grouped together. Inevitably, therefore, we have made some adaptations to the Kiel classification. These consist only of inclusion of diseases not recognized in this classification (such as true histiocytic lymphomas) and

Table 5.4 Lukes and Collins functional classification of malignant lymphomas (Lukes and Collins, 1977)

U-cell (Undefined)

T-cell
- Small lymphocyte
- Convoluted lymphocyte
- Sezary cell-mycosis fungoides
- Immunoblastic sarcoma
- Lennert's lymphoma

B-cell
- Small lymphocyte
- Plasmacytoid lymphocyte
- Follicle centre cell lymphoma
  - Follicular or diffuse with or without sclerosis
    - Small cleaved
    - Large cleaved
    - Small non-cleaved
    - Large non-cleaved
- Immunoblastic sarcoma
- Hairy cell leukaemia

Histiocytic

a change of order to facilitate discussion; principally the grouping together of follicle centre cell lymphomas and of T-cell lymphomas. Without in any way offering a classification of our own we will discuss NHL in the order shown in Table 5.5.

5.1 B-cell lymphomas

5.1.1 *Lymphocytic/plasmacytic lymphomas*

(1) *Malignant lymphoma, lymphocytic.*
Kiel: B-CLL;
Lukes and Collins: B-cell type, small lymphocyte (CLL);
Rappaport: ML, lymphocytic, well differentiated, diffuse.
Lymphoma composed of small B-lymphocytes with variable numbers of prolymphocytes and lymphoblasts. The latter may be aggregated to form 'proliferation centres'. Involvement of bone marrow and peripheral blood present or develops in most cases.

(2) *Malignant lymphoma, prolymphocytic (B).*
Tumour composed of prolymphocytes. Splenomegaly and large numbers of tumour cells in peripheral blood are characteristic.

Table 5.5 Categorization of non-Hodgkin's lymphomas used in this book

I *B-cell lymphomas*
- (a) Lymphocytic/plasmacytic lymphomas
  - (1) ML lymphocytic (B-CLL)
  - (2) ML prolymphocytic (B)
  - (3) ML lymphoplasmacytoid
  - (4) ML lymphoplasmacytic
  - (5) ML plasmacytic
- (b) Follicle centre cell lymphomas
  - (1) ML centrocytic
  - (2) ML centroblastic – centrocytic
    - (i) Follicular
    - (ii) Follicular and diffuse
    - (iii) Diffuse
  - (3) ML centroblastic
- (c) ML immunoblastic
- (d) Burkitt's lymphoma and tumours of similar morphology

II *T-cell lymphomas*
- (1) ML lymphocytic (T-CLL)
- (2) ML prolymphocytic (T)
- (3) Cutaneous T-cell lymphomas
  - (i) Mycosis fungoides
  - (ii) Sezary's syndrome
- (4) Pleomorphic T-cell lymphoma
- (5) Monomorphic T-cell lymphoma
- (6) Other T-cell lymphomas
  - (i) Multilobated type
  - (ii) Lennert's lymphoma

III *Malignant lymphoma of B- and T-cell precursors*
- (1) ML lymphoblastic T-cell type
- (2) ML lymphoblastic 'null-cell' type

IV *Neoplasms of the monocyte/macrophage system*
- (1) Histiocytic lymphoma
- (2) Malignant histiocytosis
- (3) Malignant histiocytosis of the intestine

V *Miscellaneous*
- (1) Hairy cell leukaemia
- (2) Granulocytic sarcoma
- (3) Systemic mastocytosis

VI *Unclassifiable*

(3) *Malignant lymphoma, lymphoplasmacytic/lymphoplasmacytoid.*
Kiel: lymphoplasmacytic immunocytoma;
Lukes and Collins: B-cell type, plasmacytoid lymphocyte;
Rappaport: ML lymphocytic with dysproteinaemia.

(i) Lymphoplasmacytic.
Lymphoma composed of mixture of small lymphocytes and mature-looking plasma cells. May be associated with Waldenström's macroglobulinaemia or other dysproteinaemia.
(ii) Lymphoplasmacytoid.
Lymphoma composed of mixture of small lymphocytes and cells intermediate between lymphocytes and plasma cells. PAS positive inclusions of immunoglobulin may be found in cells. Often associated with Waldenström's macroglobulinaemia.
(4) *Malignant lymphoma, plasmacytic.*
Extramedullary plasmacytoma usually involving naso- or oropharynx or lymph nodes. Composed of uniform sheets of relatively mature-looking plasma cells.

5.1.2 *Follicle centre cell lymphomas*

(1) *Malignant lymphoma, centrocytic.*
Lukes and Collins: B-cell type, cleaved cell, diffuse;
Rappaport: ML, lymphocytic, poorly differentiated, diffuse.
Diffuse lymphoma composed of centrocytes. Varying degrees of sclerosis common.
(2) *Malignant lymphoma, centroblastic/centrocytic.*
Lukes and Collins: B-cell, FCC types, cleaved and non-cleaved;
Rappaport: ML, lymphocytic, poorly differentiated, nodular/diffuse.
Lymphoma composed of mixtures of centroblasts and centrocytes.

May be: (i) Follicular
(ii) Follicular and diffuse
(iii) Diffuse
(3) *Malignant lymphoma, centroblastic.*
Lukes and Collins: B-cell type, FCC, large non-cleaved;
Rappaport: ML, histiocytic.
High grade lymphoma that may arise in patients with pre-existing centroblastic/centrocytic lymphoma (secondary centroblastic lymphoma) or *de novo* (primary centroblastic lymphoma). Tumour composed predominantly of centroblasts with smaller numbers of centrocytes and immunoblasts. Pleomorphic forms of centroblastic lymphoma occur.

5.1.3 *Malignant lymphoma, immunoblastic*

Lukes and Collins: immunoblastic sarcoma of B-cells;
Rappaport: ML, histiocytic, diffuse.

High grade lymphoma in which immunoblasts are the predominant cell, not always clearly defined from centroblastic lymphoma. Pleomorphic forms of immunoblastic sarcoma occur.

5.1.4 *Burkitt's lymphoma*

Kiel: lymphoblastic lymphoma, Burkitt type;
Lukes and Collins: FCC lymphoma, small non-cleaved;
Rappaport: ML, undifferentiated, Burkitt type.

A high grade B-cell lymphoma first recognized in Africa where it has a defined geographic distribution. In Africa the tumour occurs predominantly in childhood, has a predilection for the jaws and abdominal viscera but tends not to involve lymph nodes. The tumour has a characteristic cytology and histology with small undifferentiated blast cells interspersed by non-neoplastic histiocytes. Morphologically similar tumours occur sporadically throughout the world but have a slightly different anatomic distribution. The separation of Burkitt's lymphoma from some other undifferentiated lymphomas of childhood can be difficult.

5.2 T-cell lymphomas

(1) *Malignant lymphoma, lymphocytic.*
Kiel: T-CLL;
Lukes and Collins: T-cell type – small lymphocytic;
Rappaport: ML, lymphocytic, well differentiated, diffuse.

Predilection for skin, may cause massive splenomegaly, neutropenia common. Bone marrow and lymph node involvement less common than in B-CLL. Tumour composed of slightly pleomorphic lymphocytes with occasional blast cells. Epithelioid venules prominent.

(2) *Malignant lymphoma, prolymphocytic.*

Tumour cells have prominent nucleoli, epithelioid venules prominent.

(3) *Cutaneous T-cell Lymphomas. Mycosis fungoides and Sezary's syndrome.*

Tumours of epidermotrophic T-cells with variable spillover of cells into peripheral blood. Dissemination to lymph nodes and viscera usually occurs late and indicates poor prognosis. Tumour cells have complex 'cerebriform' nuclei. Blast cell transformation sometimes accompanies dissemination.

(4) *Pleomorphic T-cell lymphoma.*
Kiel: T-zone lymphoma;
Lukes and Collins: T-cell type, immunoblastic sarcoma.
Tumour starts in paracortex of lymph node and may be associated with follicular hyperplasia. Neoplastic T-cells vary from small lymphoid cells with irregular nuclei to pleomorphic blast cells. Epithelioid venules are prominent, eosinophils, plasma cells and epithelioid histiocytes occur in variable numbers.
(5) *Monomorphic T-cell lymphoma, small and large cell types.*
(6) *Other node based T-cell lymphomas.*
(i) T-cell lymphoma of multilobated type.
Lymphoma composed of large cells with polylobated nuclei.
(ii) Lymphoma with high content of epithelioid cells (Lennert's lymphoma).
Histology dominated by clusters of epithelioid histiocytes. Tumour cells composed of small irregular T-lymphoid cells with occasional blast cells that may be multinucleated. (NB: Large numbers of epithelioid histiocytes may occur in Hodgkin's disease and some other non-Hodgkin's lymphomas).

5.3 Malignant lymphoma of B- and T-cell precursors

(1) *Malignant lymphoma, lymphoblastic.*
Kiel: ML, lymphoblastic, convoluted cell type;
Lukes and Collins: T-cell type, convoluted lymphocyte;
Rappaport: ML, lymphoblastic.
High grade lymphoma composed of relatively monomorphic lymphoblasts. Some have characteristics of T-cells and some of 'null cells'. Some, but not all, of the T-cell type have convoluted nuclei. Disease usually becomes leukaemic.

5.4 Neoplasms of the monocyte/macrophage system

(1) *Histiocytic lymphoma.*
Rappaport: ML, histiocytic, diffuse.
Tumours composed of a range of cells from histioblasts to more mature looking histiocytes. Difficult tumours to recognize. Have not been well characterized.
(2) *Malignant histiocytosis.*
Neoplasm of histiocytes in which the tumour cells may be monomorphic or pleomorphic. Tumour cells disseminate widely in sinusoids of bone marrow, liver and spleen and sinuses of lymph nodes. Solid

tumours may occur and in such cases distinction from histiocytic lymphoma may be difficult.

(3) *Malignant histiocytosis of the intestine.*

Lymphoma that develops in patients with malabsorption and villous atrophy of the upper small intestine. Tumour may be monomorphic or pleomorphic. Dissemination occurs in an intrasinusoidal pattern similar to that seen in malignant histiocytosis.

5.5 Miscellaneous

(1) *Hairy cell leukaemia*

Neoplasm of B-lymphocytes with characteristic hairy surfaces and tartrate resistant acid phosphatase. Monomorphic infiltrate in spleen and bone marrow, less frequent in lymph nodes, with distinctive angiomatous formations.

(2) *Granulocytic sarcoma.*

Solid tumours that develop in patients with granulocytic leukaemia. May precede onset of leukaemia by months or years.

(3) *Systemic mastocytosis.*

Patients usually, but not always, have cutaneous mastocytosis with urticaria pigmentosa. Gastrointestinal symptoms, hepatosplenomegaly and osteopenia are common features. Some patients develop leukaemia.

References

Lennert, K. (1978), Malignant lymphomas other than Hodgkin's disease. In *Handbuch der Speziellen Pathologischen Anatomie und Histologie*, Springer-Verlag, Berlin (in collaboration with M. Mohri, H. Stein, E. Kaiserling and H. K. Muller-Hermelink).

Lukes, R. J. and Collins, R. D. (1977), Lukes–Collins classification and its significance. *Cancer Treat. Rep.*, **61**, 971–9.

Nathwani, B. N. (1979), A critical analysis of the classifications of non-Hodgkin's lymphoma. *Cancer*, **44**, 347–8.

Rappaport, H. (1966), *Tumors of the Hematopoietic System. Atlas of Tumor Pathology* (Sec. 3, Fasc. 8), Armed Forces Institute of Pathology, Washington D.C.

6 Lymphocytic-plasmacytic lymphomas

6.1 Malignant lymphoma: lymphocytic (B-CLL)

Lymphocytic lymphoma is frequently associated with chronic lymphocytic leukaemia and is regarded as the tissue phase of this disease in the Kiel classification (Lennert, 1981). Patients with chronic lymphocytic leukaemia frequently have some degree of generalized lymphadenopathy although there is rarely any clinical indication for biopsy of these nodes. Lymph node biopsy is more likely to be performed in those patients with lymphocytic lymphoma who present with substantial localized or generalized lymphadenopathy. Such patients may have blood and bone marrow disease at the time of biopsy or develop this after a variable period (Galton, 1964), although a number of patients have been recorded who have been followed for many years after the diagnosis of lymphocytic lymphoma and who have not developed leukaemia (Pangalis *et al.*, 1977). A small proportion of patients with chronic lymphocytic leukaemia develop an aggressive lymphoma with pleomorphic cytology that may cause nodal or extranodal tumour masses (Richter's syndrome) (Richter, 1928). There is increasing evidence from careful immunohistological studies that the pleomorphic lymphoma that characterizes Richter's syndrome is of the same clonal origin as the small lymphocytes of the original lymphocytic lymphoma (Delsol *et al.*, 1981; Harousseau *et al.*, 1981). Lymphocytic lymphoma occurs most frequently in the sixth and seventh decades of life, is rare in young adults and is usually generalized at the time of diagnosis.

6.1.1 Histology

Lymph node biopsies from patients with established chronic lymphocytic leukaemia and moderate lymphadenopathy show diffuse infiltration of the node by leukaemic cells with preservation of much of the underlying nodal architecture. The infiltrating leukaemic cells are slightly larger than the residual small lymphocytes and are interspersed with occasional prolymphocytes and lymphoblasts (Fig. 6.1). Nodal biopsies from patients with lymphocytic lymphoma presenting primarily as lymphadenopathy usually show a rather different histological appearance.

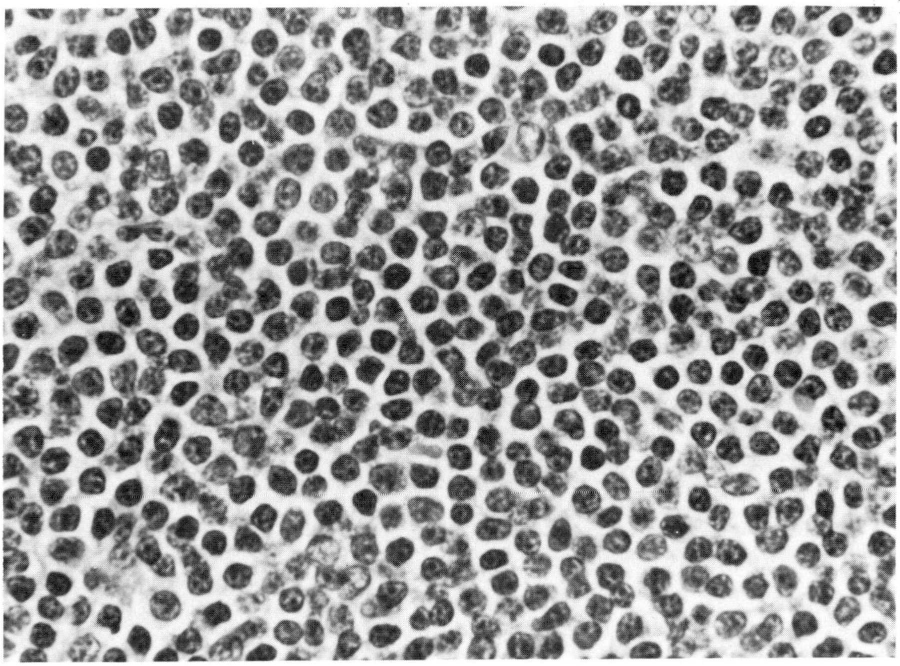

Fig. 6.1 Malignant lymphoma, lymphocytic. The tumour consists predominantly of small lymphocytes with occasional nucleolated prolymphocytes and lymphoblasts, × 480.

The tumour infiltration appears to be more destructive with obliteration of the pre-existing nodal architecture. Prolymphocytes and lymphoblasts may occur singly throughout the sheets of small lymphocytes but are commonly aggregated into small groups designated as proliferation centres (Lennert, 1978). These collections of paler staining cells may give the tumour a pseudofollicular appearance (Figs 6.2, 6.3 and 6.4). Mitotic figures are frequent within the proliferation centres whereas the surrounding small lymphocytes do not appear to divide.

Lymphocytic lymphoma induces little new fibre formation and the reticulin pattern is either scanty or reflects that of the tissue being infiltrated. The PAS stain is negative, and is useful in separating lymphocytic lymphoma from some cases of lymphoplasmacytoid lymphoma. The methyl green pyronin stain shows weak cytoplasmic

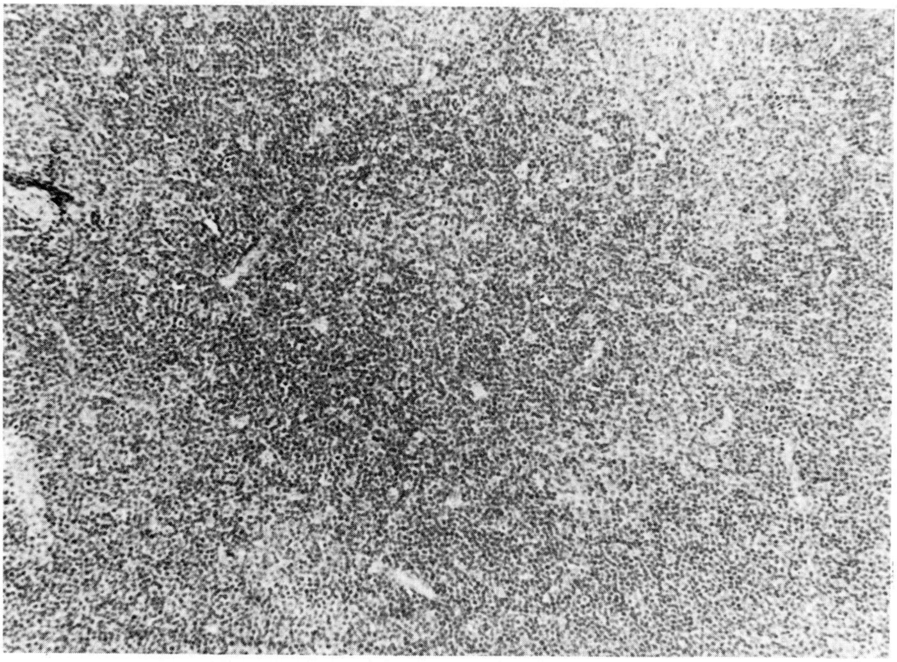

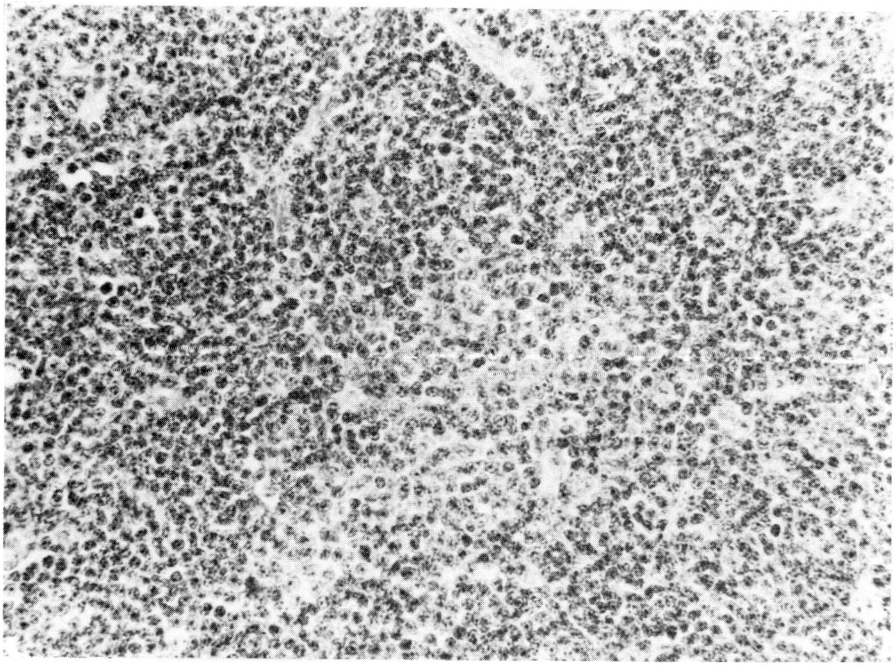

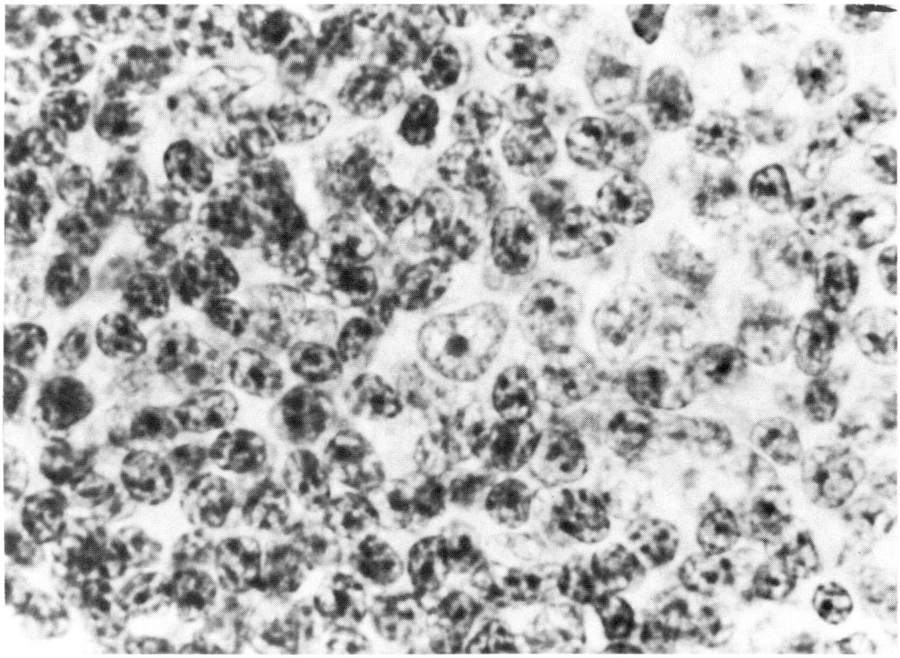

Fig. 6.4 Higher power view of proliferation centre showing nucleolated prolymphocytes and lymphoblasts, × 1000.

pyroninophilia of the small lymphocytes but highlights the prolymphocytes and lymphoblasts which show strong pyroninophilia of their cytoplasm and nucleoli. These cells are also well seen in sections of plastic embedded tissue where their large size, abundant cytoplasm and pale-staining nuclei with prominent nucleoli clearly distinguish them from the surrounding small lymphocytes (Fig. 6.5).

Immunoperoxidase stains for cytoplasmic immunoglobulin are negative in lymphocytic lymphoma. Weak monotypic surface immunoglobulin can be detected in frozen sections.

In patients with lymphocytic lymphoma the spleen shows diffuse infiltration by predominantly small lymphocytes. The lymphoid follicles are effaced and small lymphocytes infiltrate both the splenic cords and sinusoids. Infiltration of the liver occurs predominantly in the portal areas and can be differentiated from inflammatory lymphoid infiltrates by

---

Fig. 6.2 Malignant lymphoma, lymphocytic showing pale-staining proliferation centres giving a vague nodular appearance to the tumour, × 80.
Fig. 6.3 Higher power view of Fig. 6.2 showing pale-staining proliferation centre containing prolymphocytes and lymphoblasts, × 250.

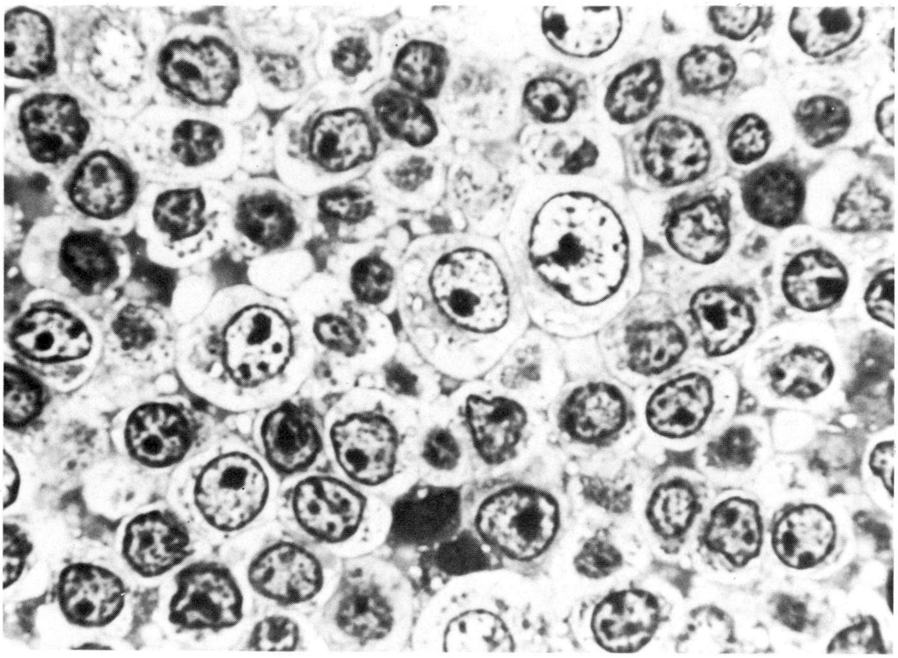

Fig. 6.5 Malignant lymphoma, lymphocytic. Plastic embedded section. The predominant cells are small lymphocytes with clumped heterochromatin. Larger prolymphocytes and lymphoblasts with prominent nucleoli are also seen. Toluidine blue, × 1200.

the monomorphism of the small lymphocytes and the absence of parenchymal cell changes.

Bone marrow infiltration is usually diffuse although in a substantial number of cases focal deposits of tumour are present (Fig. 6.6) (Rozman *et al.*, 1981). In the latter circumstances separation from follicle centre cell lymphoma is based upon the morphology of the individual tumour cells (Fig. 6.7).

6.1.2 Differential diagnosis

Poor fixation and thick sectioning tend to make many lymphoma cells look like small lymphocytes. In good quality sections lymphocyte-

---

Fig. 6.6 Bone marrow trephine biopsy from a patient with malignant lymphoma, lymphocytic. Focal islands of lymphoma cells can be seen, × 30.
Fig. 6.7 Higher power view of Fig. 6.6 showing that the tumour cells consist predominantly of small lymphocytes, × 300.

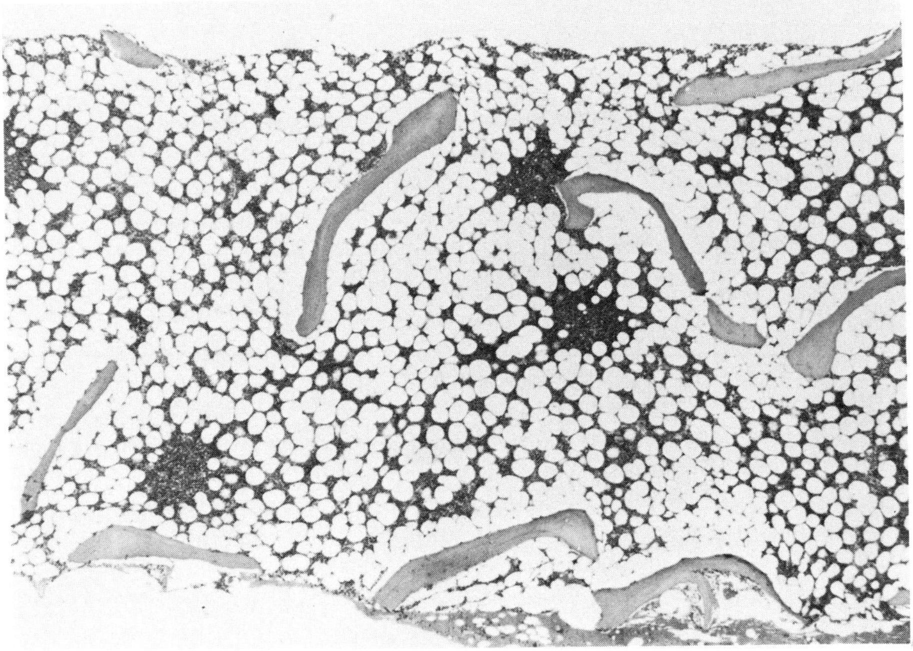

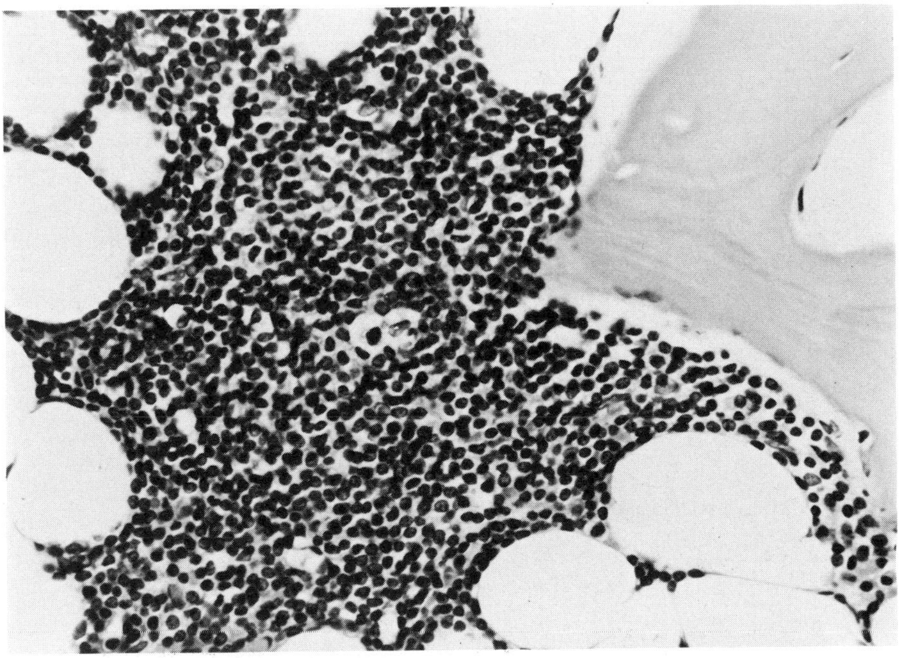

predominant Hodgkin's disease may occasionally resemble lymphocytic lymphoma and vice versa (Colby *et al.*, 1981) and should be seriously considered in any patient under 50 with a diffuse small lymphocytic tumour. Apart from the presence of Reed–Sternberg cells (essential for the diagnosis of Hodgkin's disease) lymphocyte-predominant Hodgkin's disease usually shows scattered clusters of epithelioid cells and occasional eosinophils. Focal condensations of reticulin, often giving an overall nodular pattern are common in Hodgkin's disease. Proliferation centres do not occur in Hodgkin's disease although the scattered lymphoblasts seen in some lymphocytic lymphomas must be distinguished from the polylobated Reed–Sternberg cells characteristic of lymphocyte-predominant Hodgkin's disease.

Diffuse small centrocytic lymphoma is frequently misdiagnosed as lymphocytic lymphoma. The differentiation between these two tumours depends essentially on the recognition of the characteristic features of small lymphocytes and small centrocytes. Centrocytic tumours are generally more destructive in their pattern of infiltration, have a coarser reticulin pattern and do not show proliferation centres. Prominent proliferation centres giving a pseudofollicular pattern in lymphocytic lymphoma occasionally cause confusion with follicular lymphoma, however, the prolymphocytes and lymphoblasts in proliferation centres are smaller and have a more delicate nuclear chromatin and smaller nucleoli than centroblasts. Proliferation centres are less well defined than the neoplastic follicles of follicular lymphomas and do not show the characteristic reticulin pattern of this tumour.

Mann *et al.* (1979) and Weisenburger *et al.* (1981) have described a lymphoma in which the morphology of the tumour cells is intermediate between lymphocytic lymphoma (CLL) and centrocytic lymphoma. These cells have surface immunoglobulin which stains at an intensity intermediate between that observed on CLL cells and centrocytes. They have C3 receptors and some stain for alkaline phosphatase. Mann *et al.* (1979) suggest that these tumours may arise from the cells of primary follicles or the mantle zones of secondary follicles. It has yet to be established whether malignant lymphoma intermediate lymphocytic type represents a distinct entity.

6.2 Malignant lymphoma: prolymphocytic (B)

Galton *et al.* (1974) separated prolymphocytic leukaemia from typical B-CLL. The characteristic cell in the peripheral blood is a large lymphoid cell with a prominent central nucleolus, relatively coarse nuclear chromatin and a moderate amount of cytoplasm. Patients typically have systemic symptoms, high white cell counts and massive splenomegaly although lymphadenopathy is not usually a prominent feature. In tissue sections thc tumour cells have rounded nuclei with prominent central nucleoli and a moderate amount of pyroninophilic cytoplasm (Fig. 6.8). The pattern of infiltration in lymph nodes is often 'nodular' (Figs 6.9 and 6.10), in the bone marrow and spleen it may be nodular or diffuse (Bearman *et al.*, 1978).

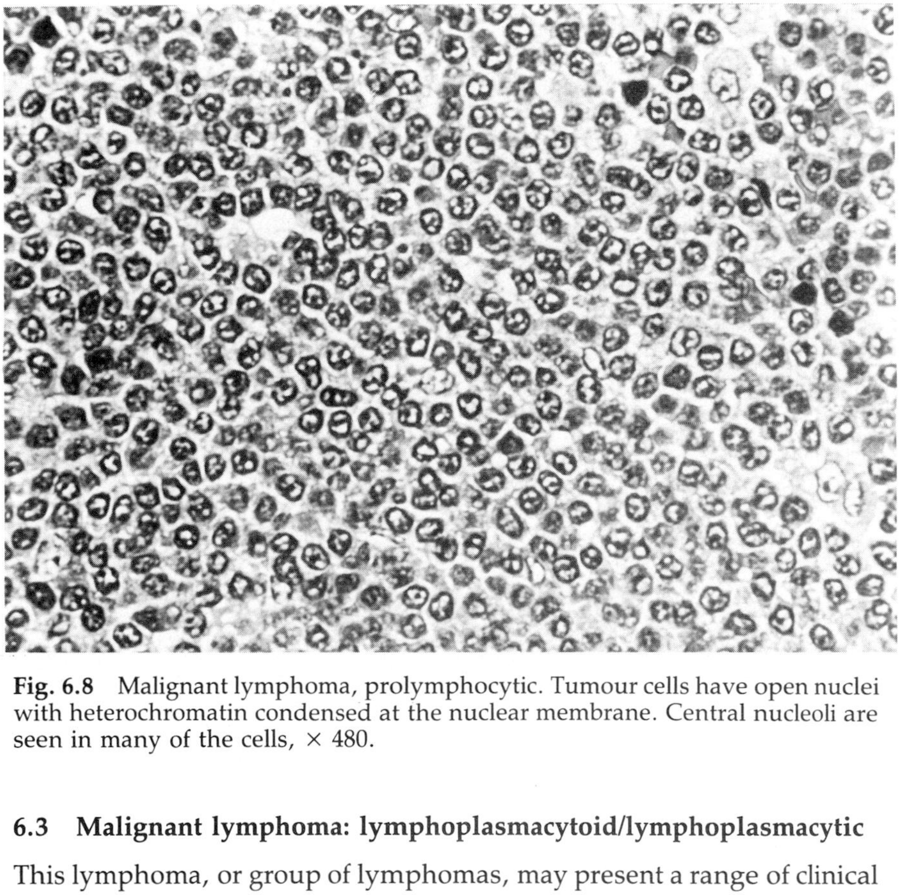

Fig. 6.8 Malignant lymphoma, prolymphocytic. Tumour cells have open nuclei with heterochromatin condensed at the nuclear membrane. Central nucleoli are seen in many of the cells, × 480.

6.3 Malignant lymphoma: lymphoplasmacytoid/lymphoplasmacytic

This lymphoma, or group of lymphomas, may present a range of clinical features and histological appearances. Essentially it is a tumour of B-lymphocytes that show varying degrees of differentiation towards plasma cells. Lennert (1978) recognized three subtypes of this lymphoma: *lymphoplasmacytoid* which shows a mixture of small lymphocytes and cells intermediate in appearance between lymphocytes and plasma cells; *lymphoplasmacytic* consisting of a mixture of small lymphocytes and plasma cells and *polymorphic* showing a mixture of centrocytes and centroblasts as well as plasmacytic cells. We would prefer to categorize

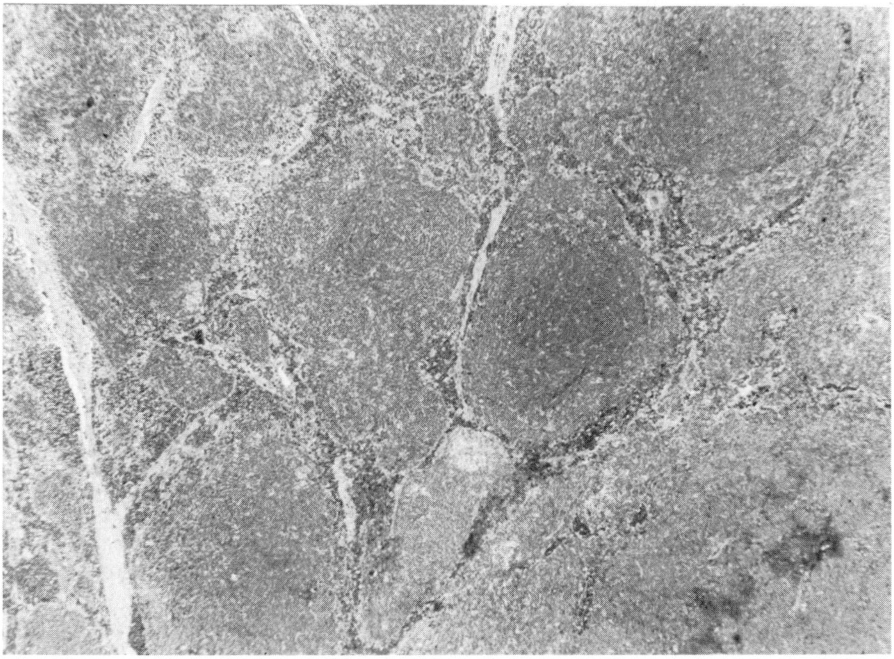

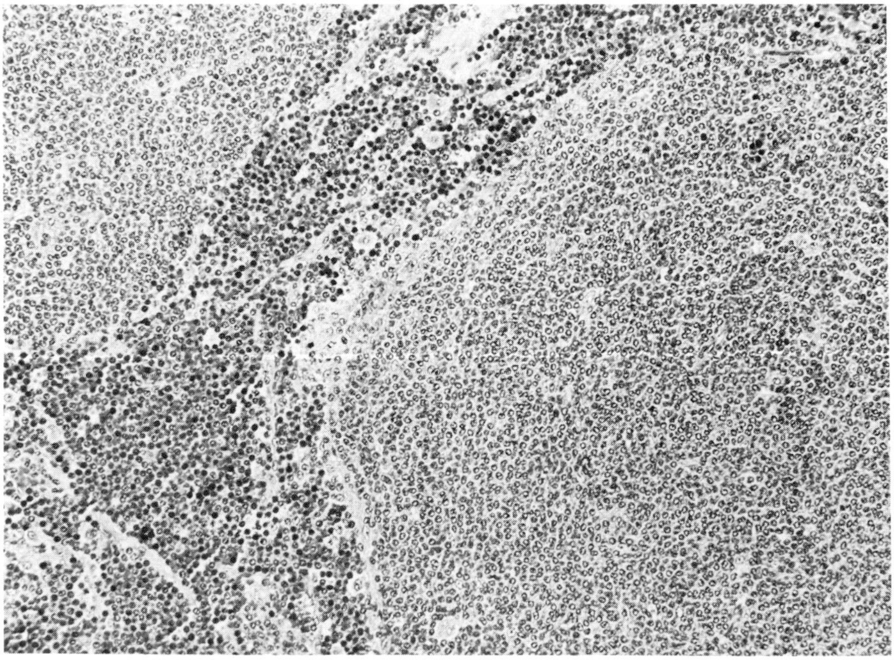

the latter group as centroblastic/centrocytic lymphoma with plasmacytic differentiation than as a variant of lymphoplasmacytoid/cytic lymphoma.

Lymphoplasmacytoid/cytic lymphoma occurs most frequently in the sixth and seventh decades. Patients may present with a variety of symptoms including fever, weakness, loss of appetite, loss of weight, night sweats and arthralgia. Many patients have a paraprotein in the blood and urine. If the tumour is secreting IgM they may have macroglobulinaemia of Waldenström, however the tumour may produce other heavy chains or be non-secretory. More than half the patients have a lymphocytosis in the peripheral blood of greater than 4000 mm^{-3} with an appearance similar to CLL although the circulating cells may show greater cytoplasmic basophilia (Lennert, 1981). In the absence of overt leukaemia a predominant monotypic B-cell population may be identified in the peripheral blood or bone marrow by surface marker techniques. Careful analysis will reveal paraproteins in the blood and urine of many patients. Coomb's-positive haemolytic anaemia occurred in 13.5% of cases studied by the Kiel Lymphoma Group (Heinz *et al.*, quoted by Lennert, 1981).

Three anatomic variants of lymphoplasmacytoid/cytic lymphoma have been described (Lennert, 1978). The lymph node type manifests generalized lymphadenopathy usually of small to moderate size. The splenomegalic group shows splenomegaly without bone marrow involvement or lymphadenopathy. Least frequently encountered in the oculocutaneous group with tumour deposits in the orbit (frequently misdiagnosed as pseudolymphoma) and skin. Overlap and transitions between these groups occur.

6.3.1 *Malignant lymphoma: lymphoplasmacytoid*

(a) *Histology*

In H and E stained sections this tumour appears similar, or identical, to lymphocytic lymphoma (Figs 6.11 and 6.12) although imprint preparations may show lymphoplasmacytoid cells (Fig. 6.13). Lymphoplasmacytoid cells are discernible in Giemsa or methyl green pyronin stained sections by their increased cytoplasmic basophilia or pyroninophilia. In approximately half the cases PAS-stained preparations will show intracytoplasmic or intranuclear PAS-positive immunoglobulin inclu-

---

Fig. 6.9 Low power view of malignant lymphoma, prolymphocytic showing nodular pattern of the infiltrate, × 30.

Fig. 6.10 Malignant lymphoma, prolymphocytic showing densely packed nodules of lymphoma cells with intervening loosely packed cells that are filling pre-existing lymph node sinuses, × 120.

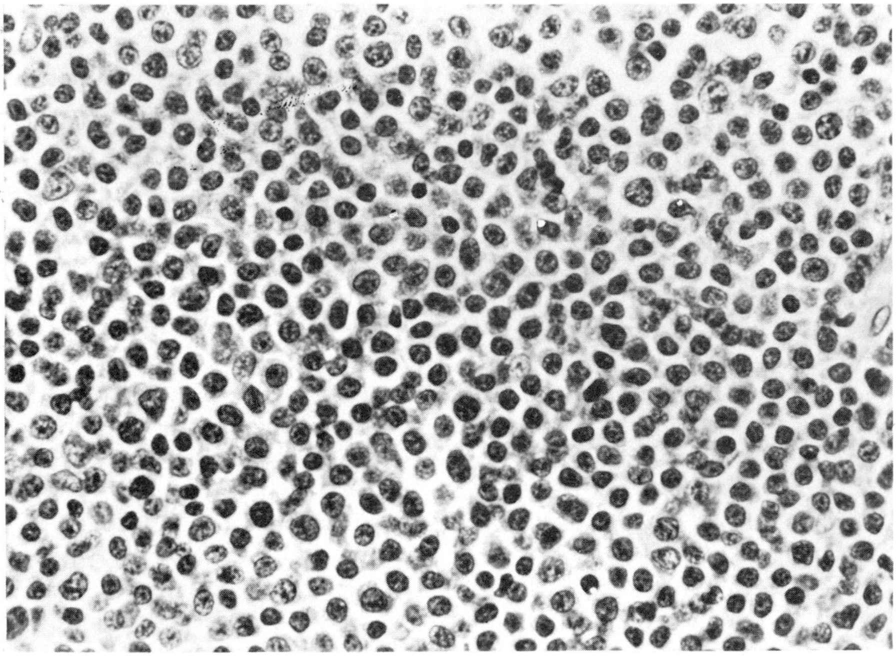

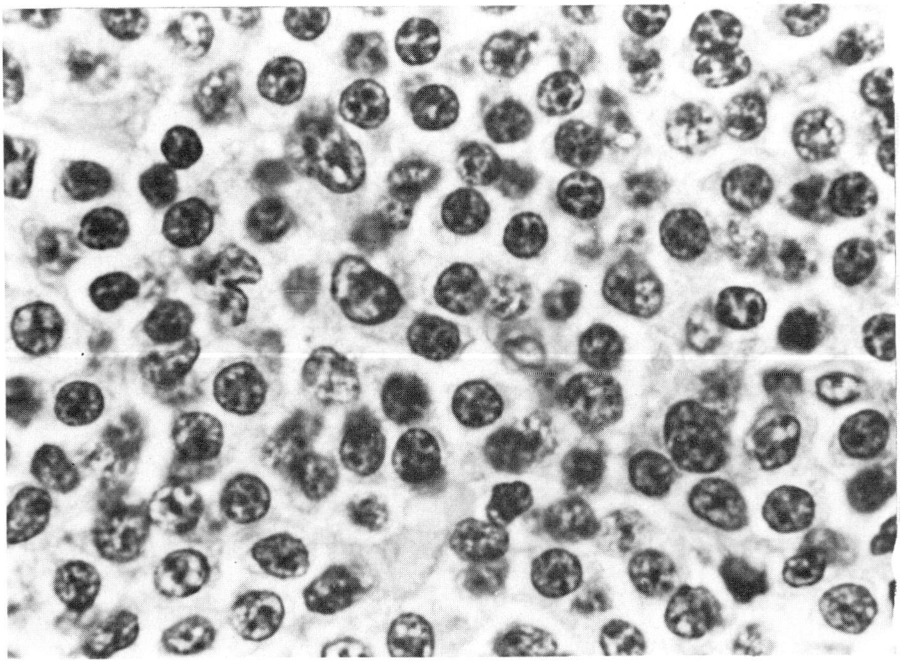

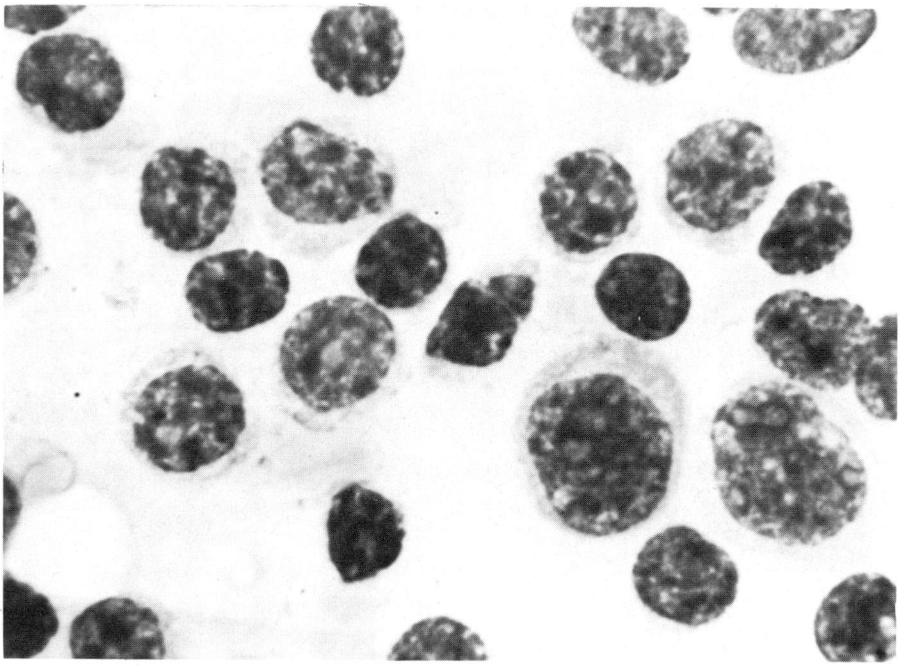

Fig. 6.13 Imprint preparation of malignant lymphoma, lymphoplasmacytoid. In this preparation some of the lymphoma cells show more abundant, darkly staining cytoplasm, i.e. plasmacytoid differentiation. Giemsa, × 1200.

sions (Fig. 6.14). The frequent intranuclear location of these inclusions is due to accumulation of immunoglobulin in the perinuclear space with protrusion into the nucleus. Pangalis *et al.* (1977) found PAS-positive cytoplasmic and intranuclear inclusions in approximately a quarter of patients with lymphocytic lymphoma or CLL although they were not as frequent as in patients with lymphoplasmacytoid lymphoma. In all cases of lymphoplasmacytoid lymphoma immunohistochemical studies will show monotypic cytoplasmic immunoglobulin in a high proportion of the lymphoplasmacytoid cells (Fig. 6.15). This is almost invariably of the IgM heavy chain class.

Scattered blast cells (paraimmunoblasts) are found in lymphoplas-

---

Fig. 6.11 Malignant lymphoma, lymphoplasmacytoid. The appearances of this tumour are similar to those of malignant lymphoma, lymphocytic. The predominant cells are small lymphocytes with scattered nucleolated cells amongst them, × 400.

Fig. 6.12 Higher power view of Fig. 6.11 showing that the majority of the tumour cells resemble small lymphocytes, × 1000.

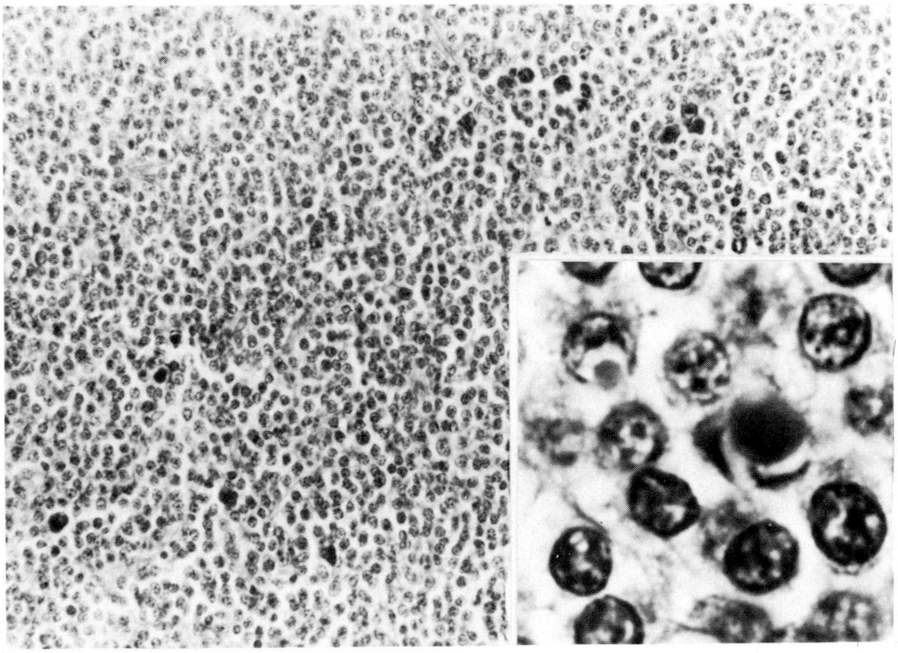

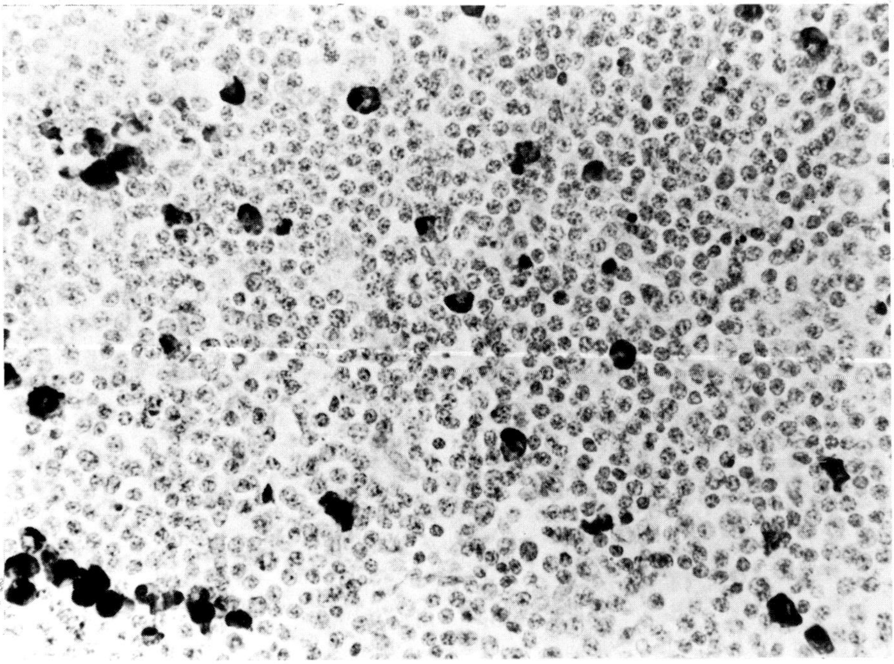

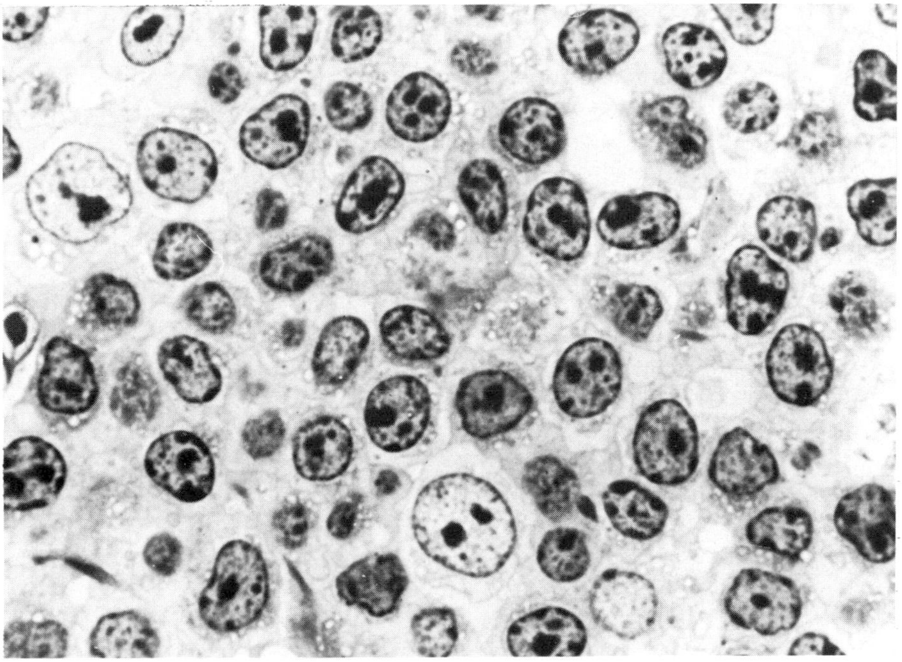

Fig. 6.16 Malignant lymphoma, lymphoplasmacytoid. Plastic embedded section. The majority of cells have the appearance of small lymphocytes, occasional nucleolated cells are seen with more abundant cytoplasm containing strands of rough endoplasmic reticulum. Toluidine blue, × 1200.

macytoid lymphomas (Fig. 6.16) and as in lymphocytic lymphoma these may be aggregated to give a pseudofollicular appearance. Transition to a high grade lymphoma, immunoblastic sarcoma, occurs in a small proportion of cases. These high grade tumours express the same immunological phenotype as the original lymphoplasmacytoid cells (Brouet *et al.*, 1976; Habeshaw *et al.*, 1979).

(b) *Differential diagnosis*

The study of Pangalis *et al.* (1977) suggests that lymphoplasmacytoid lymphoma cannot be differentiated from CLL and lymphocytic lymphoma in H and E stained sections alone. The detection of lymphoplas-

---

Fig. 6.14 PAS stain of tumour shown in Fig. 6.11. Many of the tumour cells show PAS-positive intranuclear and cytoplasmic inclusions. Inset high power view showing two cells with intranuclear PAS-positive immunoglobulin inclusions, × 250 (inset, × 1200).

Fig. 6.15 Section of the tumour illustrated in Fig. 6.11 stained for kappa light chains by the immunoperoxidase technique. Many of the tumour cells show positive cytoplasmic and intranuclear staining for immunoglobulin, × 300.

macytoid cells with the Giemsa or methyl green pyronin stains or of immunoglobulin inclusions with the PAS stain will aid in the identification of lymphoplasmacytoid lymphoma. Immunohistochemical studies provide the most reliable means of identifying lymphoplasmacytoid lymphoma in tissue sections although even with this technique the differentiation from lymphocytic lymphoma is not always clear cut (Papadimitriou, 1979).

6.3.2 *Malignant lymphoma: lymphoplasmacytic*

(a) *Histology*

This lymphoma is composed of small lymphocytes, plasma cells and cells intermediate between these (Figs 6.17, 6.18 and 6.19). The tumour may

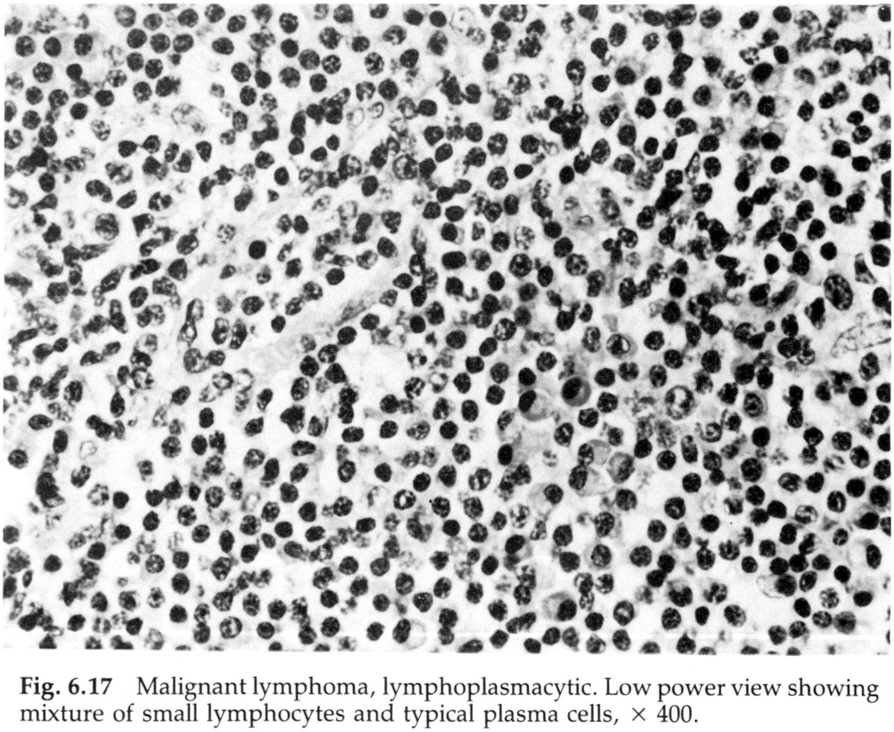

Fig. 6.17 Malignant lymphoma, lymphoplasmacytic. Low power view showing mixture of small lymphocytes and typical plasma cells, × 400.

Fig. 6.18 Higher power view of Fig. 6.17 showing a mixture of small lymphocytes and typical plasma cells, × 1000.

Fig. 6.19 Malignant lymphoma, lymphoplasmacytic. Plastic embedded section showing mixture of small lymphocytes and plasma cells. One tumour cell top right contains numerous intracytoplasmic inclusions of immunoglobulin giving it a granulated appearance. Toluidine blue, × 1200.

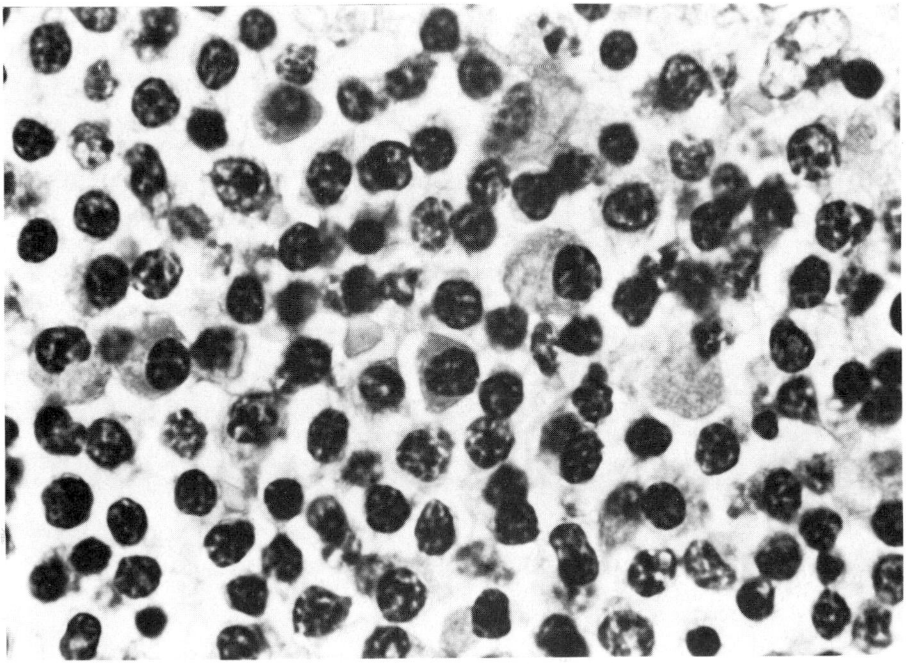

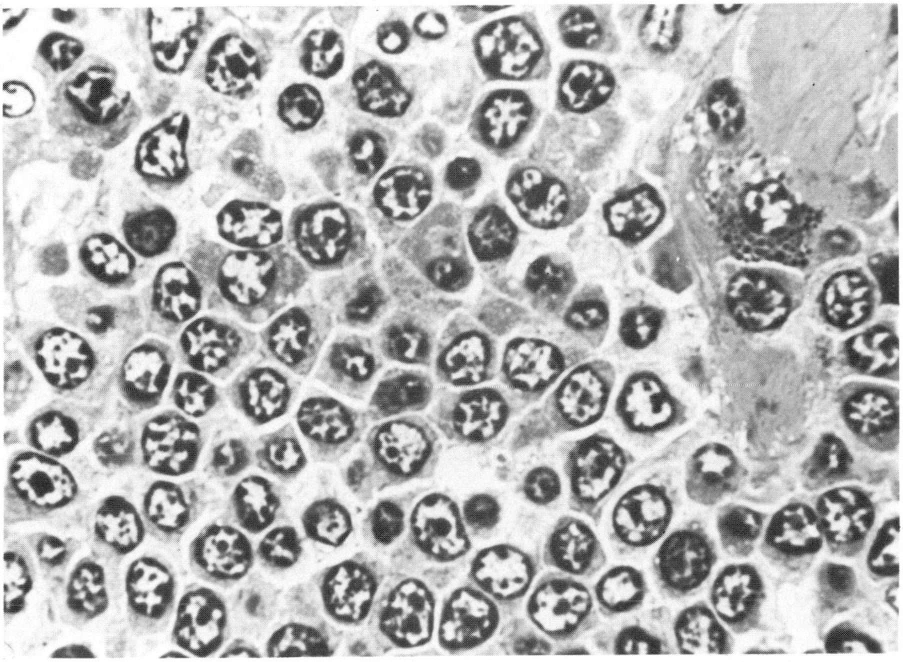

form solid infiltrating masses but in lymph nodes characteristically infiltrates the medullary cords and paracortex leaving the sinuses intact. These may be distended by eosinophilic PAS-positive proteinaceous material (Fig. 6.20).

PAS-positive inclusions of immunoglobulin may be seen in the plasma cells and these sometimes appear crystalline. Immunohistochemical studies will always show monotypic staining of the plasma cells for immunoglobulin (Fig. 6.21). Occasionally extracellular accumulations of PAS-positive inspissated proteinaceous material are seen and less commonly amyloid deposits are found in the tumour; both of these materials may evoke a giant cell reaction. Scattered clusters of epithelioid histiocytes are not infrequently seen in these tumours, sometimes giving the appearance of 'Lennert's lymphoma'. Increased numbers of mast cells have been reported in lymphoplasmacytic lymphomas (Harrison, 1972).

(b) *Differential diagnosis*

The presence of large numbers of small lymphocytes in lymphoplasmacytic lymphoma scattered amongst the plasma cells as an integral part of the tumour serves to differentiate it from plasmacytoma.

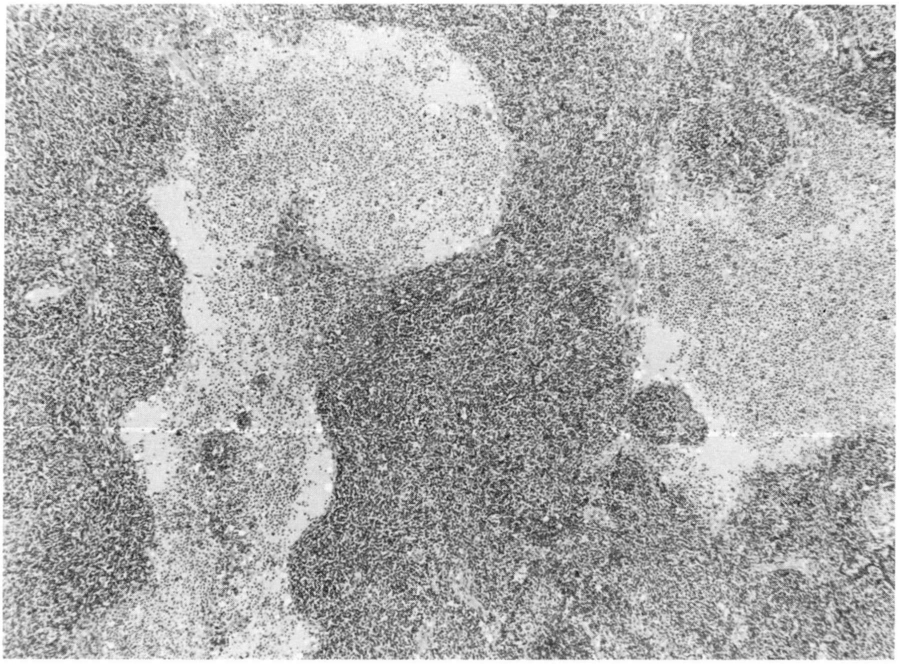

Fig. 6.20 Malignant lymphoma, lymphoplasmacytic. Low power view showing distention of lymph node sinuses by proteinaceous fluid, × 30.

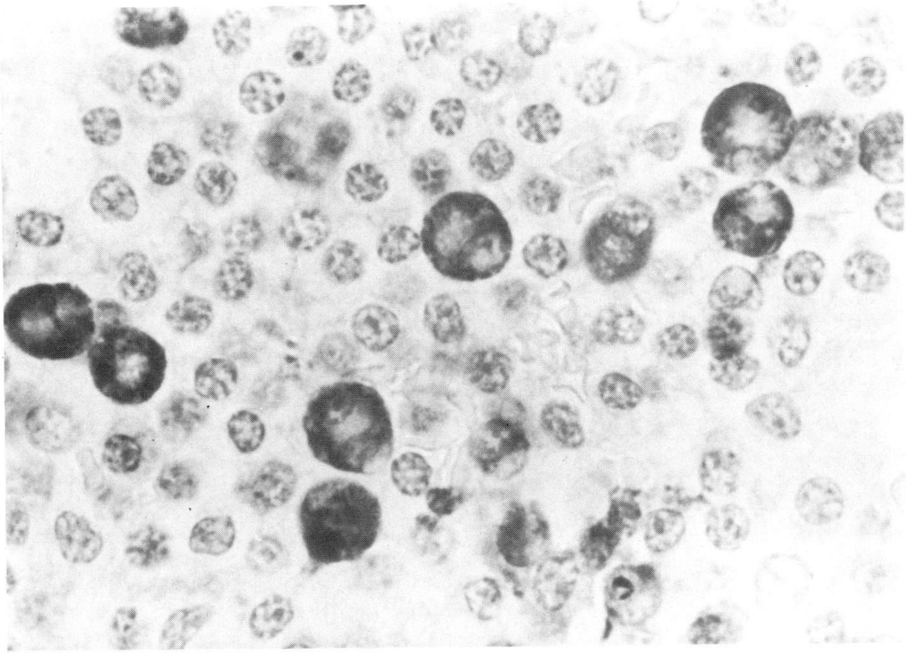

Fig. 6.21 Malignant lymphoma, lymphoplasmacytic stained for kappa chain by the immunoperoxidase technique. The plasma cells in the tumour show strong positive cytoplasmic staining. The pale-staining area in the cytoplasm corresponds to the position of the Golgi apparatus, × 1000.

6.4 Malignant lymphoma: plasmacytic

Plasmacytomas usually arise in the bone marrow and compared with this involvement of the lymph nodes is rare. Extramedullary plasmacytomas occur most frequently in the paranasal air sinuses, naropharynx and oropharynx, other locations include the salivary glands, lung, breast, thyroid and gonads. In contrast to the report of Henry and Farrer-Brown (1977) that plasmacytoma accounted for over 50% of primary intestinal lymphoma, we have seen very few cases at this site. Primary lymph node plasmacytoma accounted for 0.8% of the non-Hodgkin's lymphomas in the Kiel lymph node registry (Lennert, 1981).

A full haematological work-up together with a skeletal survey should be performed to determine whether the plasmacytoma is indeed localized or part of generalized myelomatosis. The blood and concentrated urine should be examined for paraproteins. Paraproteinaemia and paraproteinuria are said to be less frequent in extramedullary plasmacytoma than in multiple myelomatosis because of the smaller bulk of the tumour.

6.4.1 Histology

Histologically most plasmacytomas show a monotonous proliferation of plasma cells (Figs 6.22 and 6.23). Varying degrees of pleomorphism may occur although multinucleate plasma cells are not of themselves necessarily indicative of malignancy. Less differentiated tumours may not show the coarse clock-face nuclear chromatin characteristic of plasma cells but have a more open nucleus, often with a single central nucleolus. The methyl green pyronin stain always shows intense cytoplasmic pyroninophilia in plasma cells with a pale area adjacent to the nucleus corresponding to the site of the Golgi apparatus. PAS positivity of the cytoplasm may be diffuse or granular and intranuclear PAS-positive inclusions may be seen. Inclusions are highlighted in plastic embedded sections (Fig. 6.24). Immunohistochemical techniques are invaluable as a

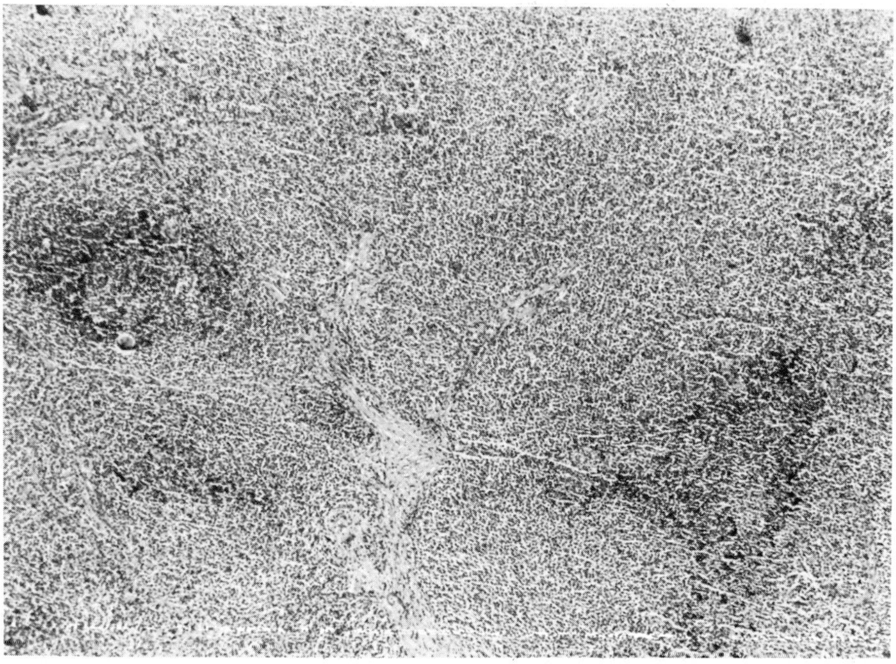

Fig. 6.22 Malignant lymphoma, plasmacytic. Low power view showing sheets of plasma cells surrounding residual lymphoid follicles, × 400.

Fig. 6.23 Higher power view of Fig. 6.22 showing a uniform proliferation of typical plasma cells, × 400.

Fig. 6.24 Plastic embedded section of a malignant lymphoma, plasmacytic. Stacks of rough endoplasmic reticulum can just be discerned in the dark-staining cytoplasm of many of the plasma cells. One cell (top right) contains intracytoplasmic inclusions of darkly staining immunoglobulin. Toluidine blue, × 1200.

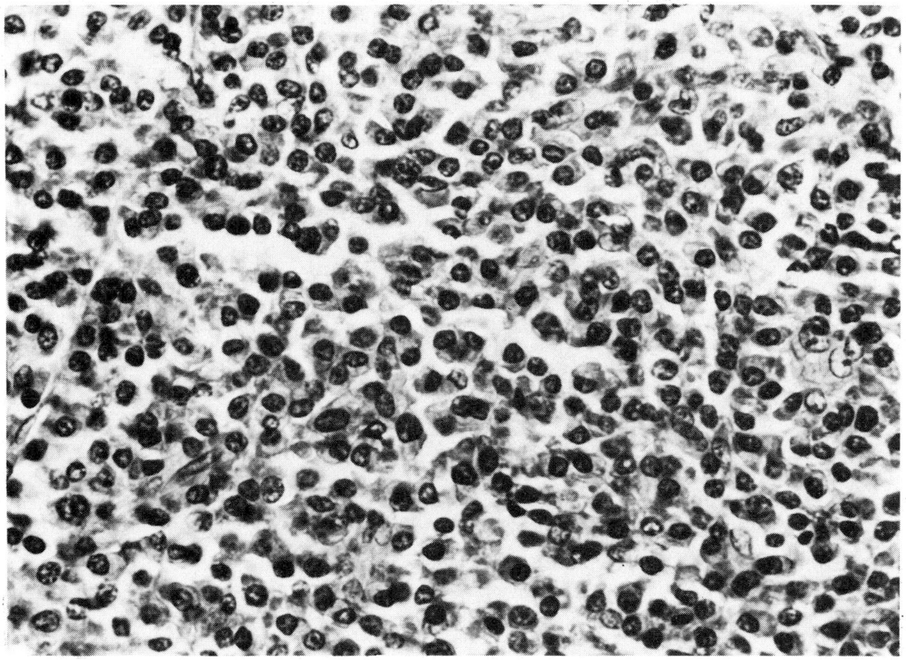

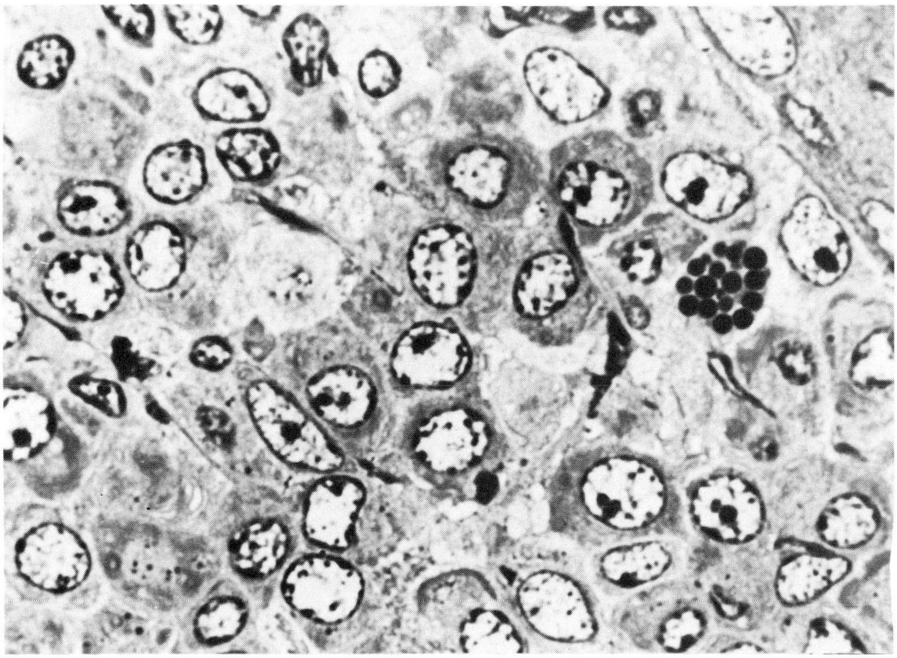

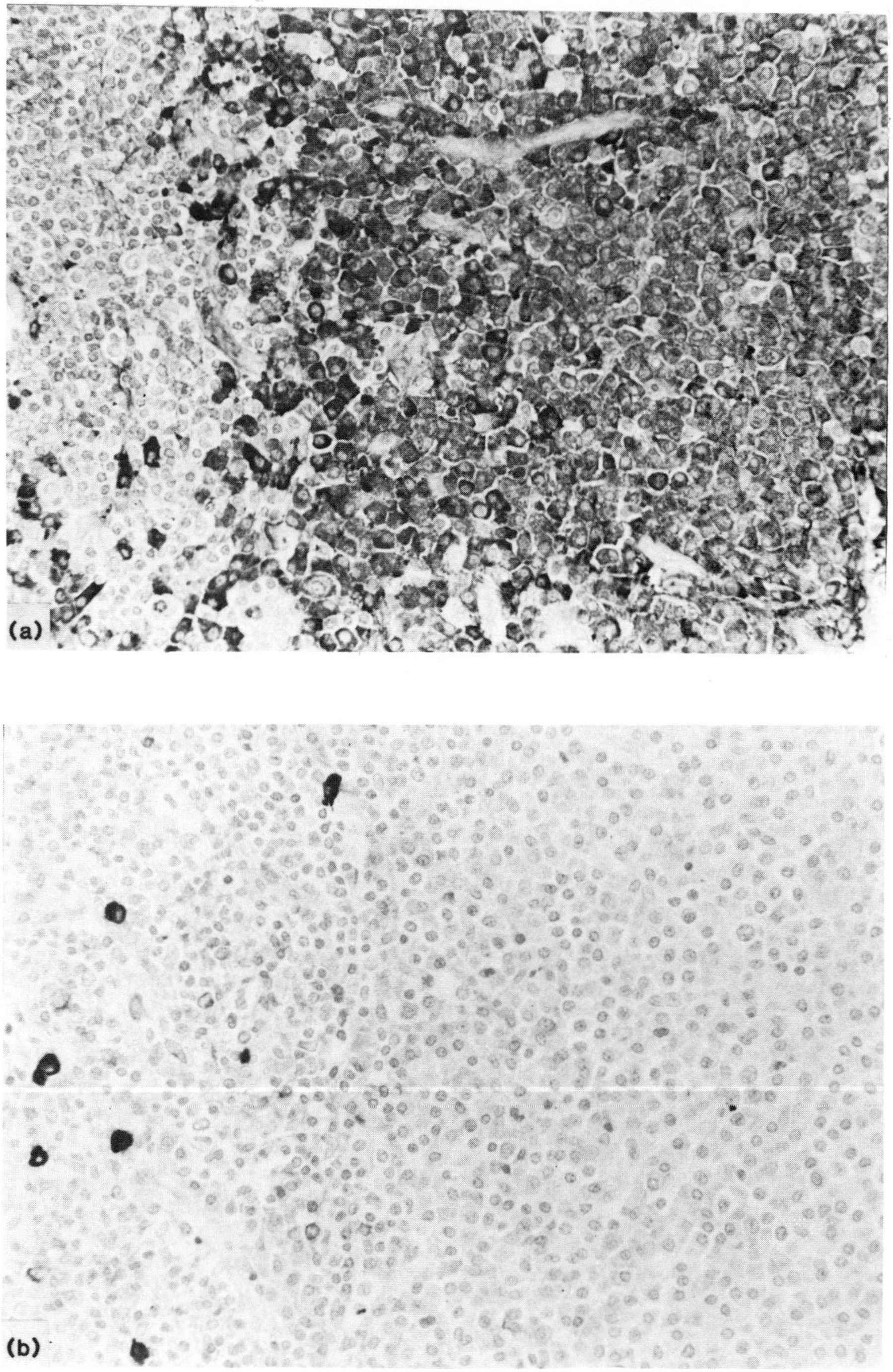

means of demonstrating the monotypia of the neoplastic plasma cells (Fig. 6.25).

In lymph nodes primarily involved by plasmacytoma the tumour often appears to start in the medullary region and spread to the cortex so that it is not unusual to see reactive lymphoid follicles marooned in a sea of plasma cells (Fig. 6.22). As in lymphoplasmacytic lymphoma and multiple myelomatosis deposits of amorphous proteinaceous material or amyloid may be seen within the tumour; these often evoke a giant cell reaction (Fig. 6.26).

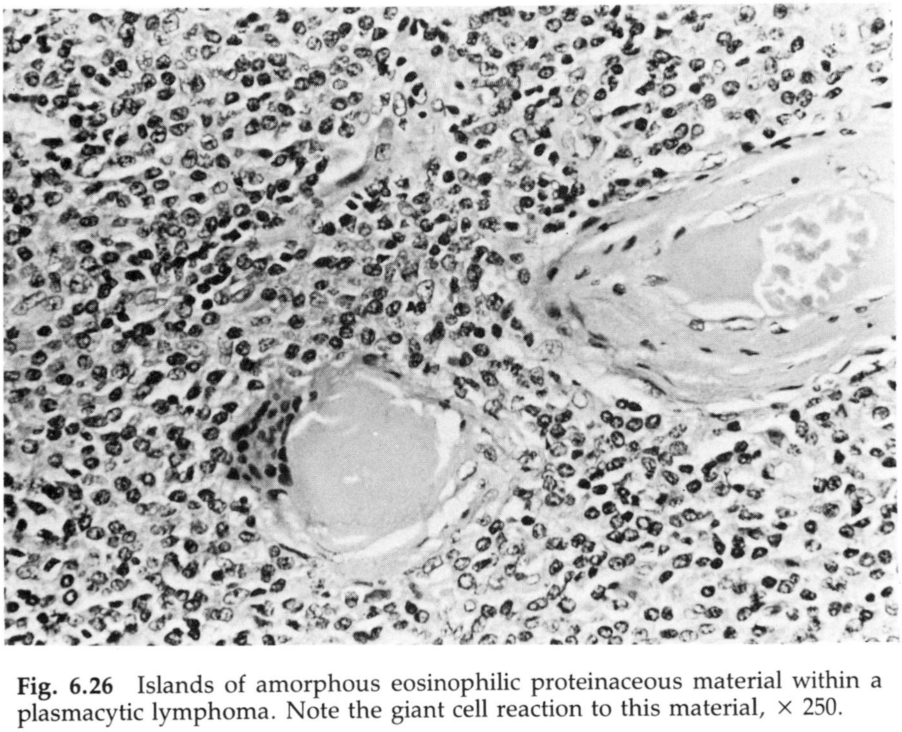

Fig. 6.26 Islands of amorphous eosinophilic proteinaceous material within a plasmacytic lymphoma. Note the giant cell reaction to this material, × 250.

6.4.2 *Differential diagnosis*

Undoubtedly many reactive plasma cell proliferations have in the past, been misdiagnosed as plasmacytomas. This can be a very difficult

---

Fig. 6.25 Malignant lymphoma, plasmacytic stained for kappa light chains (a) and lambda light chains (b) by the immunoperoxidase technique. There is monotypic staining for kappa chain only. The unstained cells to the left are part of a pre-existing lymphoid follicle. The scanty cells that have stained for lambda chain are residual, non-neoplastic plasma cells, × 250.

differential diagnosis, particularly on small biopsies. Immunohistochemical techniques which can demonstrate whether the cells are polytypic (reactive) or monotypic (neoplastic) are particularly valuable in such cases.

Malignant lymphoma lymphoplasmacytic and follicle centre cell lymphomas showing marked plasmacytic differentiation can usually be readily separated from malignant lymphoma plasmacytic by their content of lymphocytes or follicle centre cells. Those cases showing large amyloid deposits might be confused with primary amyloidosis of the lymph nodes and a search should be made for residual tumour between the islands of amyloid. Immunohistochemical methods may be helpful in these cases in identifying a monotypic neoplastic population of plasma cells.

6.5 Heavy chain disease

6.5.1 γ-Chain disease and μ-chain disease

The morphological features of these rare conditions have not been well described. It would appear that the majority of cases are lymphoplasmacytic lymphomas or follicle centre cell lymphomas in which the tumour cells are secreting an incomplete heavy chain in the absence of light chain production.

6.5.2 α-Chain disease

This condition is discussed in Chapter 13.

References

Bearman, R. M., Pangalis, G. A. and Rappaport, H. (1978), Prolymphocytic leukemia. Clinical, histopathological and cytochemical observations. *Cancer*, **42**, 2360–72.

Brouet, J. C., Preud'homme, J. L., Flandrin, G. *et al.* (1976), Membrane markers in 'histiocytic' lymphomas (reticulum cell sarcomas). *J. Natl Cancer Inst.*, **56**, 631–3.

Colby, T. V., Warnke, R. A., Burke, J. S. and Dorfman, R. F. (1981), Differentiation of chronic lymphocytic leukemia from Hodgkin's disease using immunologic marker studies. *Am. J. Surg. Pathol.*, **5**, 707–10.

Delsol, G., Laurent, G., Kuhlein, E. *et al.* (1981), Richter's syndrome. Evidence for the clonal origin of the two proliferations. *Am. J. Clin. Pathol.*, **76**, 308–15.

Galton, D. A. G. (1964), Chronic lymphocytic leukaemia. Its pathogenesis and relationship to lymphosarcoma. In *Symposium on Lymphoreticular Tumours in Africa*, Paris, 1963 (ed. F. C. Roulet), S. Karger AG, Basel, New York, pp. 163–72.

Galton, D. A. G., Goldman, J. M., Wiltshaw, E. *et al.* (1974), Prolymphocytic leukaemia. *Br. J. Haematol.*, **27**, 7–23.

Habeshaw, J. A., Catley, P. F., Stansfeld, A. G. and Brearley, R. L. (1979), Surface phenotyping, histology and the nature of non-Hodgkin lymphoma in 157 patients. *Br. J. Cancer*, **40**, 11–34.

Harousseau, J. L., Flandrin, G., Tricot, G. *et al.* (1981), Malignant lymphoma supervening in chronic lymphocytic leukemia and related disorders. Richter's syndrome. A study of 25 cases. *Cancer*, **48**, 1302–8.

Harrison, C. V. (1972), The morphology of the lymph node in the macroglobulinaemia of Waldenström. *J. Clin. Pathol.*, **25**, 12–16.

Henry, K. and Farrer-Brown, G. (1977), Primary lymphomas of the gastrointestinal tract. I. Plasma cell tumours. *Histopathology*, **1**, 53–76.

Lennert, K. (1978), Malignant lymphomas other than Hodgkin's disease. In *Handbuch der Speziellen Pathologischen Anatomie und Histologie*, Springer-Verlag, Berlin (in collaboration with N. Mohri, H. Stein, E. Kaiserling and H. K. Müller-Hermelink).

Lennert, K. (1981), *Histopathology of Non-Hodgkin's Lymphomas (based on the Kiel Classification)*, Springer-Verlag, Berlin.

Mann, R. B., Jaffe, E. S. and Berard, C. W. (1979), Malignant lymphomas – a conceptual understanding of morphologic diversity. *Am. J. Pathol.*, **94**, 105–75.

Pangalis, G. A., Nathwani, B. N. and Rappaport, H. (1977), Malignant lymphoma well differentiated lymphocytic. Its relationship with chronic lymphocytic leukemia and macroglobulinemia of Waldenström. *Cancer*, **39**, 999–1010.

Papadimitriou, C. S., Muller-Hermelink, U. and Lennert, K. (1979), Histologic and immunohistochemical findings in the differential diagnosis of chronic lymphocytic leukemia of B-cell type and lymphoplasmacytic/lymphoplasmacytoid lymphoma. *Virchows Arch. (Pathol. Anat.)*, **384**, 149–58.

Richter, M. N. (1928), Generalised reticular cell sarcoma of lymph nodes associated with lymphatic leukemia. *Am. J. Pathol.*, **4**, 285–99.

Rozman, C., Hernandez-Nieto, L., Montserrat, E. and Brugues, R. (1981), Prognostic significance of bone marrow patterns in chronic lymphocytic leukaemia. *Br. J. Haematol.*, **47**, 529–37.

Weisenburger, D. D., Nathwani, B. N., Diamond, L. W. *et al.* (1981), Malignant lymphoma, intermediate lymphocytic type: A clinicopathologic study of 42 cases. *Cancer*, **48**, 1415–25.

7 Malignant lymphomas derived from follicle centre cells and malignant lymphoma: immunoblastic

The great majority of nodal and extranodal non-Hodgkin's lymphomas are derived from cells of the follicle centre and a clear understanding of this group of tumours is central to the histological diagnosis of malignant lymphoma. The cells that constitute the reactive follicle centre have been described and illustrated in Chapter 1 and reference to this normal cell population is of great help in the diagnosis of follicle centre cell lymphomas.

A minority of follicle centre cell lymphomas consist overwhelmingly of a single cell type but the majority, even when one cell is predominant will contain a mixture of centrocytes and centroblasts. Together with these two cell types, which within themselves show a range of sizes, other elements of the follicle centre are present. Dendritic reticulum cells can be demonstrated by electron microscopy and immunohistochemistry, and varying numbers of macrophages are also present. T-lymphocytes are often present in large numbers.

Cytoplasmic immunoglobulin synthesis is a normal function of small numbers of centrocytes and centroblasts in reactive follicle centres and may be exaggerated in follicle centre cell lymphomas. Follicle centre cells engaged in cytoplasmic immunoglobulin synthesis have pyroninophilic cytoplasm and may contain PAS-positive immunoglobulin inclusions. These cells should not be confused with plasma cells which may be present rarely as an integral part of the tumour or more commonly as a reactive component.

Another cell type found in small numbers in reactive follicle centres but seen more frequently in follicle centre cell lymphomas is the so-called immunoblast. Some lymphomas consist almost entirely of these large cells which have open nuclei, prominent central nucleoli and pyroninophilic cytoplasm. This type of tumour is designated an immunoblastic lymphoma and is not usually included among the group of follicle centre cell lymphomas. Large numbers of immunoblasts may, however, be seen in follicle centre cell lymphomas intimately mixed with centroblasts and centrocytes.

Follicle centre cell lymphomas may grow in a follicular or in a diffuse pattern or show a mixture of these two patterns of growth. Recognition of a follicular growth pattern is important since it helps firmly to categorize the tumour as of follicle centre cell type and also has prognostic implications (Warnke *et al.*, 1977; Meuge *et al.*, 1978; Herrmann *et al.*, 1982). Distinction must be drawn between the terms follicular and nodular when describing patterns of growth of malignant lymphomas. The former refers to a growth pattern of a malignant lymphoma that reproduces, albeit incompletely, the structure of normal lymphoid follicles; the latter refers to a nodular growth pattern which may be imposed on the tumour by such factors as the structure of the tissue being invaded or by reactive fibrosis. Even if such a lymphoma had arisen from follicle centre cells it should not be categorized as follicular on the basis of this type of nodularity. The follicles produced by follicle centre cell lymphoma sometimes closely resemble benign reactive follicle centres and the differential diagnosis between follicular lymphoma and reactive hyperplasia can be one of the most difficult problems of lymph node histopathology. This will be discussed in detail later in this chapter. Follicle centre cell lymphomas may show varying, and sometimes extreme, degrees of plasma cell differentiation, sclerosis and epithelioid cell infiltration. These features can cause the tumour to mimic other malignant lymphomas such as lymphoplasmacytic, plasmacytic and lymphoepithelioid lymphoma (Lennert's lymphoma).

7.1 Malignant lymphoma: centrocytic

The evidence that this lymphoma is of follicle centre cell origin is based partly on the morphological and immunological similarity of the tumour cells to centrocytes. These cells have a similar immunological phenotype to normal follicle centre cells in that they exhibit dense surface immunoglobulin and express both complement receptor subtypes (C3b and C3d) (Tolksdorf *et al.*, 1980). Dendritic reticulum cells can be demonstrated in a high proportion of tumours by electron microscopy (Kaiserling, 1978) and by immunohistochemical staining using monoclonal antibodies.

Lukes and Collins (1974; 1975) do not separate malignant lymphoma centrocytic (cleaved FCC lymphoma) from diffuse centroblastic/centrocytic tumours in which centrocytes are the predominant cells. Lennert (1981) makes this separation on the grounds that in histological sections malignant lymphoma centrocytic consists exclusively of centrocytes and contains no centroblasts; centroblasts may, however, be seen in lymph node imprints and in electron micrographs (Lennert, 1978). Lennert (1981) further states that the borderline between centrocytic lymphoma and centroblastic/centrocytic lymphoma is not sharp and that both tumours may co-exist in the same patient or even in the same biopsy. It would seem rational to conclude that although centrocytic lymphoma is a reasonably well-defined histopathological entity it represents one extreme of the spectrum of centroblastic/centrocytic lymphoma.

Malignant lymphoma centrocytic has a significantly worse prognosis than centroblastic/centrocytic lymphoma follicular (Brittinger *et al.*, 1976). Like this tumour it occurs most frequently in the sixth and seventh decades. Lymphadenopathy is the commonest presenting feature with splenomegaly in approximately half the cases. Bone marrow infiltration occurs in two-thirds of the cases with a variable spillover of neoplastic cells into the peripheral blood. Full haematological investigation with a bone marrow trephine biopsy should, therefore, be performed on all cases. Lymphoma cells in the peripheral blood have the morphological characteristics of centrocytes with irregular and cleaved nuclei. Even when they cannot be detected in blood smears these cells may be identified with immunological marker techniques by their monotypic surface immunoglobulin. Radiological investigations including lymphangiograms are valuable in determining the extent of the disease but staging laparotomy is not indicated.

7.1.1 Histology and cytology

The tumour most frequently shows sheets of monomorphic small centrocytes with characteristic irregular contorted nuclei (Fig. 7.1) but tumours composed of larger centrocytes may show considerable nuclear pleomorphism (Fig. 7.2). The nuclear diameters in centrocytic lymphoma range in size from 4.6–8.2 μm forming a continuous curve and not two separate populations of small and large cells (Satodate, 1978). There are approximately 0–2 mitotic figures per high power field with, in general, a higher mitotic rate in the large cell tumours. The methyl green pyronin stain shows weaker pyroninophilia of the cytoplasm of centrocytes and small inconspicuous nucleoli. Sclerosis is present in 40% of diffuse centrocytic lymphomas and is more prominent in the large cell than in the small cell type (Bennett, 1975). Blood vessels in these tumours are generally scanty but characteristically show perivascular dense hyaline

---

Fig. 7.1 Follicle centre cell lymphoma (FCCL) centrocytic-diffuse showing a monomorphic infiltration of small centrocytes, × 250.

Fig. 7.2 Centrocytic lymphoma of large cell type. Note irregular contorted nuclei, × 480.

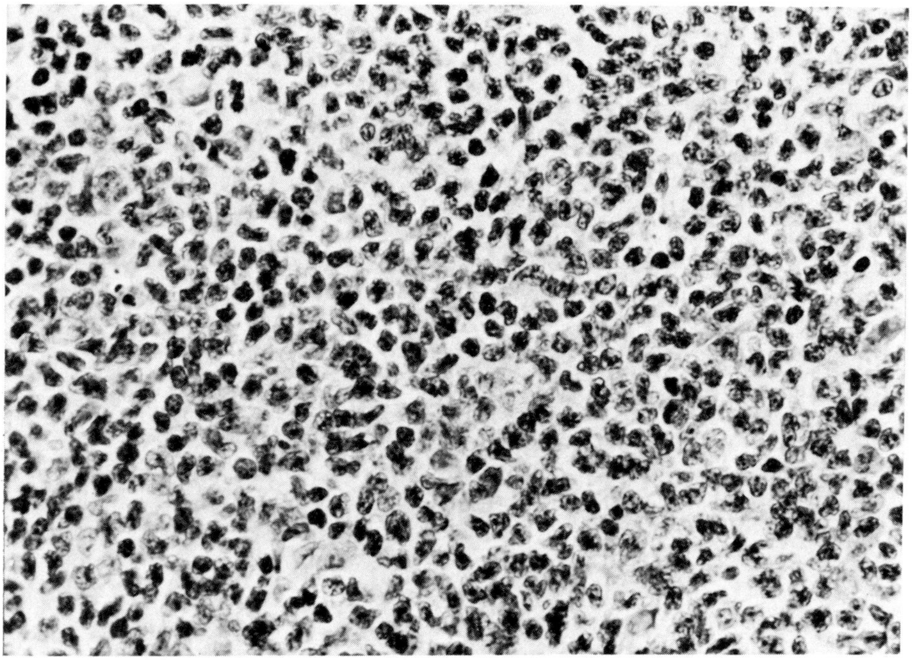

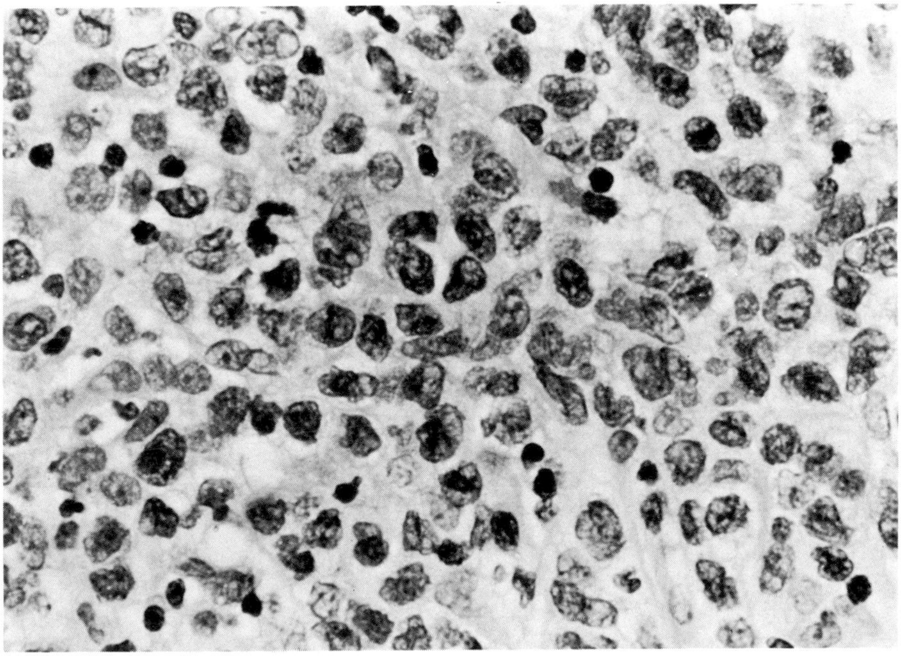

collagen. This is well delineated by the reticulin stains which show coarse short strands of reticulin radiating out from the vessels sometimes producing a fine compartmentalization of the tumour (Fig. 7.3). In imprint preparations (Fig. 7.4) the malignant centrocytes are larger than small lymphocytes and their nuclei have an irregular outline. The characteristic clefting of centrocytic nuclei is seen only in peripheral blood and bone marrow films (Fig. 7.5).

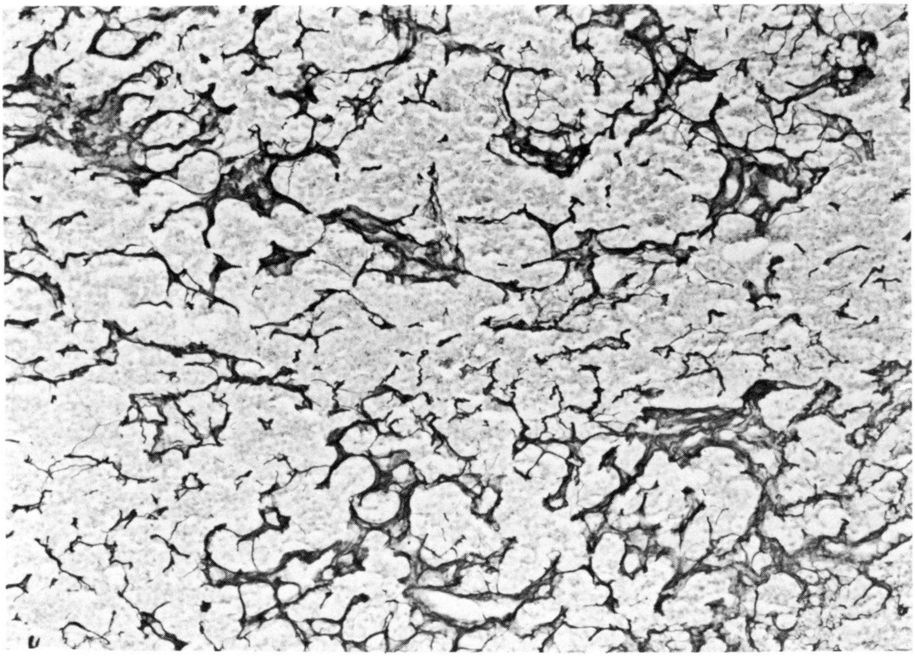

Fig. 7.3 Centrocytic lymphoma stained to show reticulin. Note dense reticulin around blood vessels with blunt short strands extending between the tumour cells, × 120.

7.1.2 Differential diagnosis

Lymphoblastic lymphoma may be misdiagnosed as diffuse centrocytic lymphoma (small cell type). There are marked cytological differences between the cells of these two tumours which are best appreciated in

---

Fig. 7.4 Imprint preparation of centrocytic tumour. In these preparations nuclear cleavages are not usually evident. Giemsa, × 1200.
Fig. 7.5 Bone marrow smear showing small centrocytes. Nuclear clefts are evident in this preparation. Giemsa, × 1200.

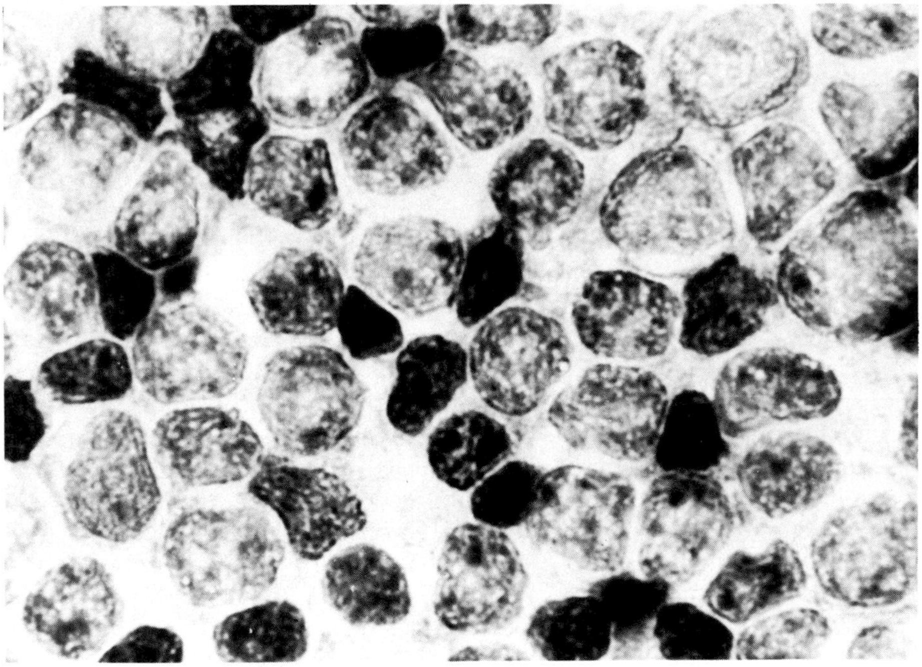

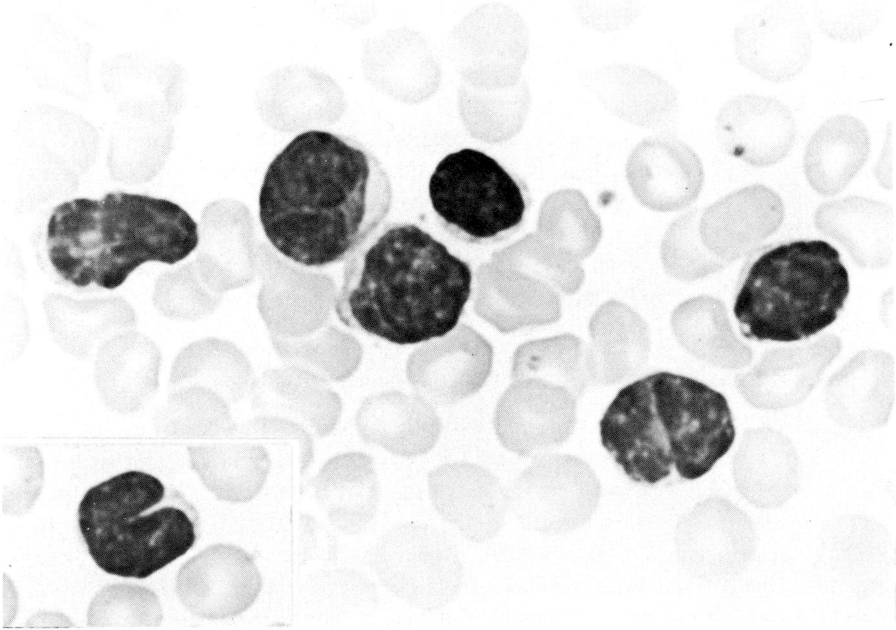

imprint preparations (Fig. 7.4). In paraffin sections, however, both tumours show a diffuse population of medium-sized lymphoid cells with varying degrees of nuclear irregularity. Lymphoblastic lymphomas infiltrate tissues in a diffuse fashion and with considerable preservation of the underlying normal reticulin pattern while centrocytic lymphomas infiltrate in a destructive manner and have a characteristic coarse reticulin pattern. Pleomorphism is greater in centrocytic than in lymphoblastic lymphomas and the methyl green pyronin stain will demonstrate a greater degree of cytoplasmic pyroninophilia and more prominent nucleoli in lymphoblastic than in centrocytic lymphomas.

In some cases of centrocytic lymphoma the cells are unusually small and contain nuclei which are only slightly irregular in outline. These cases may correspond to the malignant lymphoma of intermediate cell type described by Mann *et al.* (1979) and Weisenburger *et al.* (1981), (see Chapter 6 page 134). These cases may resemble lymphocytic lymphoma and in such instances the reticulin stain may be helpful in that reticulin is characteristically extremely sparse in lymphocytic lymphoma.

The considerable pleomorphism and nuclear irregularity of some large centrocytic lymphomas may cause confusion with histiocytic lymphoma. In general, centrocytes have coarser nuclear chromatin and smaller nucleoli than malignant histiocytes. Although centrocytes may have contorted nuclei they do not show the marked nuclear indentations and prominent nucleoli nor the giant cell forms seen in many histiocytic lymphomas. Reactive plasma cells, eosinophils and histiocytes are usually much more abundant in histiocytic than in centrocytic lymphomas.

Monocytic leukaemia may rarely be confused with centrocytic lymphoma. Haematological and cytochemical studies will usually readily separate these two entities. In histological sections monocytic leukaemia infiltrates in a relatively non-destructive leukaemic fashion and does not show the characteristic coarse reticulin fibres of centrocytic lymphomas. The cells of monocytic leukaemia are more uniform and have a finer nuclear structure than those of centrocytic lymphoma.

7.2 Malignant lymphoma: centroblastic/centrocytic

Malignant lymphoma, centroblastic/centrocytic is the commonest non-Hodgkin's lymphoma accounting for between one-quarter and one-half of all cases in Europe and North America (Lennert, 1981). It is composed of a variable mixture of neoplastic centroblasts and centrocytes together with non-neoplastic cells that are found in the normal germinal centre, namely dendritic reticulum cells, histiocytes and T-lymphocytes.

Malignant lymphoma, centroblastic/centrocytic is subdivided on the basis of its growth pattern into follicular, follicular and diffuse and diffuse. The purely follicular pattern is seen most frequently followed by the follicular and diffuse pattern with entirely diffuse tumours accounting for less than 10% of the total (Lennert, 1981). It may be further subcategorized according to the proportions of centrocytes and centroblasts in the tumour.

There is a tendency for malignant lymphoma, centroblastic/centrocytic, follicular, to progress to diffuse histology and centroblast predominance. Cullen *et al.* (1979) found that four of 21 patients with follicular lymphoma in relapse had developed diffuse centroblastic or centroblastic/centrocytic lymphoma. Lennert (1981) reported that 40% of patients with centroblastic/centrocytic lymphoma coming to autopsy had converted to a high grade (centroblastic) lymphoma and Risdall *et al.* (1979) noted a similar high incidence of histological conversion at autopsy. Lennert (1978) categorizes these high grade tumours as secondary centroblastic lymphomas. They show greater degrees of pleomorphism than centroblastic lymphomas arising in patients without preceding centroblastic/centrocytic lymphoma and have a worse prognosis.

The relationship between histology and prognosis in follicle centre cell lymphomas has undergone a change in recent years with advances in chemotherapy. It is generally accepted that any degree of follicularity imparts a favourable prognosis (Warnke *et al.*, 1977; Lennert, 1981; Herrmann *et al.*, 1982) and that those follicle centre cell lymphomas containing a large proportion of centroblasts have a worse prognosis than those composed mainly of centrocytes (Rappaport *et al.*, 1956; Jones *et al.*, 1973; Warnke *et al.*, 1977). Transformation from low grade to high grade lymphomas is associated with a worsening of prognosis. Longo *et al.* (1982) reported histological progression in 41% of 114 patients with 'good prognosis' lymphoma and that these patients survived about half as long (46 months) as those with unchanged histology (96 months). Nevertheless he found that the chances of obtaining a sustained complete remission with combination chemotherapy were greater with 'bad prognosis' than the 'good prognosis' subtypes. Paradoxically, then, it may be that the 'good prognosis' lymphomas have their best prognosis when they convert to 'bad prognosis' histology (Longo *et al.*, 1982). The poor outlook of many secondary centroblastic lymphomas as reported by Lennert (1978) may be due to preceding 'conservative' chemotherapy selecting more aggressive or resistant clones or compromising the bone marrow.

Centroblastic/centrocytic lymphomas are often widely disseminated with approximately two-thirds of patients in Stage III or IV at presentation (Jones *et al.*, 1973; Lennert, 1981; Herrmann *et al.*, 1982). Despite this widespread disease most patients do not have systemic symptoms (Lennert, 1981). Leukaemia has been reported in from 5–15% of patients with centroblastic/centrocytic lymphoma (Lennert, 1981). This may resemble chronic lymphocytic leukaemia (Spiro *et al.*, 1975) although the leukaemic cells are frequently clefted (Reider cells). Lesser degrees of spillover into the blood occur in a much higher proportion of patients and even when this cannot be detected morphologically immunological marker studies will frequently reveal a monotypic B-cell population. A full haematological investigation should thus be performed in all patients with centroblastic/centrocytic lymphoma and include a trephine biopsy of the bone marrow. As in the peripheral blood immunological analysis of bone marrow cells may reveal a tumour cell population even in the absence of morphological evidence of disease. There appears to be no justification for staging procedures in this disease beyond the investigations mentioned above and a lymphangiogram. Occasional patients with malignant lymphoma centroblastic/centrocytic, follicular, develop massive splenomegaly, often with bone marrow infiltration but without significant lymphadenopathy. A diagnostic splenectomy is sometimes performed in these patients.

7.2.1 *Histology and cytology*

(a) *Malignant lymphoma, centroblastic/centrocytic, follicular*

The nature of this tumour is often apparent on low power scanning of the section. The lymph node architecture is effaced and replaced by neoplastic follicles that extend throughout the node (Fig. 7.6). These follicles are usually relatively uniform in size and regular in shape. They are often ill-defined with blurred margins (Fig. 7.7). In contrast reactive follicles usually show a sharp line of demarcation between the reactive centre and the surrounding mantle of small lymphocytes (Fig. 7.8). A very helpful diagnostic feature is the presence of neoplastic follicles in the perinodal fat (Fig. 7.9), or in the fat in the hilum of the node. Although reactive lymphoid proliferations may extend beyond the capsule of the node, this feature is much more characteristic of follicle centre cell lymphomas.

Within the neoplastic follicle the full range of follicle centre cells may be represented but in most instances centrocytes predominate (Fig. 7.10). This is in contrast to reactive follicle centres which contain a high proportion of centroblasts (Fig. 7.11). The sizes of the centrocytes form a continuous spectrum from small to large rather than two distinct

---

Fig. 7.6 FCCL, centroblastic/centrocytic, follicular. Note relatively uniform rounded neoplastic follicles extending throughout the lymph node, × 20.

Fig. 7.7 FCCL, centroblastic/centrocytic, follicular. The neoplastic follicles are poorly defined, × 40.

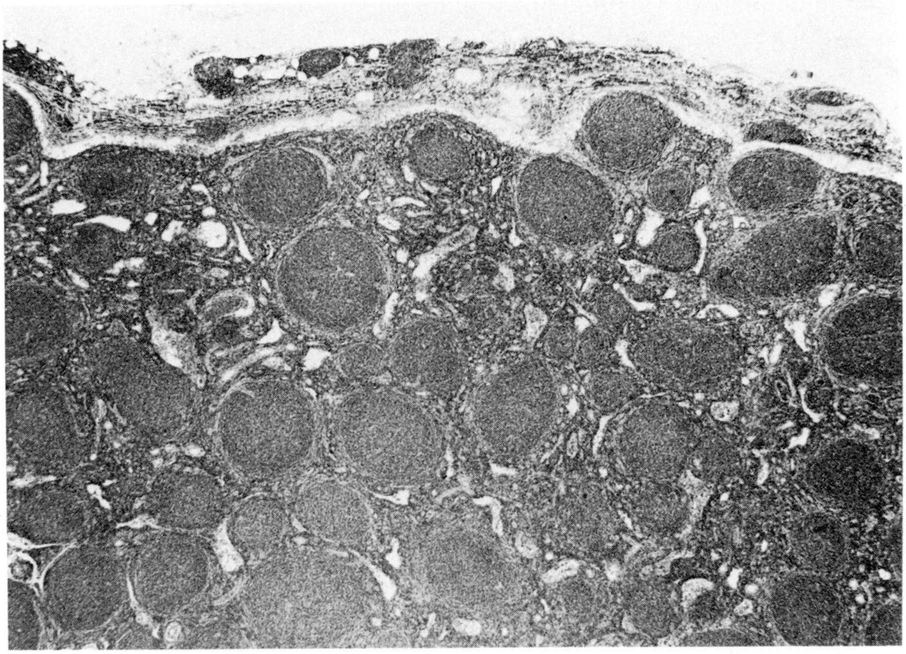

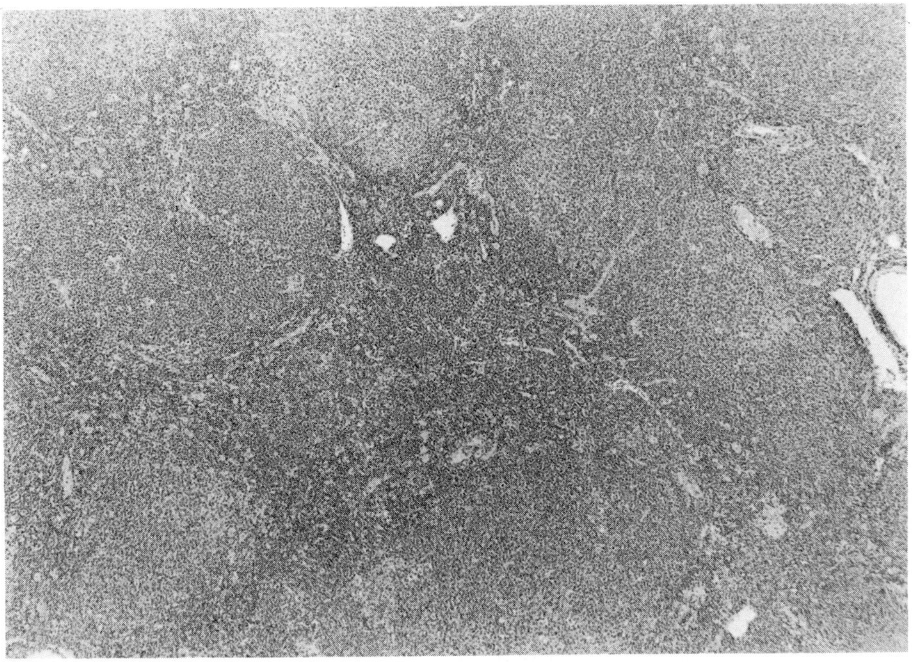

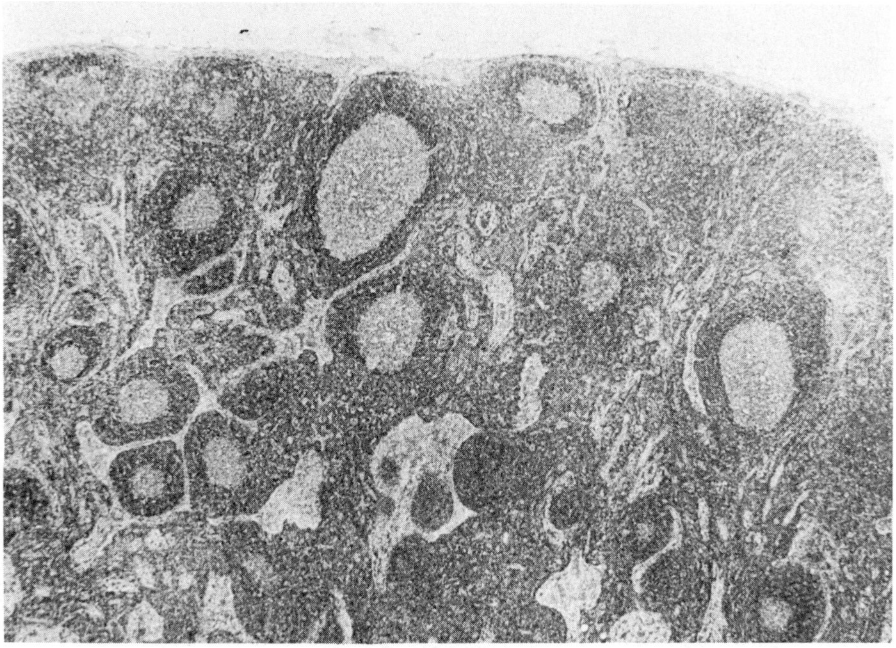

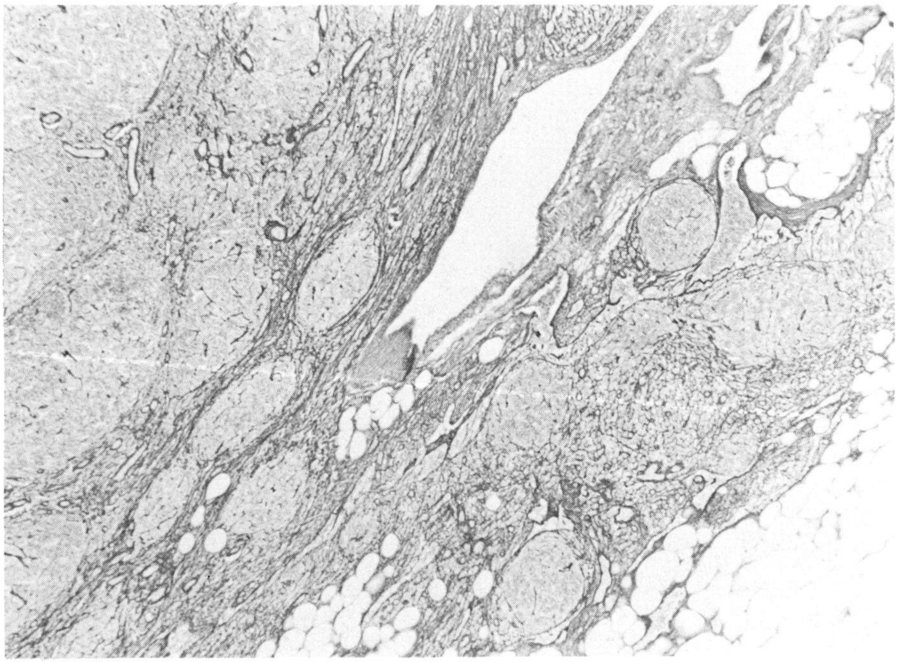

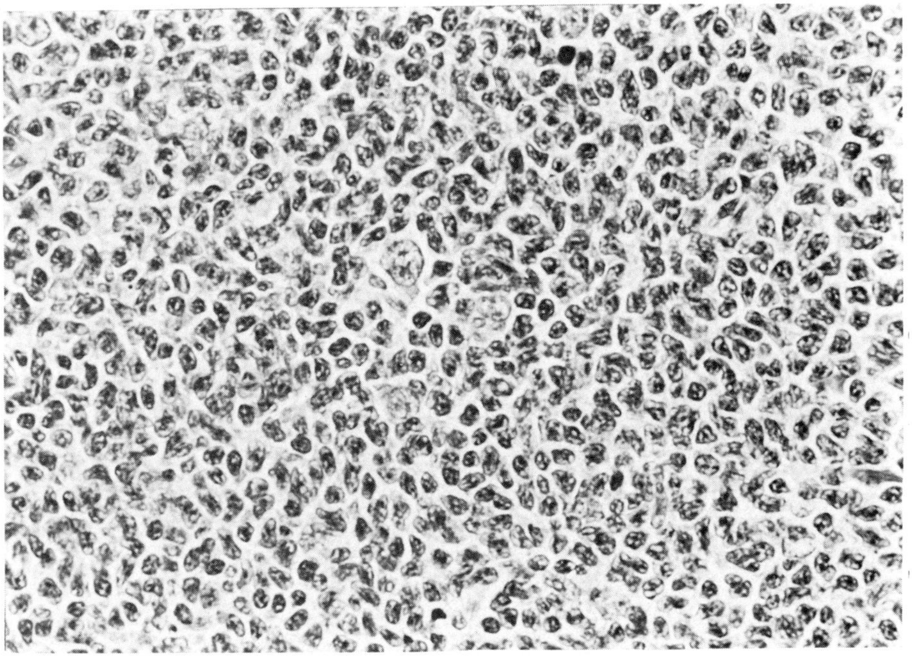

Fig. 7.10 FCCL, centroblastic/centrocytic, follicular. High power view of a neoplastic follicle showing that the cells consist predominantly of small centrocytes. Two centroblasts are seen towards the centre of the photograph, × 400.

populations of small and large cells. The irregular and often triangular centrocytic nuclei contrast with those of small lymphocytes which are round and smaller (Fig. 7.12). Centrocytic nuclei also show less clumping of chromatin than small lymphocytes and may contain 1–3 small nucleoli (Fig. 7.12). Larger and more conspicuous nucleoli are found in cells intermediate between centrocytes and centroblasts. The cytoplasm of centrocytes is scanty, indistinct and not strongly pyroninophilic. Interspersed amongst the centrocytes are varying numbers of centroblasts. These are frequently a relatively inconspicuous minority population but may sometimes be present in large numbers (Fig. 7.13). In some

---

Fig. 7.8 Lymph node showing reactive follicular hyperplasia for comparison with Figs 7.6 and 7.7. The reactive follicles have sharply defined reactive centres with well-developed lymphocyte mantles. Lymph node sinuses are clearly seen, × 20.

Fig. 7.9 FCCL, centroblastic/centrocytic, follicular stained to show reticulin. Note extension of neoplastic follicles into perinodal fat, × 30.

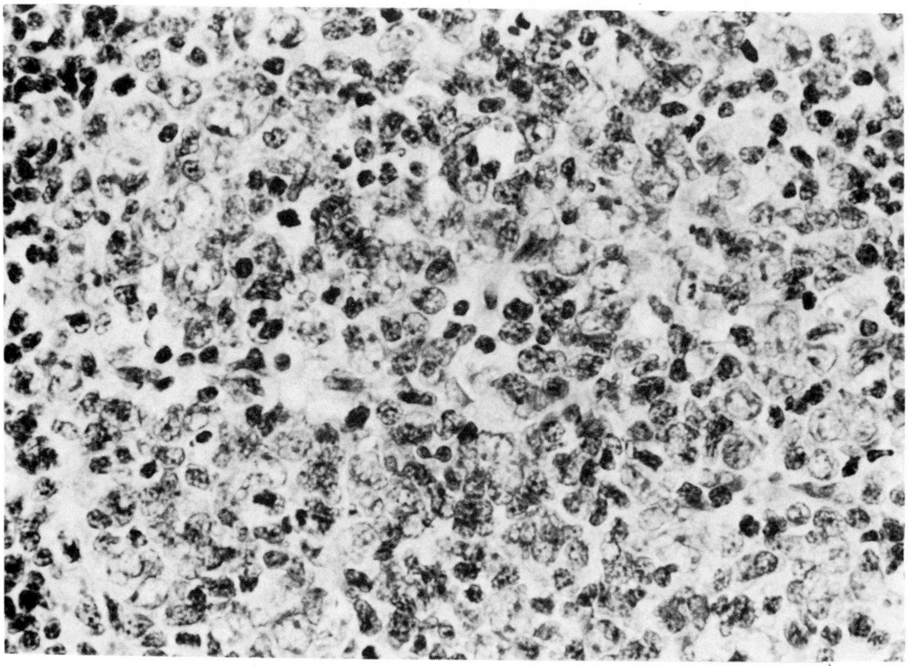

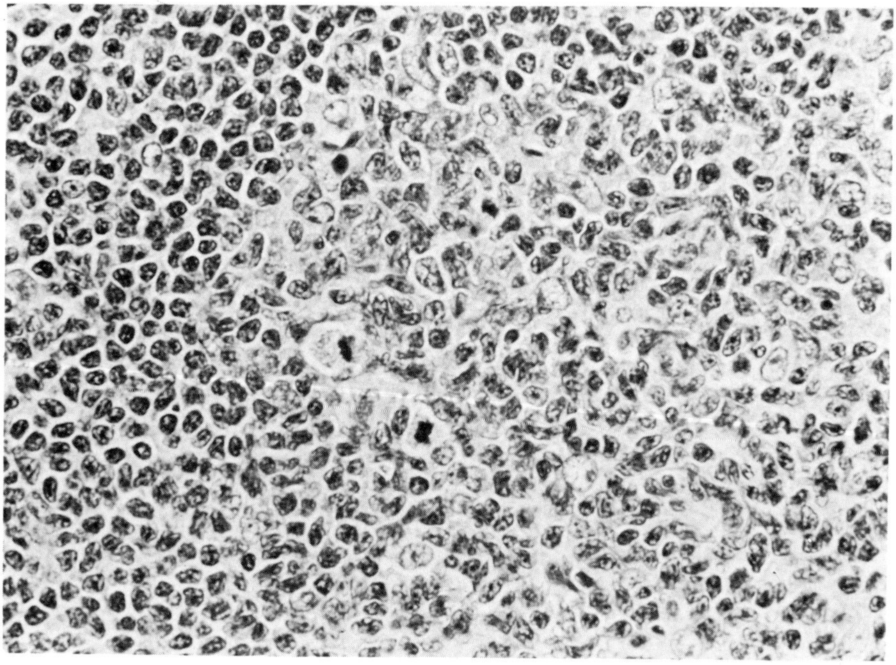

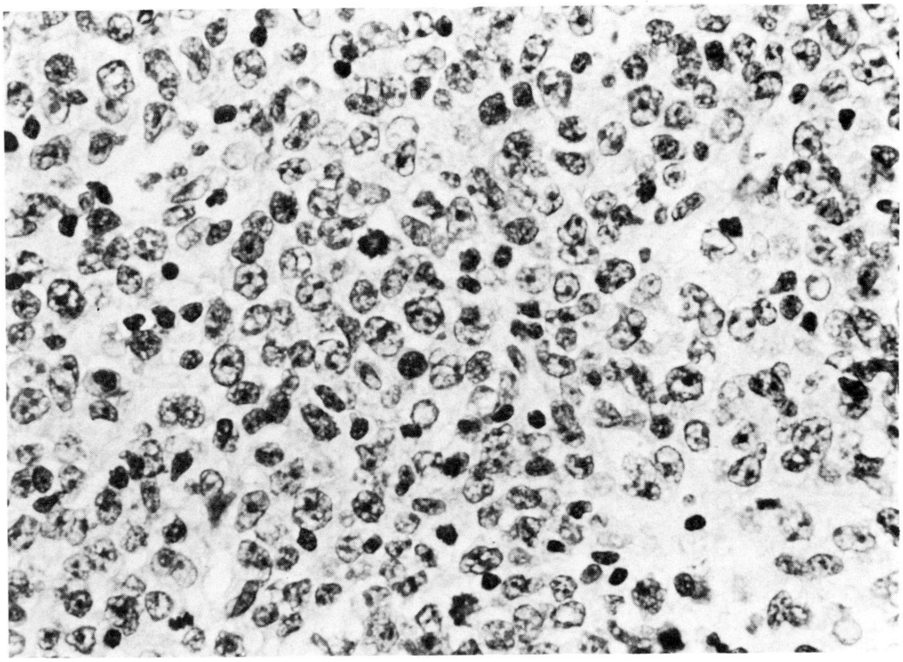

Fig. 7.13 FCCL, centroblastic/centrocytic, follicular. High power view of a follicle showing that in this lymphoma a high proportion of the tumour cells are centroblasts, × 400.

classifications, but not the Kiel classification, malignant lymphoma, centroblastic/centrocytic is further subcategorized on the basis of the relative proportions of centroblasts and centrocytes. Centroblasts have rounded vesicular nuclei with 2–4 conspicuous nucleoli often apposed to the nuclear membrane (Fig. 7.13). The cytoplasm of these cells, which is amphophilic in H and E stained sections is strongly pyroninophilic.

Very occasionally inclusions of immunoglobulin may be demonstrated in the cytoplasm or nucleus of tumour cells by the PAS stain. More frequently this stain highlights amorphous eosinophilic PAS-positive extracellular material in the centre of the neoplastic follicles (Rosas-Uribe *et al.*, 1973). Occasional histiocytes can be demonstrated within the

---

Fig. 7.11 High power view of a reactive follicle centre for comparison with Fig. 7.10. Note the predominance of centroblasts, × 400.
Fig. 7.12 FCCL, centroblastic/centrocytic, follicular. The irregular centrocytes of the neoplastic follicle can be compared with the small lymphocytes of the interfollicular tissue (left), × 400.

follicles by enzyme histochemistry or immunochemical methods but these are not usually very prominent in routine paraffin sections.

Reticulin stains confirm the follicular pattern already apparent from the haematoxylin and eosin section (Fig. 7.14). Often the reticulin appears compressed at the edge of the follicle and serves as a point of differentiation from reactive follicular hyperplasia (Figs 7.15 and 7.16), but this is an inconstant feature. Reticulin stains also assist in the assessment of sclerosis in the tumour. This may consist of fine compartmentalization of the node by collagen bundles, coarse sclerosis or hyalinization of the neoplastic follicles (Fig. 7.17). Sclerosis has been shown to be a feature of favourable prognostic significance (Bennett, 1975).

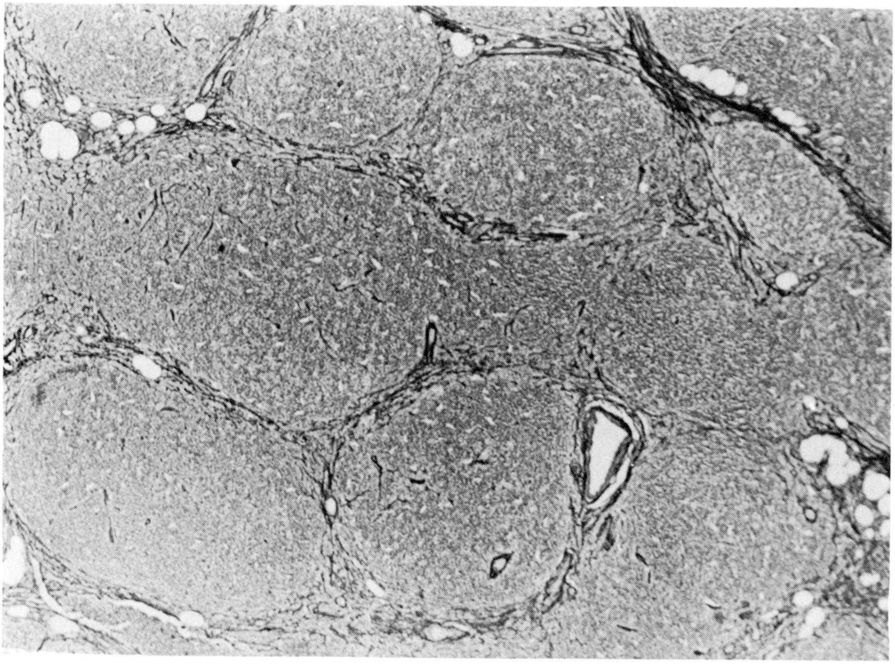

Fig. 7.14 FCCL, centroblastic/centrocytic, follicular stained for reticulin. Note compressed reticulin at periphery of follicles, × 40.

Fig. 7.15 Higher power view of Fig. 7.14 showing compressed reticulin at the periphery of a neoplastic follicle, × 100.

Fig. 7.16 Reticulin-stained section of a lymph node showing reactive follicular hyperplasia for comparison with Figs 7.14 and 7.15. The reticulin is not compressed and is seen mostly outside the lymphocyte mantle. There is no reticulin between the germinal centre and the lymphocyte mantle, × 100.

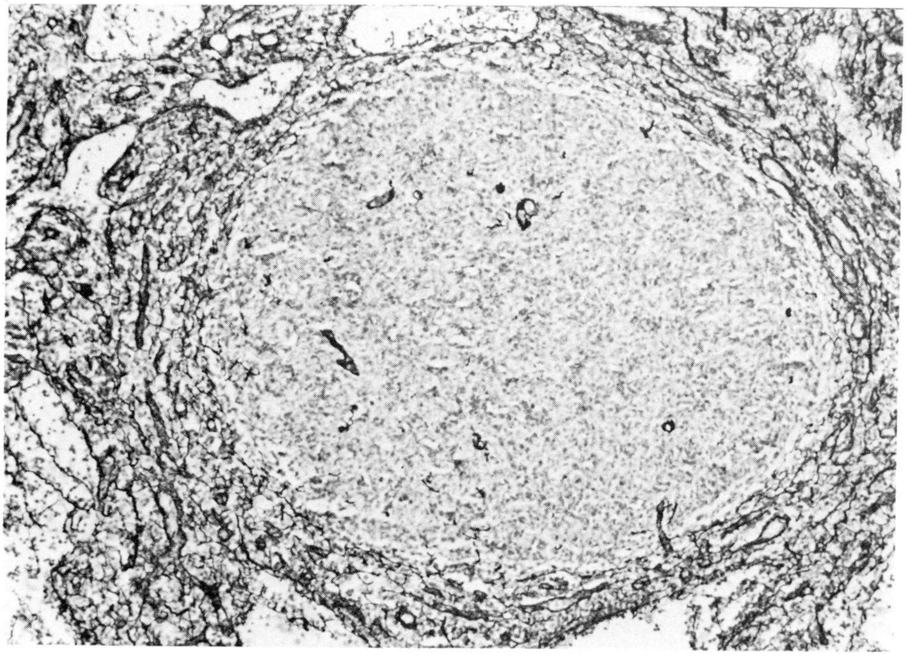

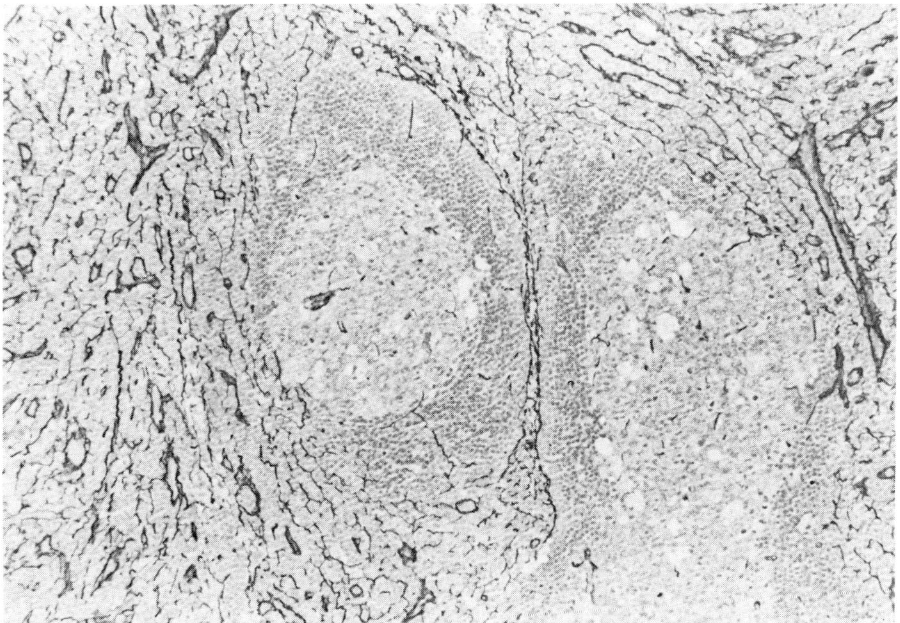

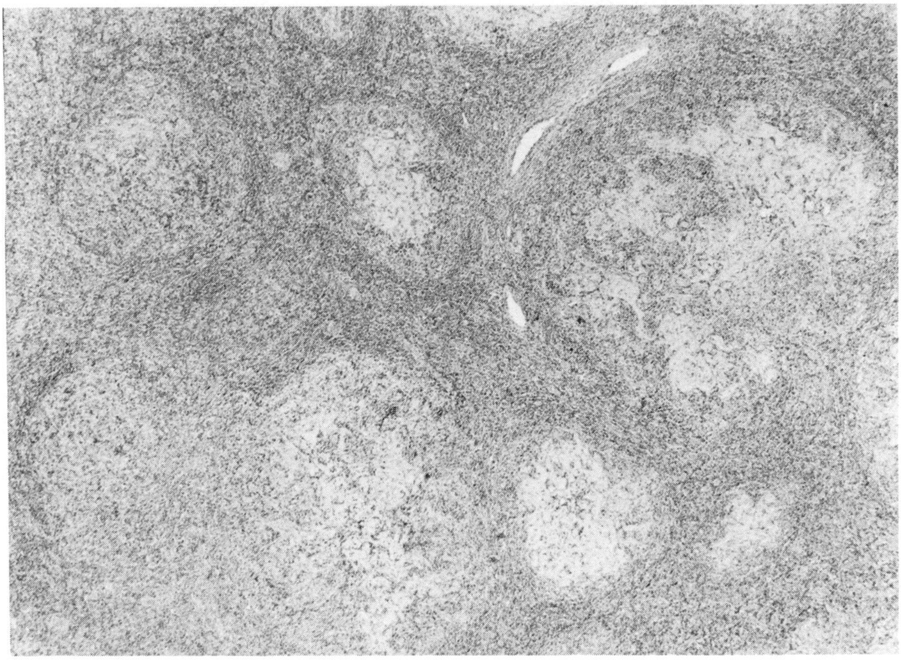

Fig. 7.17 FCCL, centroblastic/centrocytic, follicular showing marked sclerosis of some of the neoplastic follicles, × 25.

The interfollicular tissue in follicular lymphoma is very variable. In some lymphomas there are broad swathes of lymphocytes containing prominent high endothelial-type venules (Fig. 7.18). The relationship of this tissue to the neoplastic follicles and its prognostic significance has not been established. In other follicular lymphomas the neoplastic follicles almost abut on each other with little intervening tissue. Occasional plasma cells can usually be identified in the interfollicular tissue although in rare instances when the tumour shows plasmacytic differentiation large numbers may be seen.

Perhaps because of the large size attained by nodes involved by follicle centre cell lymphoma these appear to be particularly prone to infarction. In such cases a search should be made for residual tumour tissue at the periphery of the node or in adjacent nodes. Reticulin stains of an infarcted area will often be helpful in demonstrating the persisting follicular pattern of the infarcted tumour.

(b) *Malignant lymphoma, centroblastic/centrocytic, follicular and diffuse*
This tumour shows both follicular and diffuse growth patterns (Fig. 7.19).

(c) *Malignant lymphoma, centroblastic/centrocytic, diffuse*
This tumour has a diffuse growth pattern and is therefore less easily

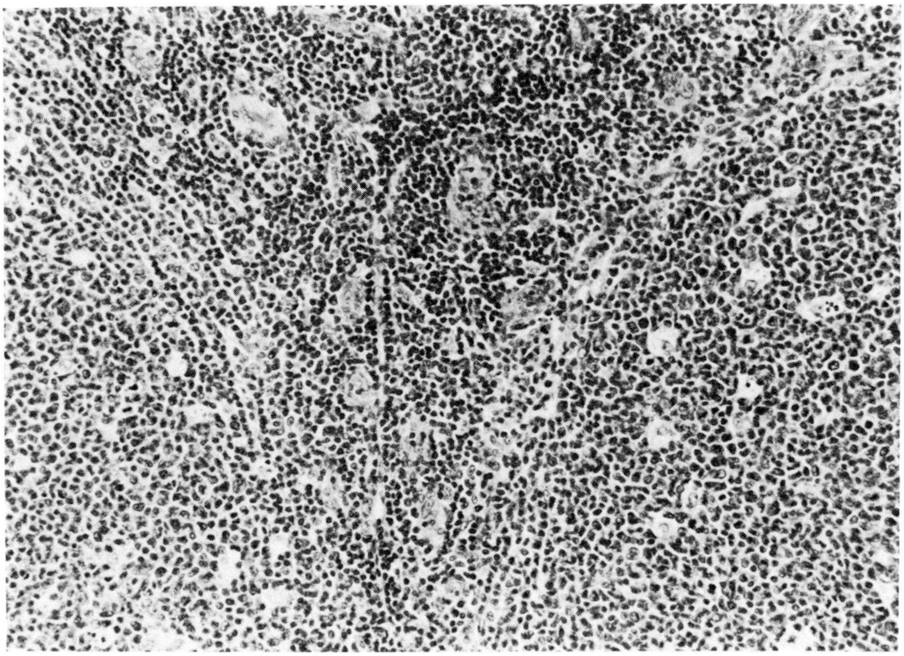

Fig. 7.18 FCCL, centroblastic/centrocytic, follicular showing interfollicular lymphocytes and high endothelial blood vessels, × 120.

recognized as a follicle centre cell lymphoma than its follicular counterpart. The tumour is, however, made up of the same neoplastic population of centroblasts and centrocytes in varying proportions and identification of the tumour rests on the recognition of these cells (Fig. 7.20). In this respect 1 μm sections of plastic embedded material are particularly helpful (Fig. 7.21). The population of follicle centre cells comprising diffuse centroblastic/centrocytic lymphoma tends to include more centroblasts than in the follicular tumours and a varying number of cells with the morphological features of immunoblasts may be seen, especially in tumours containing a high proportion of centroblasts. Difficulty in the diagnosis of diffuse centroblastic/centrocytic lymphoma may be caused by varying degrees of sclerosis and epithelioid cell infiltration which may accompany these tumours.

Imprints are helpful in the diagnosis of centroblastic/centrocytic lymphomas. Although nuclear cleavages of centrocytes are not as well seen in these preparations as they are in blood-films of patients with peripheral blood involvement, the slight irregularity of the nuclei and their larger size serve to distinguish centrocytes from small lymphocytes. Centroblasts are quite distinctive, being considerably larger than the

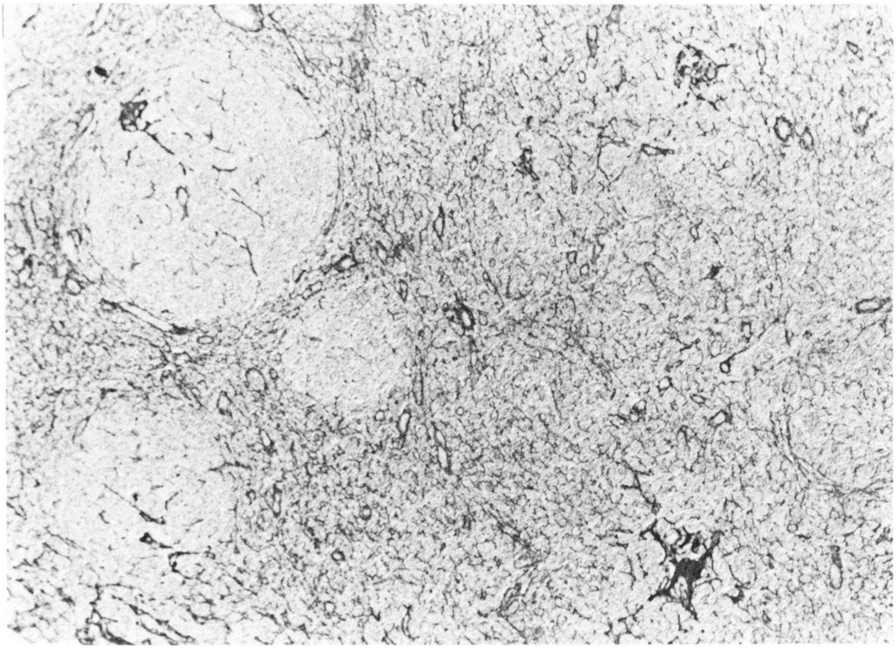

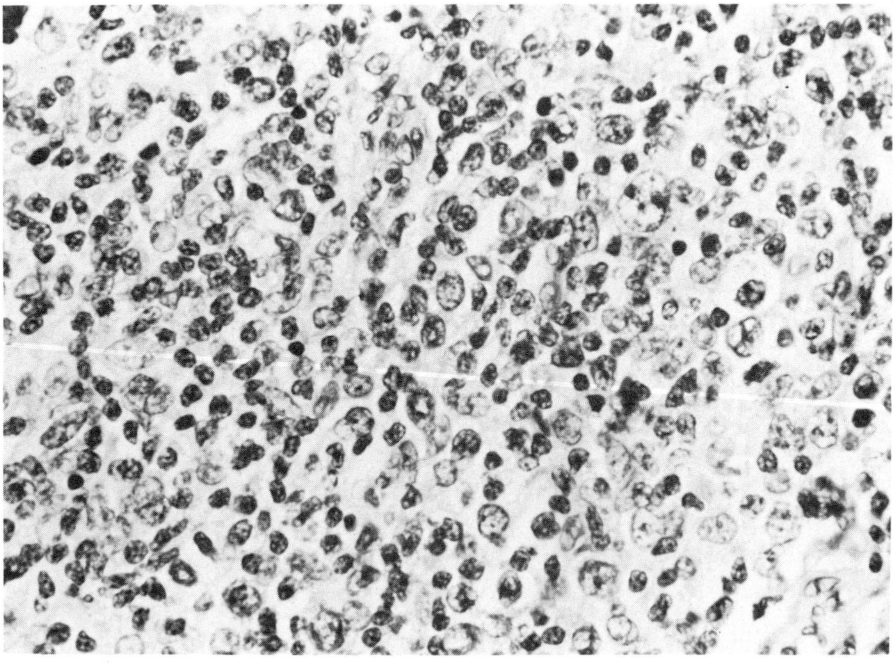

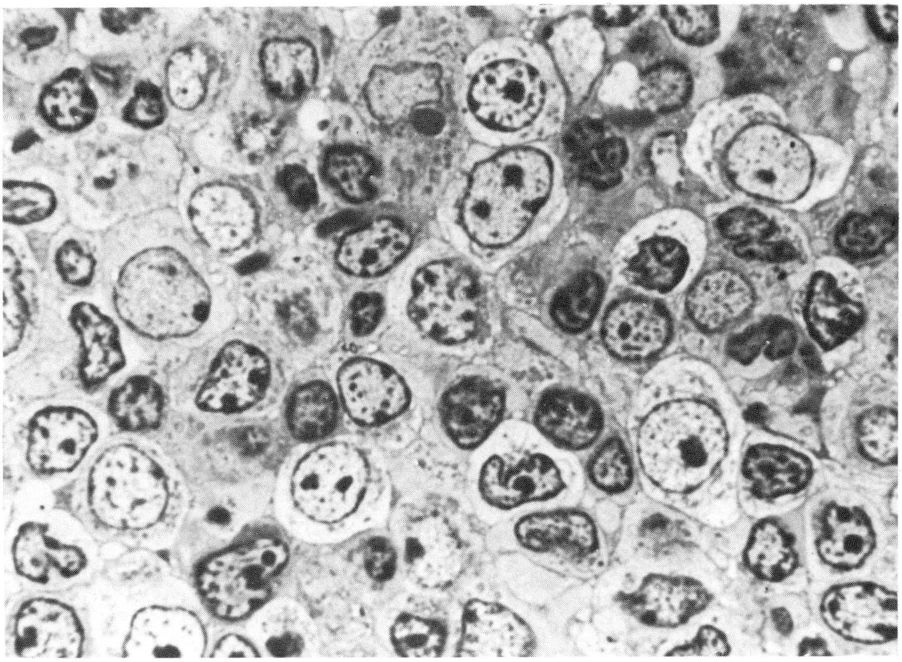

Fig. 7.21 Plastic embedded section of FCCL, centroblastic/centrocytic, diffuse showing a mixture of centrocytes with their smaller, darkly staining nuclei, and centroblasts. Toluidine blue, × 1200.

centrocytes and showing prominent nucleoli and deeply basophilic cytoplasm (Fig. 7.22).

7.2.2 Differential diagnosis

The main differential diagnosis of malignant lymphoma centroblastic/centrocytic, follicular is reactive follicular hyperplasia. Table 7.1 and its accompanying illustrations set out the main features that differentiate these two conditions. Each histological feature listed should be carefully sought in difficult cases.

Spiro *et al.* (1975) observed that a number of patients eventually

---

Fig. 7.19 FCCL, centroblastic/centrocytic, follicular and diffuse. Reticulin stain showing both follicular and diffuse growth patterns, × 100.
Fig. 7.20 FCCL, centroblastic/centrocytic, diffuse. The tumour is composed predominantly of centrocytes with scattered centroblasts, × 400.

diagnosed as having follicular lymphoma had recurrent lymphadenopathy for many years before the diagnosis was established and that earlier lymph node biopsies frequently showed reactive follicular hyperplasia or were considered to be border-line between hyperplasia and follicular lymphoma. It would appear that some, and possibly all patients, with follicular lymphoma pass through a phase of follicular hyperplasia and that at some stages of this progression the separation of these two conditions is not possible. Immunological marker studies on dispersed lymph node cells and immunohistochemistry on frozen or paraffin sections to look for a monotypic B-cell population may be particularly helpful in such patients. In any case in which the distinction between reactive and neoplastic follicular proliferation cannot be made with certainty, the patient should be kept under observation and further biopsies taken if indicated. Therapy should be withheld until the diagnosis is established with certainty.

A rare morphological variant of follicle centre cell lymphoma has been designated signet ring lymphoma (Kim *et al.*, 1978; Harris *et al.*, 1981). In this variant which may occur in either follicular or diffuse tumours the lymphoma cells accumulate large quantities of cytoplasmic immunoglo-

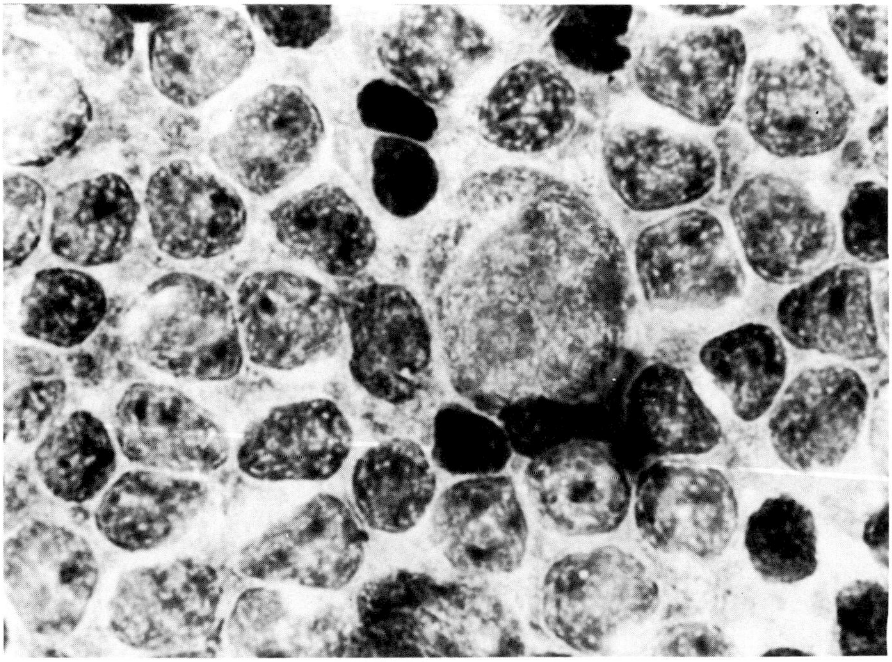

Fig. 7.22 Imprint preparation of FCCL, centroblastic/centrocytic, diffuse showing a centroblast surrounded by centrocytes. Giemsa, × 1200.

Table 7.1 Differential diagnosis of malignant lymphoma centroblastic/centrocytic follicular and follicular hyperplasia

Histological feature	Follicular lymphoma	Follicular hyperplasia	Figure number
Lymph node architecture	Destroyed	Preserved but may be distorted	7.6, 7.7, 7.8
Sinus histiocytosis	Absent	May be present	7.6, 7.7, 7.8
Distribution of follicles	Throughout node	Mainly in cortex	7.6, 7.7, 7.8
Follicles in perinodal fat and in hilum	Often	Unusual	7.9
Boundaries of follicles	Indistinct	Sharply defined	7.7, 7.8
Size and shape of follicles	Regular – small	May be irregular and large	7.6, 7.8
Lymphocyte mantle	Poorly developed or absent	Present	7.6, 7.8
Reticulin pattern	Compressed at periphery of follicle	Outside lymphocyte mantle. Not compressed	7.15, 7.16
Cytology of follicles	Centrocytes usually predominate, centroblasts may be inconspicuous	Centroblasts usually prominent	7.10,7.11
Polar distribution of centroblasts and centrocytes in follicles	Not seen	Usually apparent	
Mitotic figures	May be scanty	Often numerous	
Phagocytic histiocytes (Tinctorial body macrophages)	Usually inconspicuous	Frequently prominant	
Interfollicular cells	Mainly lympocytes occasional cases show plasmacytic differentiation, sclerosis or large number of epithelioid histiocytes	Mainly lymphocytes but frequently includes plasma cells and granulocytes	
Immunohistochemistry	Strong monotypic surface immunoglobulin	Polytypic surface immunoglublin with strong polytypic network of immunoglobulin	7.32
	Monotypic cytoplasmic immunoglobulin in some cases	Polytypic cytoplasmic immunoglobulin	
	Randomly distributed T-cells	Polar distribution of T-cells	7.35

bulin. When this immunoglobulin is of the IgG class the cytoplasm of the cells appears clear or vacuolated giving an appearance that may mimic signet ring carcinoma or liposarcoma (Fig. 7.23). Immunohistochemistry may be useful in identifying these cases although much of the IgG appears to leach out of the tissues so that the staining reaction appears as a faint rim at the periphery of the vacuole.

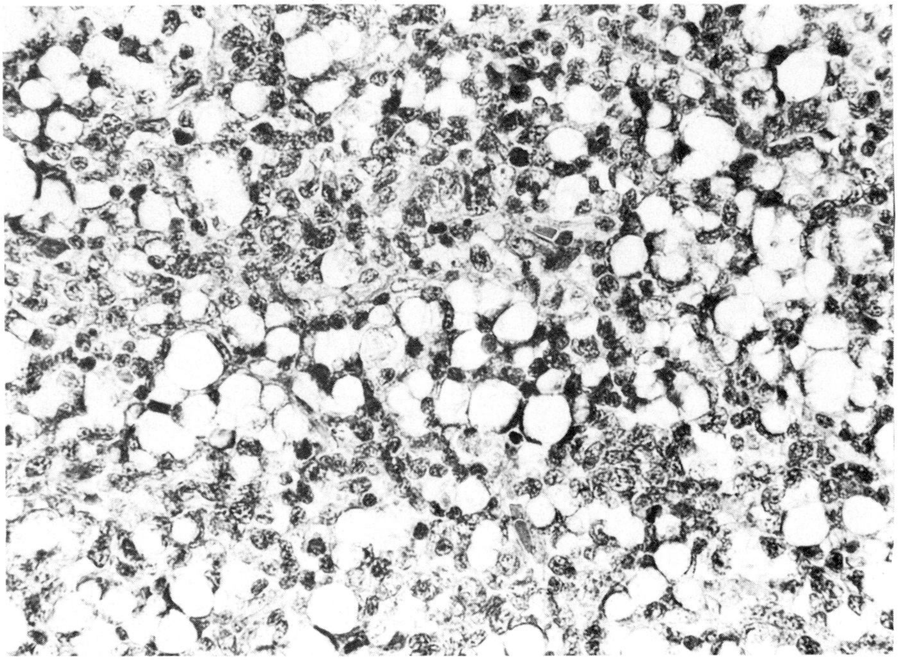

Fig. 7.23 Signet ring variant of FCCL. Many of the neoplastic centrocytes have a signet ring appearance associated with the accumulation of cytoplasmic immunoglobulin G, × 300.

7.3 Malignant lymphoma: centroblastic

This tumour accounts for approximately 5% of non-Hodgkin's lymphomas. It may develop in patients previously diagnosed as having centroblastic/centrocytic lymphoma follicular (secondary centroblastic lymphoma; Lennert, 1978) or arise *de novo*. We have no means of knowing whether the latter group had occult centroblastic/centrocytic lymphoma previously. Centroblastic lymphoma is usually categorized as a 'poor prognosis' lymphoma. However, sustained remission may be obtained with aggressive chemotherapy (Longo *et al.*, 1982).

Patients with centroblastic lymphoma usually present with lymphadenopathy but involvement of the spleen, liver and bone marrow is frequent. Leukaemic spillover into the blood is seen less frequently than in centroblastic/centrocytic lymphoma. A high proportion of cases of centroblastic lymphoma synthesize immunoglobulin and, therefore, the serum and urine should be carefully investigated for the presence of a paraprotein. Full haematological work-up with a bone marrow trephine should be performed. Radiological staging procedures should be carried out but staging laparotomy is rarely indicated. Chemotherapy is the usual treatment of choice.

7.3.1 Histology

Centroblastic lymphomas occasionally exhibit a follicular growth pattern but are more usually follicular and diffuse (Fig. 7.24) or diffuse. They are usually composed of a mixture of centroblasts and immunoblasts with scanty centrocytes (Fig. 7.25). Almost pure centroblastic tumours are occasionally seen. Dendritic reticulum cells can be demonstrated within these tumours by electron microscopy (Kaiserling, 1978) and immunohistochemistry giving support to the concept that they are related to normal follicle centre cells.

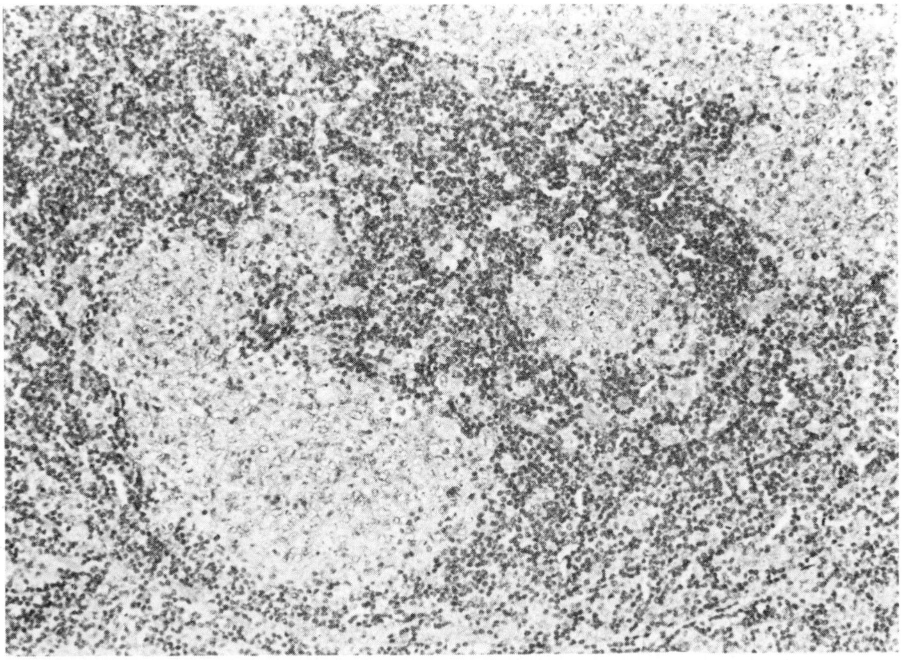

Fig. 7.24 FCCL, centroblastic showing a partially follicular pattern, × 120.

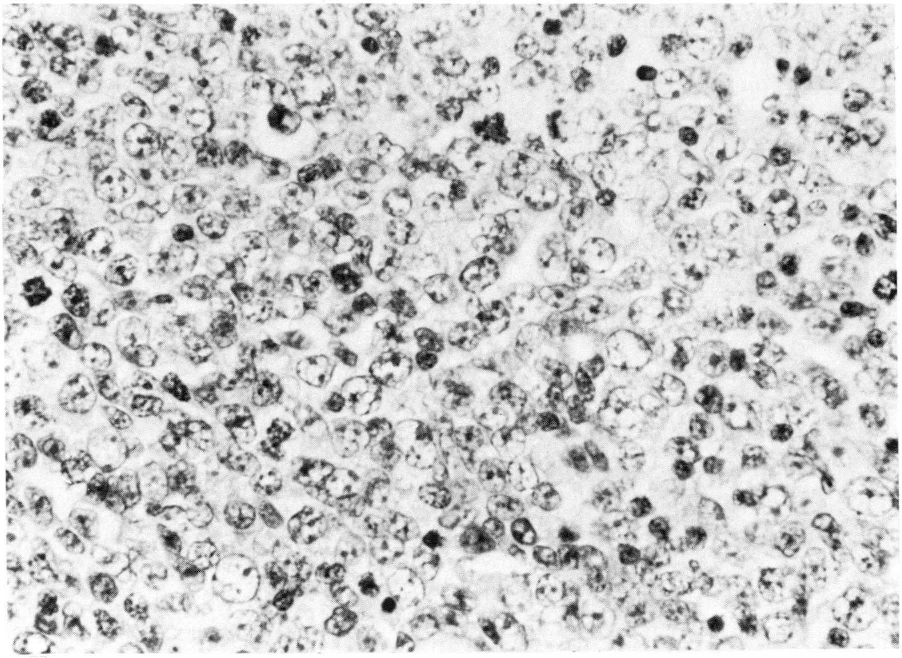

Fig. 7.25 FCCL, centroblastic. The tumour is composed predominantly of centroblasts. Occasional cells with central nucleoli may be categorized as immunoblasts, × 400.

Centroblasts are large cells with rounded nuclei containing 2–5 eosinophilic nucleoli that are frequently apposed to the nuclear membrane. They have a narrow rim of amphophilic cytoplasm that is moderately pyroninophilic. These features are well illustrated in imprint preparations (Fig. 7.26) and sections of plastic embedded tissue (Fig. 7.27). Immunoblasts are of similar size to centroblasts but have a prominent single central nucleolus and better defined, more abundant and more intensely pyroninophilic cytoplasm. In centroblastic lymphomas transitions between these cell types occur. The lymphoma cells are sometimes much more pleomorphic than normal centroblasts and multinucleate forms may be seen (Fig. 7.28).

Fig. 7.26 Imprint preparation of FCC, centroblastic. Most tumour cells have three or four nucleoli and a narrow rim of darkly basophilic cytoplasm. Giemsa, × 1200.

Fig. 7.27 Plastic embedded section of FCCL, centroblastic. There is a homogenous population of centroblasts. Compare with Fig. 7.21. Toluidine blue, × 1200.

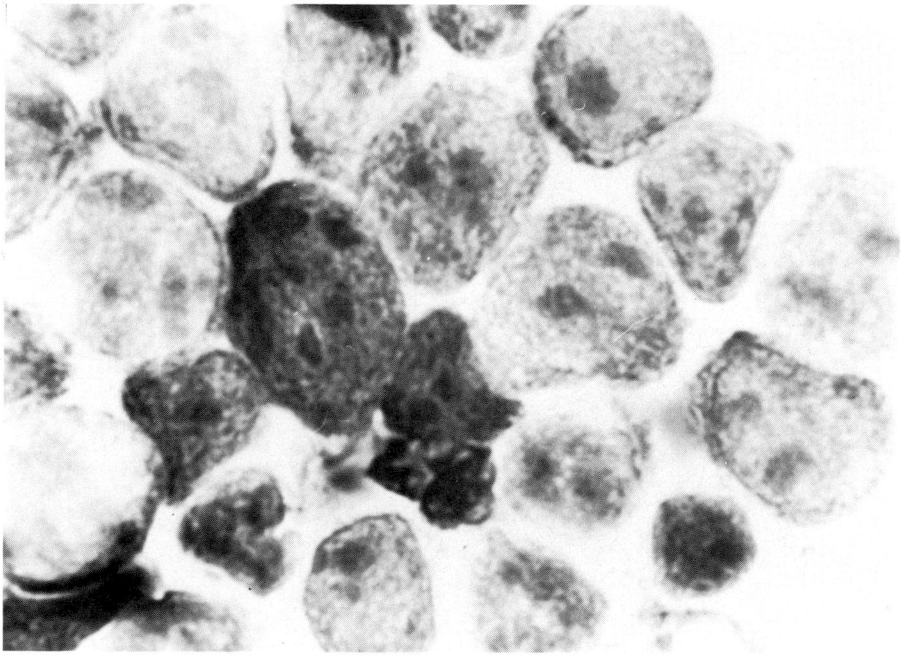

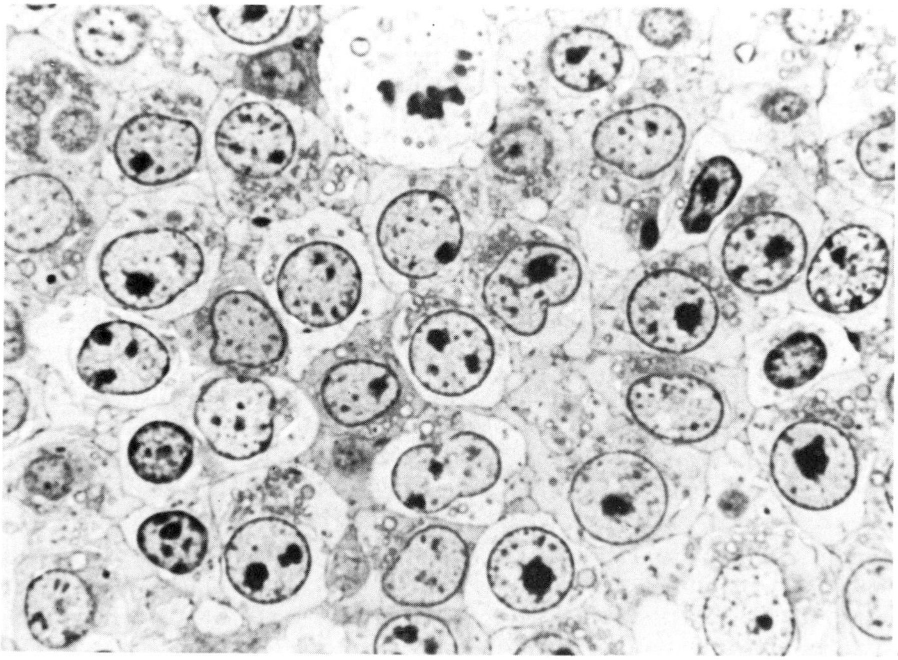

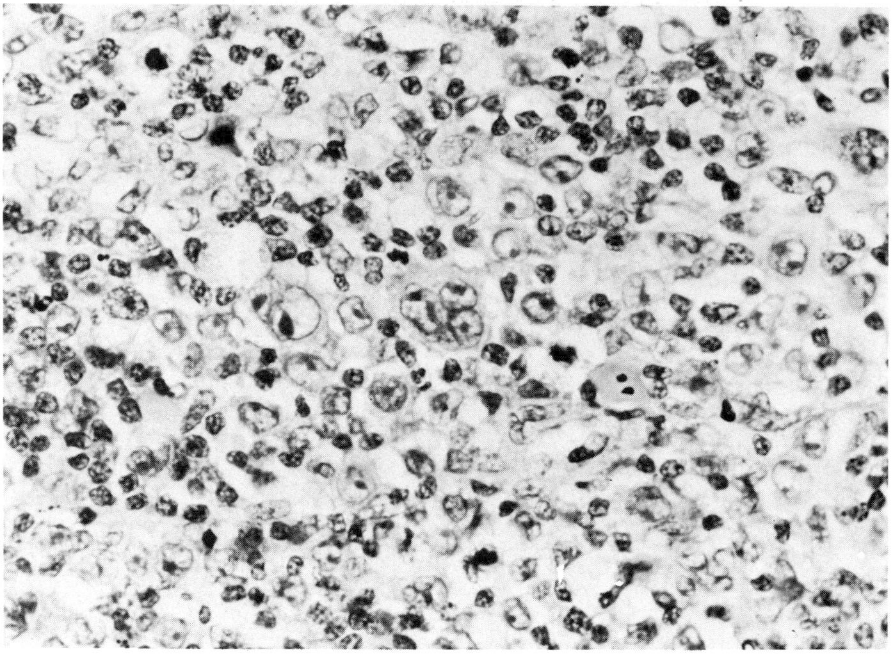

Fig. 7.28 FCCL, centroblastic showing pleomorphism. Note multinucleated 'Reed–Sternberg-like' cell at centre, × 400.

Many of these tumours synthesize immunoglobulin and in about one-third of cases PAS-positive inclusions can be demonstrated in the cytoplasm or nucleus of a small proportion of cells. Silver stains usually show a sparse and diagnostically unhelpful reticulin pattern.

7.3.2 Differential diagnosis

Centroblastic lymphomas are rarely completely monomorphic and usually contain a mixture of large and small centrocytes and of immunoblasts. They thus have to be differentiated from centroblastic/centrocytic lymphomas at one end of the spectrum and from B-immunoblastic lymphomas at the other.

Pleomorphic forms of centroblastic lymphoma may be confused with Hodgkin's disease. This is particularly so since tumours in this group frequently contain a large population of non-neoplastic histiocytes and may sometimes be infiltrated by eosinophils. The pleomorphic multinucleated centroblasts (Fig. 7.28) that are sometimes present can resemble the polylobated type of Reed–Sternberg cell usually associated with lymphocyte predominant Hodgkin's disease but rarely mimic classic

Reed–Sternberg cells. The diagnosis of Hodgkin's disease can be excluded by the fact that although some of the multinucleate cells may resemble Reed–Sternberg cells the background population, containing large numbers of centroblasts, is not appropriate for any type of Hodgkin's disease.

The separation of centroblastic lymphoma from large T-cell lymphomas can be difficult and may require the application of immunological methods for its resolution. The presence of eosinophils, epithelioid cells and high endothelial venules should raise suspicions of a T-cell lymphoma. Marked polylobation of tumour cell nuclei and small serpiginous lymphocytes are characteristic of some T-cell lymphomas (see Chapter 9).

Centroblastic lymphoma, particularly when it has a follicular growth pattern may resemble metastatic anaplastic carcinoma (Fig. 7.24). Separation of these two neoplasms must be based on a careful evaluation of the cytology of the tumour cells. Immunological and immunohistochemical studies, and electron microscopy, can be of particular value in such cases.

7.4 Malignant lymphoma: immunoblastic

The category immunoblastic lymphoma has been adopted into most of the new classifications of malignant lymphoma. Unfortunately this term has not been well defined morphologically and like the term reticulum cell sarcoma which it has to some extent replaced, it is interpreted in many different ways. In his review of lymphoma classifications Nathwani (1979) states 'the variation in incidence of immunoblastic lymphomas reported by those using this term suggests that the criteria employed are not uniform and need to be reconciled'.

There are two major reasons for this confusion. Firstly, the term immunoblastic lymphoma is often applied indiscriminately to all large cell lymphomas arising in patients with chronic immune disorders, immune suppressed patients and those with a variety of lymphoproliferative disorders. The assumption that all of these tumours will be of a single histogenetic type is, we believe, unjustified. The second reason is that immunoblastic lymphomas have not been clearly delineated from centroblastic lymphomas. Lukes and Collins (1974; 1975) defined immunoblastic sarcomas as having pyroninophilic cytoplasm and often showing plasmacytoid features or differentiation. They described the nuclei of these cells as similar to those of the large non-cleaved follicular centre cell (centroblast). Lennert (1978) states that as a rule immunoblastic lymphomas reveal a great increase in immunoglobulin in the tumour tissue and/or blood. Clearly they cannot be separated from centroblastic lymphomas on these criteria. In the most recent version of the Kiel classification immunoblastic lymphomas are divided into those with plasmacytoid differentiation (B-cell) and those without (B- or T-cell).

We believe that immunoblastic sarcoma should be defined in morphological and immunological terms. The cells have round or oval nuclei with a single prominent central nucleolus and well-defined pyroninophilic cytoplasm. They show varying degrees of plasmacytic differentiation at the light microscope and ultrastructural level. Centroblastic lymphomas contain a variable number of these cells and we only use the term immunoblastic sarcoma when they predominate to give a fairly monomorphous tumour. In our experience such tumours are uncommon, accounting for less than 5% of all large cell lymphomas. We are not sure whether the separation of this group from diffuse centroblastic lymphoma has clinical significance. Nathwani *et al.* (1978) found no survival difference between patients with immunoblastic lymphoma showing plasmacytoid differentiation and patients with large follicle centre cell lymphomas. However, in an analysis of diffuse large cell lymphomas Strauchen *et al.* (1978) found that follicle centre cell lymphomas had a better prognosis than 'blastic' or 'pleomorphic pyroninophilic' lymphomas. This appeared to be due mainly to the relatively good prognosis of the diffuse large centrocytic group.

Serum and urine from patients with immunoblastic lymphoma should be carefully examined for the presence of paraprotein. Full haematological investigation including bone marrow trephine may reveal focal marrow infiltration but spillover into the peripheral blood is unusual. Non-invasive staging techniques are indicated in determining the extent and distribution of the disease in those patients who are not clearly in Stage IV at presentation.

7.4.1 *Histology and cytology*

Immunoblastic lymphoma is usually a monomorphic tumour composed of large cells with oval or rounded nuclei. The heterochromatin is often clumped at the nuclear membrane and most cells have a single prominent central nucleolus (Fig. 7.29) although occasional cells show two or three nucleoli. The cytoplasm is well defined, has an amphophilic staining quality in H and E stained sections and is intensely pyroninophilic. These features are clearly demonstrated in imprint preparations (Fig. 7.30) and

---

Fig. 7.29 Malignant lymphoma immunoblastic. Most of the tumour cells have a prominent central nucleolus and dark-staining (amphophilic) cytoplasm, × 480.
Fig. 7.30 Imprint preparation of immunoblastic lymphoma. Note prominent central nucleoli and deeply basophilic rim of cytoplasm. Giemsa, × 1200.

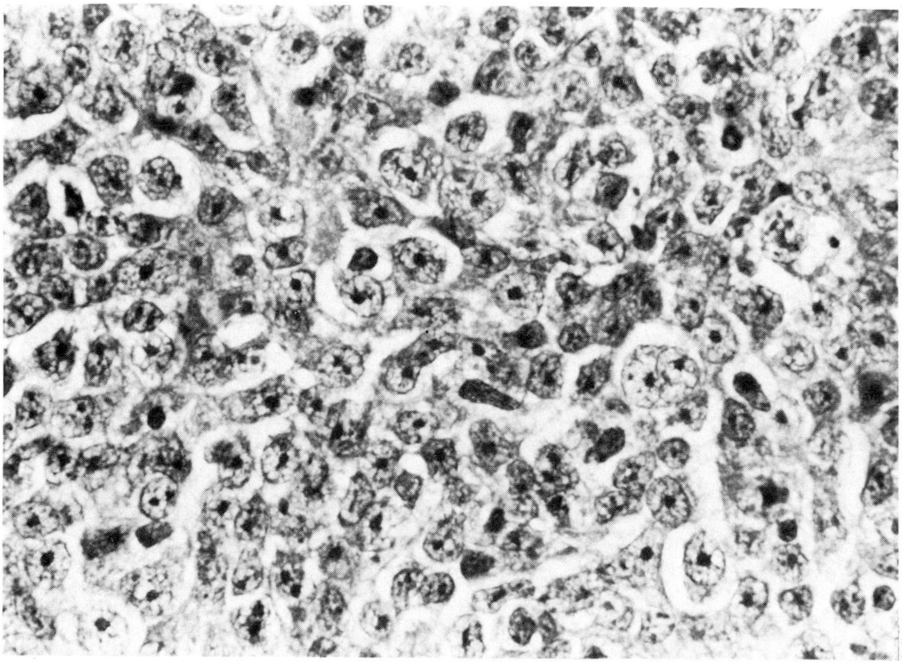

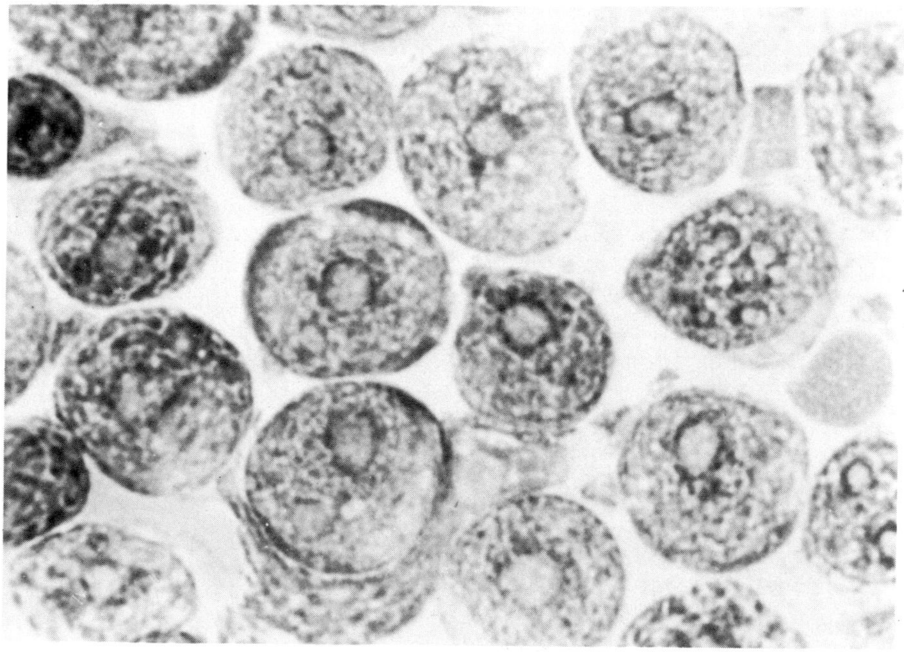

sections of plastic embedded tissue (Fig. 7.31). In most tumours some of the cells show plasmacytic differentiation, i.e. they are smaller, have more clumped nuclear chromatin and may show a pale area in the cytoplasm adjacent to the nucleus corresponding to the position of the Golgi apparatus. These cells are frequently aggregated around blood vessels and fibrous trabeculae.

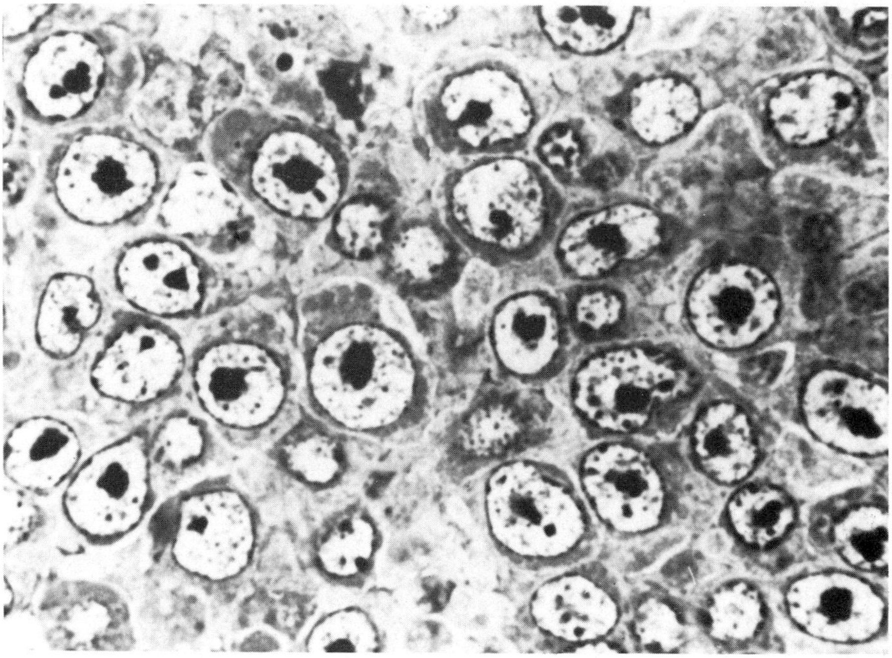

Fig. 7.31 Plastic embedded section of immunoblastic lymphoma shown in Fig. 7.29. The darkly staining cytoplasm and eccentrically placed nuclei give some of the cells a 'plasmacytoid' appearance. Toluidine blue stain, × 1200.

B-immunoblastic lymphomas synthesize immunoglobulin and PAS-stained sections show diffuse weak positivity of the cytoplasm of the tumour cells and in a high proportion of cases will also reveal intracytoplasmic and intranuclear droplets or globules of immunoglobulin. Immunoperoxidase studies will usually show strong positivity of the more plasmacytic cells for monotypic immunoglobulin. Scattered phagocytic non-neoplastic macrophages may be present throughout the tumour.

Occasional immunoblastic lymphomas show marked pleomorphism of some of the tumour cells with multinucleate giant cell forms. Binucleate giant cells may resemble Reed–Sternberg cells because of their prominent nucleoli. These pleomorphic tumours are frequently infiltrated by large numbers of non-neoplastic histiocytes and sometimes also by lymphocytes, plasma cells and granulocytes. In this respect they resemble the pleomorphic forms of diffuse centroblastic lymphoma.

7.4.2 *Differential diagnosis*

As discussed above, centroblastic lymphomas and some immunoblastic lymphomas appear to be part of a spectrum and the exact point at which the separation of these tumours is made is to some extent arbitrary.

Immunoblastic lymphoma sometimes develops in patients with chronic lymphocytic leukaemia and lymphoplasmacytic/cytoid lymphomas. Residual elements of the pre-existing lymphoma may be seen in these patients. Undifferentiated plasmacytomas (plasmablastomas) show prominent central nucleoli and have intensely basophilic/pyroninophilic cytoplasm, thus resembling immunoblastic lymphoma. We are unsure of the relationship between these tumours. Plasmablastomas usually involve extranodal sites and in our experience have more delicate nuclear chromatin than immunoblastic lymphoma. Perhaps of greater significance is the observation that plasma cell tumours show relatively uniform staining of all the tumour cells for cytoplasmic immunoglobulin whereas in immunoblastic lymphomas immunoglobulin is found mainly in those cells showing plasmacytoid differentiation.

Amelanotic melanomas and anaplastic postnasal space carcinomas may closely simulate immunoblastic lymphomas. The metastatic pattern of lymph node involvement together with fine cytological differences will usually differentiate these tumours. Since, in our experience, B-immunoblastic lymphomas always synthesize immunoglobulin they may be identified and separated from anaplastic tumours by immunohistochemical techniques.

Pleomorphic variants of B-immunoblastic lymphoma may simulate Hodgkin's disease with binucleate B-immunoblasts that closely mimic classic Reed–Sternberg cells. The clue to the true nature of the neoplasm is given by the background infiltrate of monomorphic immunoblasts which is inappropriate for any type of Hodgkin's disease. The immunoblasts may, however, be mistaken for mononuclear Hodgkin's cells and therefore lead to a diagnosis of lymphocyte-depleted (reticular) Hodgkin's disease. In our experience reticular Hodgkin's disease exhibits much more pleomorphism than is ever seen in B-immunoblastic lymphomas. Immunohistochemical studies by identifying monotypic immunoglobulin production by B-immunoblastic lymphomas may be diagnostically helpful in these cases.

7.5 Immunohistochemistry of follicle centre cell and immunoblastic lymphomas

Immunohistochemistry is not only of considerable value in the diagnosis of malignant lymphomas of follicle centre cell origin but also helps to explain and justify the classification of this histologically diverse group of tumours as a single broad entity. The essential immunohistochemical feature of these B-cell tumours is the presence of monotypic (i.e. single light chain) immunoglobulin on the surface (Fig. 7.32) or in the cytoplasm (Figs 7.33 and 7.34) of centrocytes, centroblasts and immunoblasts.

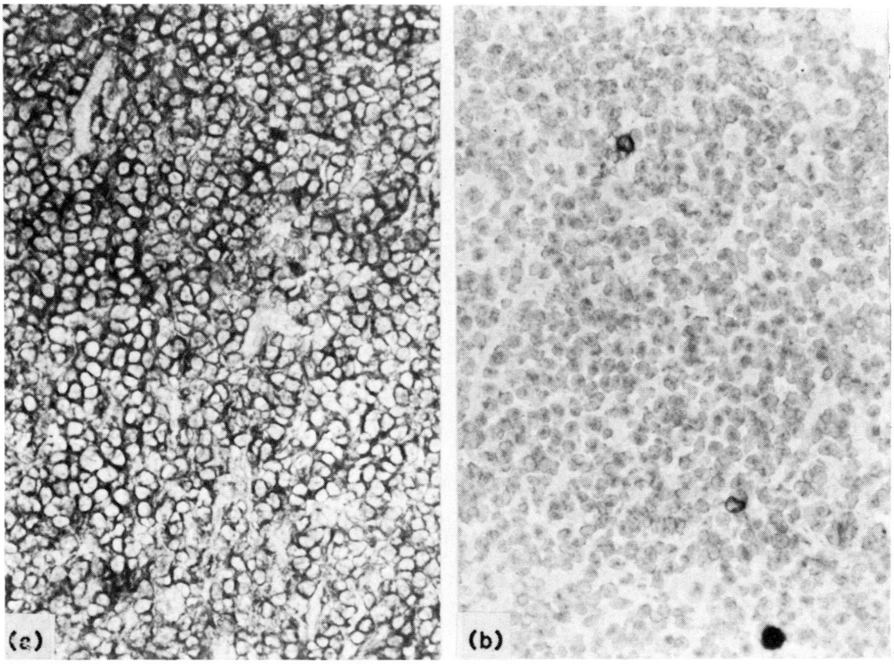

Fig. 7.32 FCCL, centroblastic/centrocytic, follicular. High power view of a neoplastic follicle in a frozen section stained to show surface immunoglobulin (lambda chain (a), kappa chain (b)). The tumour cells show monotypic staining for lambda chain. Immunoperoxidase technique, × 250.

Fig. 7.33 FCCL, centroblastic/centrocytic. Paraffin section stained to show cytoplasmic immunoglobulin (lambda chain (a), kappa chain (b)). A proportion of the tumour cells show monotypic staining for kappa chain. Immunoperoxidase technique, × 300.

Fig. 7.34 Immunoperoxidase stain for kappa light chains on immunoblastic lymphoma shown in Fig. 7.29. The cells showing strong staining for cytoplasmic immunoglobulin tend to be focally aggregated around blood vessels and fibrous trabeculae. Stains for lambda chains were negative, × 120.

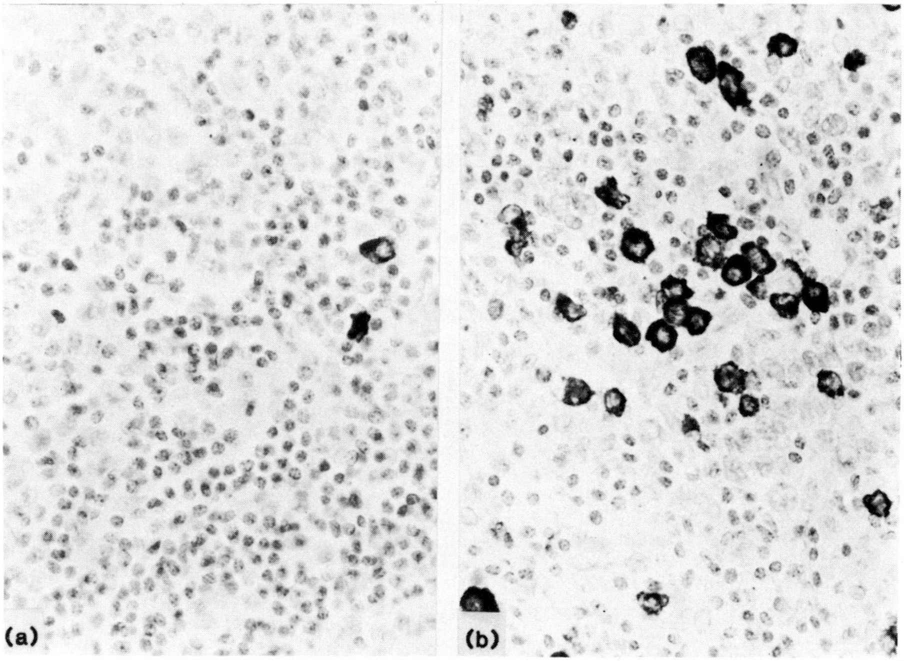
(a)
(b)

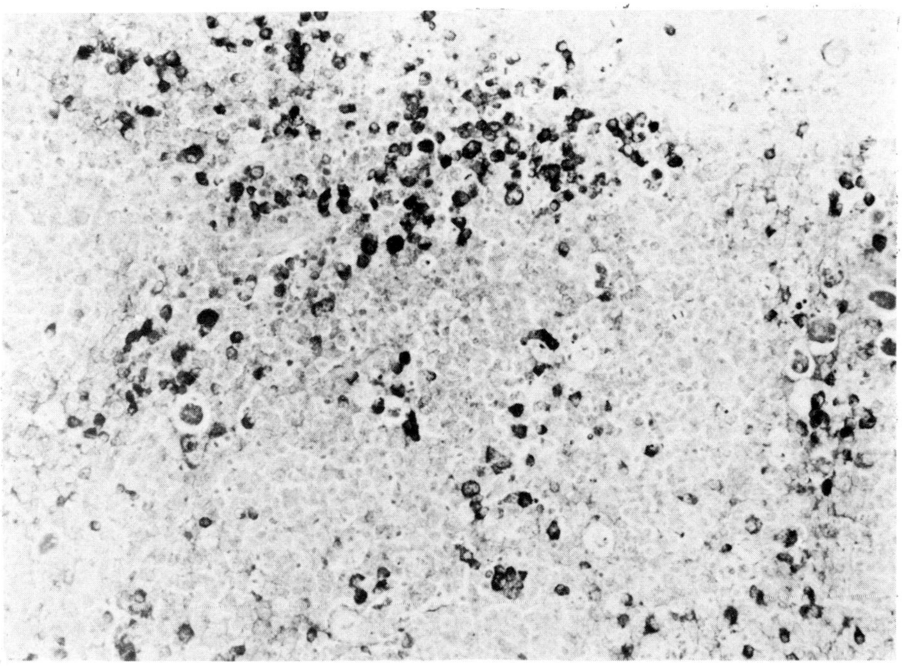

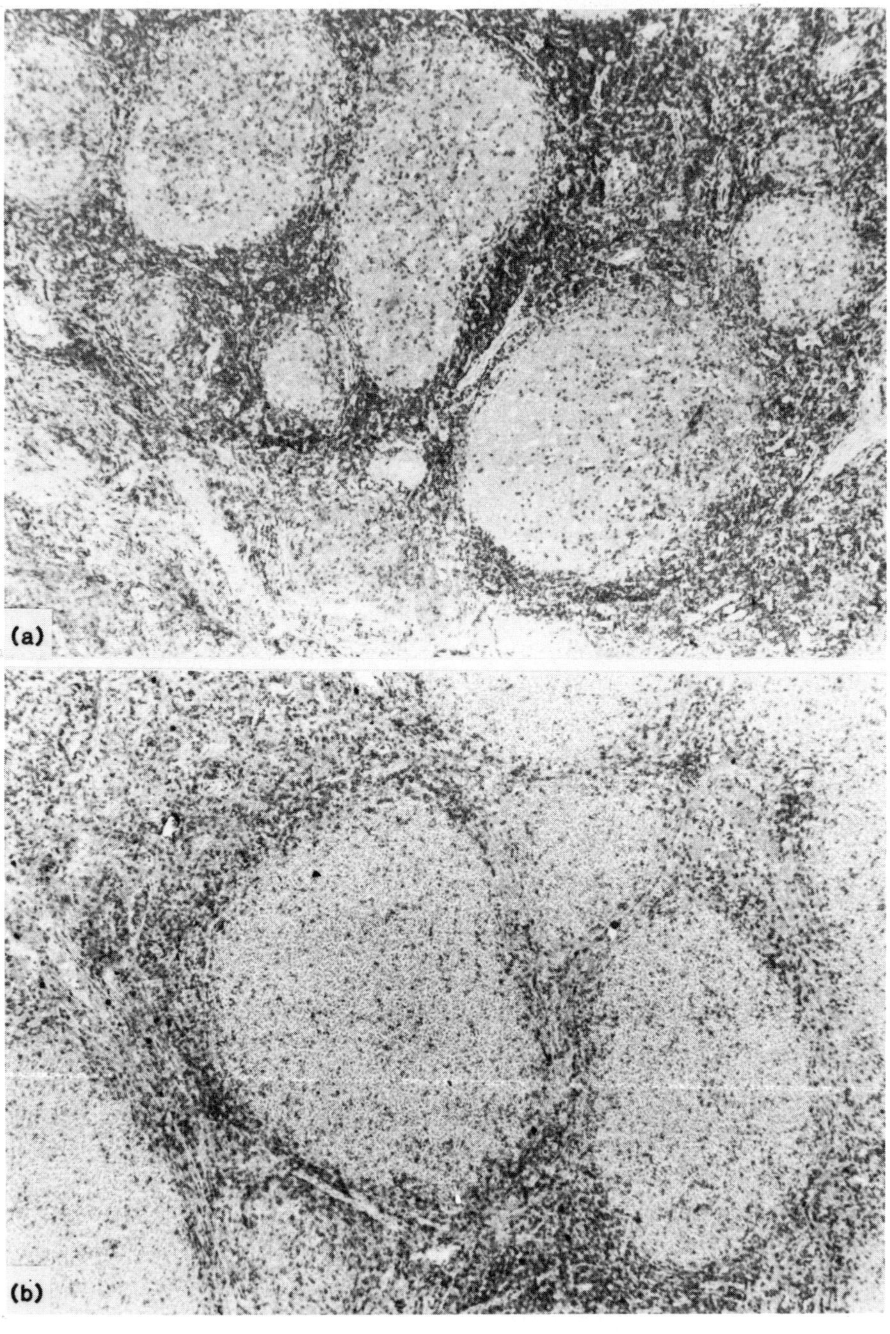
(a)
(b)

Surface immunoglobulin can be detected in almost all centroblastic/centrocytic lymphomas using frozen sections while cytoplasmic immunoglobulin can be demonstrated in paraffin sections of up to two-thirds of cases. The presence of other components of the follicle centre can also be demonstrated in these tumours. Like the normal follicle, T-cells (mostly of the helper variety) are found in the tumour, often in large numbers (Fig. 7.35) and the demonstration of dendritic reticulum cells serves to highlight the follicular pattern (Fig. 7.36). Even in diffuse centroblastic/centrocytic lymphomas small aggregates of dendritic reticulum cells can be demonstrated in contrast to other diffuse lymphomas.

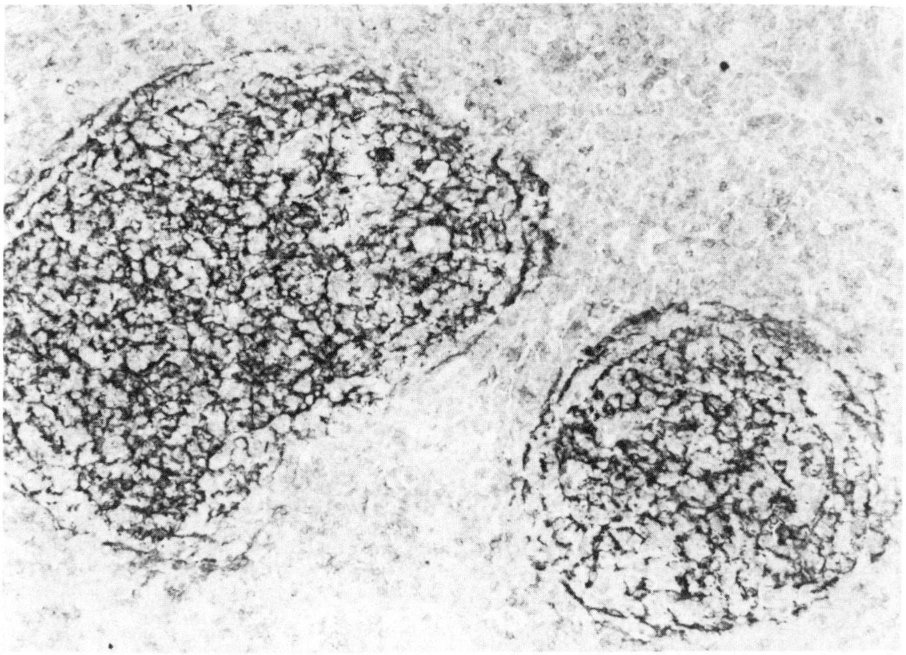

Fig. 7.36 Frozen section of FCCL, centroblastic/centrocytic, follicular stained by the immunoperoxidase technique with a monoclonal antibody (E 11) that identifies dendritic reticulum cells and hence serves to highlight the follicular pattern, × 120.

Fig. 7.35 Frozen sections of reactive lymph node (a) and FCCL, centroblastic/centrocytic, follicular (b) stained with a monoclonal antibody ($UCHT_1$) to show T-cells. There are large numbers of T-cells in the interfollicular areas of both sections. Scattered T-cells are also seen in the reactive and the neoplastic follicles. In the former, they have a polar distribution best seen in the follicle at lower right. Immunoperoxidase technique, × 40.

References

Bennett, M. H. (1975), Sclerosis in non-Hodgkin's lymphomata. *Br. J. Cancer*, **31**, (Suppl. II), 44–52.

Brittinger, G., Bartels, H., Bremer, K. *et al.* (1976), in *Maligne Lymphome und Monoklonale Gammopathien* (ed. H. Löffler), Lehmanns, München, pp. 211–23.

Cullen, M. H., Lister, T. A., Brearley, R. L. *et al.* (1979), Histological transformation of non-Hodgkin's lymphomas. A prospective study. *Cancer*, **44**, 645–51.

Harris, M., Eyden, B. and Read, G. (1981), Signet-ring lymphoma: a rare variant of follicular lymphoma. *J. Clin. Pathol.*, **34**, 884–91.

Herrmann, R., Barcos, M., Stutzman, L. *et al.* (1982), The influence of histologic type on the incidence and duration of response in non-Hodgkin's lymphoma. *Cancer*, **49**, 314–22.

Jones, S. E., Fuks, Z., Bull, M. *et al.* (1973), Non-Hodgkin's lymphomas. *IV.* Clinicopathological correlation in 405 cases. *Cancer*, **31**, 806–23.

Kaiserling, E. (1978), Ultrastructure of non-Hodgkin's lymphomas. In *Handbuch der Speziellen Pathologischen Anatomie und Histologie* (ed. K. Lennert), Springer-Verlag, Berlin, pp. 471–528.

Kim, H., Dorfman, R. F. and Rappaport, H. (1978), Signet-ring lymphoma. A rare morphologic and functional expression of nodular (follicular) lymphoma. *Am. J. Surg. Pathol.*, **2**, 119–32.

Lennert, K. (1978), Malignant lymphomas other than Hodgkin's disease. In *Handbuch der Speziellen Pathologischen Anatomie und Histologie*, Springer-Verlag, Berlin (in collaboration with M. Mohri, H. Stein, E. Kaiserling and H. K. Muller-Hermelink).

Lennert, K. (1981), *Histopathology of non-Hodgkin's Lymphomas (Based on the Kiel Classification)*, Springer-Verlag, Berlin.

Longo, D. L., Young, R. C., DeVita, V. T. (1982), What is so good about the 'good prognosis' lymphomas? In *Recent Advances in Clinical Oncology I* (eds C. J. Williams and J. M. A. Whitehouse), Churchill Livingstone, Edinburgh, pp. 223–31.

Lukes, R. J. and Collins, R. D. (1974), Immunologic characterization of human malignant lymphomas. *Cancer*, **34**, 1488–1503.

Lukes, R. J. and Collins, R. D. (1975), New approaches to the classification of the lymphomata. *Br. J. Cancer*, **31** (Suppl. II), 1–28.

Mann, R. B., Jaffe, E. S. and Berard, C. W. (1979), Malignant lymphomas – A conceptual understanding of morphologic diversity. *Am. J. Pathol.*, **94**, 105–92.

Meuge, C., Hoerni, B., DeMascarel, A. *et al.* (1978), Non-Hodgkin malignant lymphomas. Clinico-pathologic correlations with the Kiel classification. Retrospective analysis of a series of 274 cases. *Eur. J. Cancer*, **14**, 587–92.

Nathwani, B. N. (1979), A critical analysis of the classifications of non-Hodgkin's lymphomas. *Cancer*, **44**, 347–8.

Nathwani, B. N., Kim, H., Rappaport, H. *et al.* (1978), Non-Hodgkin's lymphomas. A clinico-pathologic study comparing two classifications. *Cancer*, **41**, 303–25.

Rappaport, H., Winter, W. J. and Hicks, E. B. (1956), Follicular lymphoma. A re-evaluation of its position in the scheme of malignant lymphoma, based on a survey of 253 cases. *Cancer*, **9**, 792–821.

Risdall, R., Hoppe, R. T. and Warnke, R. (1979), Non-Hodgkin's lymphoma. A study of the evolution of the disease based upon 92 autopsied cases. *Cancer*, **44**, 529–42.

Rosas Uribe, A., Variakojis, D. and Rappaport, H. (1973), Proteinaceous precipitate in nodular (follicular) lymphomas. *Cancer*, **31**, 534–42.

Satodate, R. (1978), Unpublished observations in *Malignant Lymphomas Other Than Hodgkin's Disease* (K. Lennert), Springer-Verlag, Berlin, pp. 293–4.

Spiro, S., Galton, D. A. G., Wiltshaw, E. and Lohmann, R. C. (1975), Follicular lymphoma: A survey of 75 cases with special reference to the syndrome resembling classic lymphatic leukaemia. *Br. J. Cancer*, **31** (Suppl. II), 60–72.

Strauchen, J. A., Young, R. C., DeVita, V. T. *et al.* (1978), Clinical relevance of histopathological subclassification of diffuse 'histiocytic' lymphoma. *New Engl. J. Med.*, **299**, 1382–7.

Tolksdorf, G., Stein, H., Lennert, K. (1980), Morphological and immunological definition of a malignant lymphoma derived from germinal-centre cells with cleaved nuclei (centrocytes). *Br. J. Cancer*, **41**, 168–82.

Warnke, R. A., Kim, H., Fuks, Z. and Dorfmann, R. F. (1977), The co-existence of nodular and diffuse patterns in nodular non-Hodgkin's lymphomas. Significance and clinicopathologic correlation. *Cancer*, **40**, 1229–33.

Weisenburger, D. D., Nathwani, B. N., Diamond, L. W. *et al.* (1981), Malignant lymphoma, intermediate lymphocytic type: A clinico-pathologic study of 42 cases. *Cancer*, **48**, 1415–25.

8 Burkitt's lymphoma and tumours of similar morphology

8.1 African Burkitt's lymphoma

The entity now recognized as Burkitt's lymphoma was first reported by Burkitt in 1959. He described the association between jaw sarcomas and visceral tumours in Ugandan children and made the first observations of the restricted geographical distribution of the tumour in Africa. Burkitt's lymphoma has a life-time incidence of approximately 1 in 1000 in those parts of Africa in which it is most common. In these areas the majority of cases occur in the first decade of life with a peak incidence at 6–7 years.

Jaw tumours, often multiple, are the most characteristic feature of Burkitt's lymphoma but occur most commonly in the younger age group and overall in only half the cases. The kidneys are the most frequently affected organs and retroperitoneal tumour masses are common (Wright, 1964). These are sometimes associated with infarction of the lower thoracic spinal cord and paraplegia. Nerve palsies and other manifestations of central nervous system involvement may occur as presenting features but are particularly common in patients in relapse (Magrath and Ziegler, 1979). Bilateral ovarian tumours, often massive, are a striking feature in approximately three-quarters of the girls with Burkitt's lymphoma, testicular tumours occur in about 10% of the boys. Breast tumours usually bilateral and sometimes massive are a feature of Burkitt's lymphoma occurring during pregnancy and lactation (Shepherd and Wright, 1967). Involvement of other abdominal and thoracic viscera and of the endocrine system is common, whereas involvement of the lymph nodes, spleen and lung is usually insignificant compared with the bulk of tumour elsewhere. Diffuse infiltration of the bone marrow with leukaemic manifestations is uncommon in African Burkitt's lymphoma (Wright and Pike, 1968).

8.1.1 Cytology

Imprint cytology is a most valuable aid to the diagnosis of Burkitt's lymphoma. The tumour is usually soft and makes excellent preparations. The tumour cells have rounded or indented nuclei with three or four nucleoli. The nuclear chromatin is granular and is usually condensed at the nuclear membrane and around the nucleoli. A narrow rim of cytoplasm surrounds the nucleus and is deeply basophilic except for a pale area at the nuclear hof. A variable number of cytoplasmic vacuoles are a characteristic, but not constant, feature of the tumour cells (Figs 8.1 and 8.2). These vacuoles correspond to lipid droplets that have been dissolved out of the cell during fixation. In formalin fixed imprints they may be stained by oil red O or other suitable neutral fat stains.

8.1.2 Histology

Burkitt's lymphoma infiltrates in an interstitial fashion but, perhaps because of its rapid growth rate, it rapidly destroys the underlying tissue

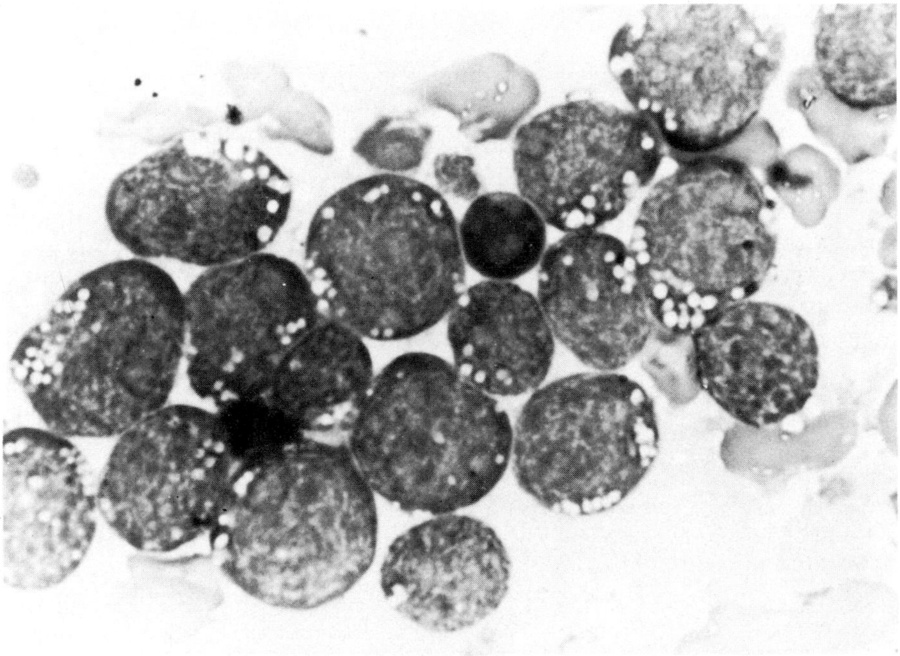

Fig. 8.1 Imprint preparation of Burkitt's lymphoma stained by May–Grunwald Giemsa. The tumour cells have a narrow rim of deeply basophilic vacuolated cytoplasm. The nuclei are rounded, have granular chromatin and show several nucleoli, × 1200.

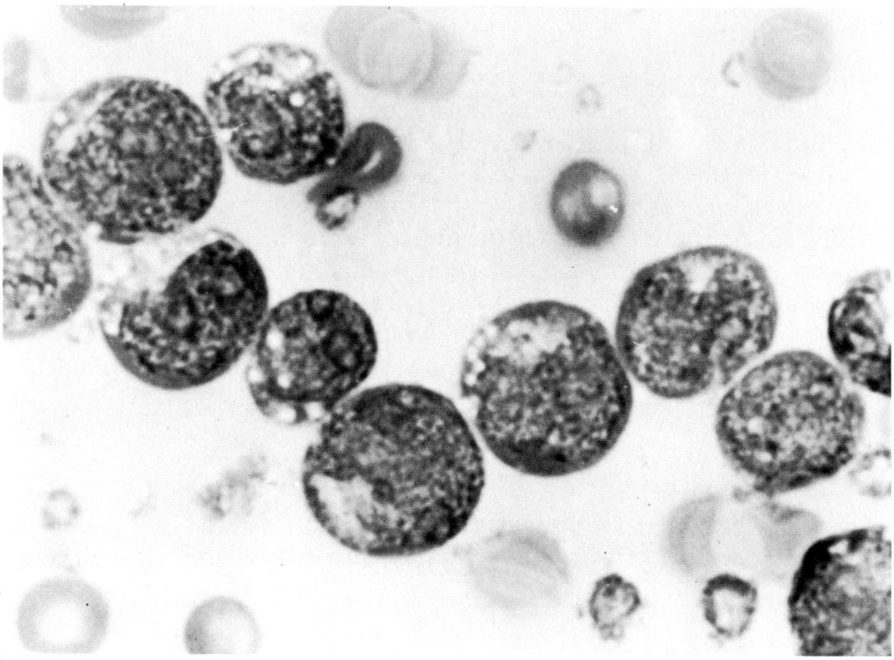

Fig. 8.2 Imprint preparation of Burkitt's lymphoma showing less prominent cytoplasmic vacuolation than the case illustrated in Fig. 8.1. The pale area in the cytoplasm adjacent to the nuclear hof corresponds to the position of the Golgi complex. Giemsa, × 1200.

architecture. An indian-file pattern of infiltration is seen when dense stroma such as that of the ovarian cortex is invaded (Fig. 8.3). The tumour is composed of sheets of monomorphic blast cells reflecting the cytological features seen in imprint preparations (Berard *et al.*, 1969) (Figs 8.4 and 8.5). Nuclei are predominantly rounded, the appearance of the chromatin varies with fixation being finely granular or homogeneous at the periphery of formalin-fixed biopsies and more vesicular towards the centre of the specimen. Most cells show three or four eosinophilic nucleoli, often near the nuclear membrane and surrounded by condensed chromatin. The cytoplasm of these cells is often ill-defined towards the centre of the biopsy but where the cells have separated from each other at the periphery appears as a well-defined amphophilic rim

---

Fig. 8.3 Ovarian cortex infiltrated by Burkitt's lymphoma. Note indian-file pattern and persistence of two primary ovarian follicles (bottom left), × 120.
Fig. 8.4 Low power view of Burkitt's lymphoma showing prominent 'starry sky' pattern, × 120.

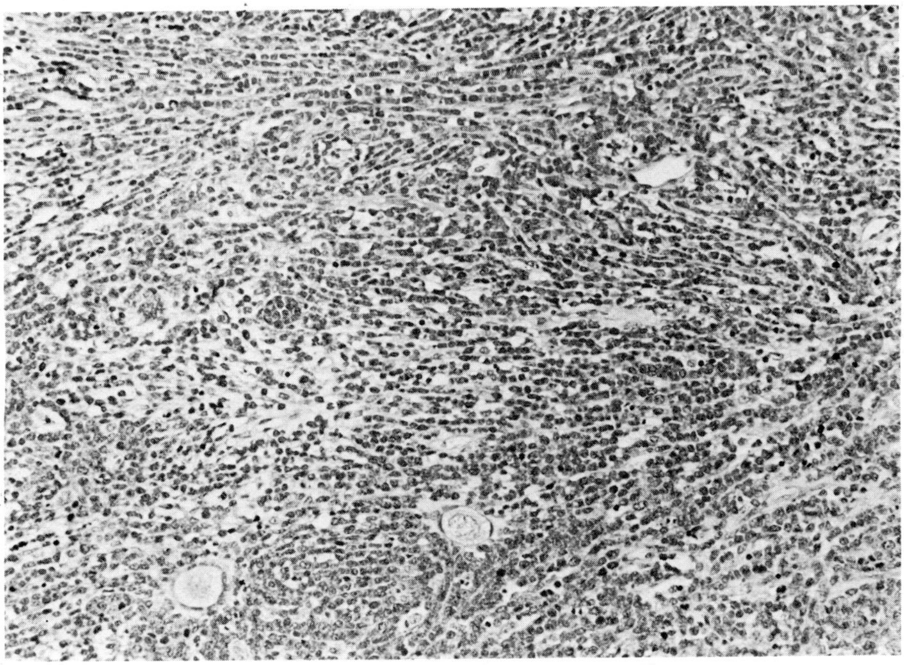

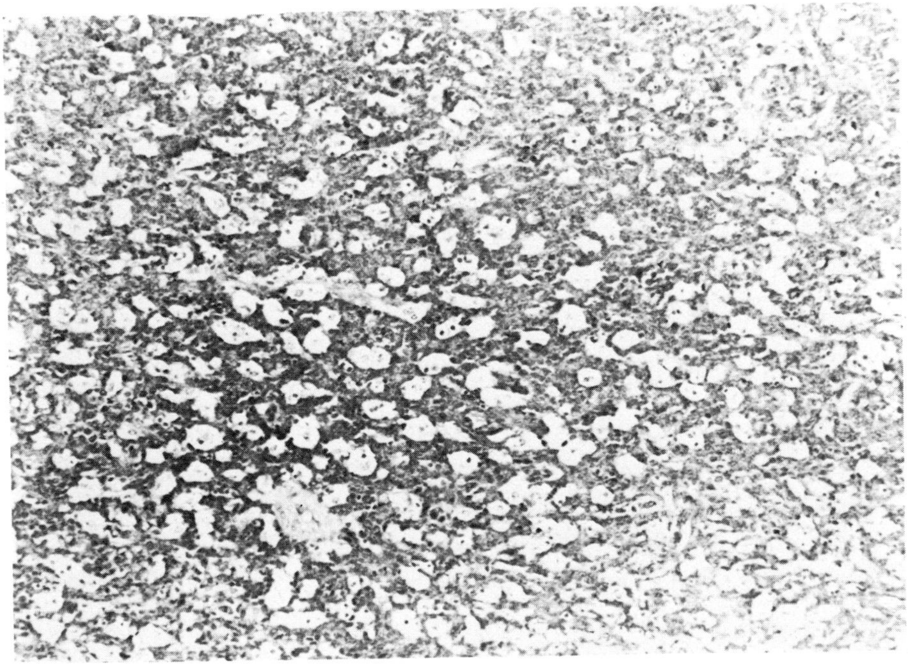

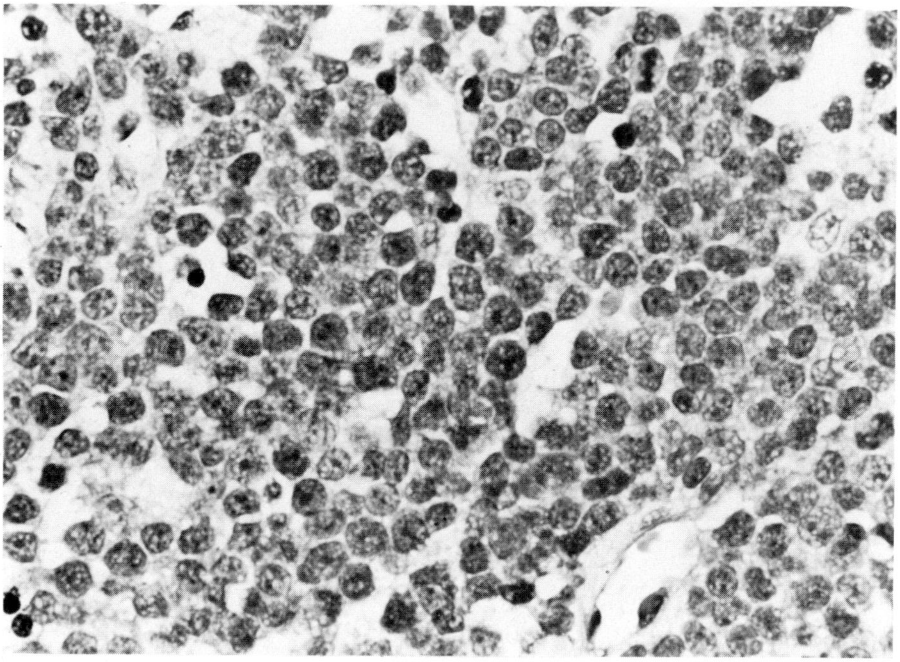

Fig. 8.5 High power photograph of Burkitt's lymphoma showing monomorphism of the tumour cells, × 480.

which stains intensely with Giemsa and pyronin. Careful inspection of this cytoplasm with an oil immersion objective usually reveals small vacuoles corresponding to dissolved fat droplets (Fig. 8.6). These droplets can be demonstrated in frozen sections of formalin-fixed tissue stained with neutral fat stains (Fig. 8.7). Burkitt's lymphoma exhibits a high mitotic rate and usually contains scattered pyknotic cells and cell remnants. In contrast to the extreme monomorphism of the tumour cells in untreated Burkitt's lymphoma recurrent tumours sometimes show marked degrees of pleomorphism. Reed–Sternberg-like cells have been described in such tumours (Wright, 1970).

A highly characteristic, though not specific, histological feature of Burkitt's lymphoma is the presence of scattered non-neoplastic macrophages between the tumour cells. These macrophages have abundant

---

Fig. 8.6 Oil immersion photograph taken at the edge of a biopsy showing the well-defined rim of darkly staining tumour cell cytoplasm containing tiny vacuoles, × 1200.

Fig. 8.7 Frozen section of Burkitt's lymphoma stained with oil-red-O showing numerous lipid droplets in the cytoplasm of the tumour cells, × 480.

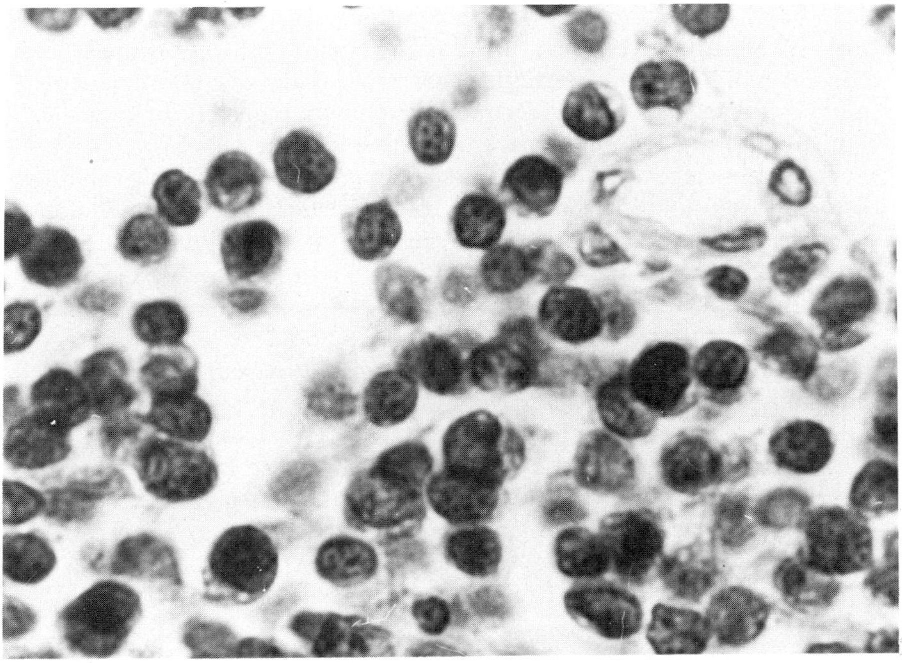

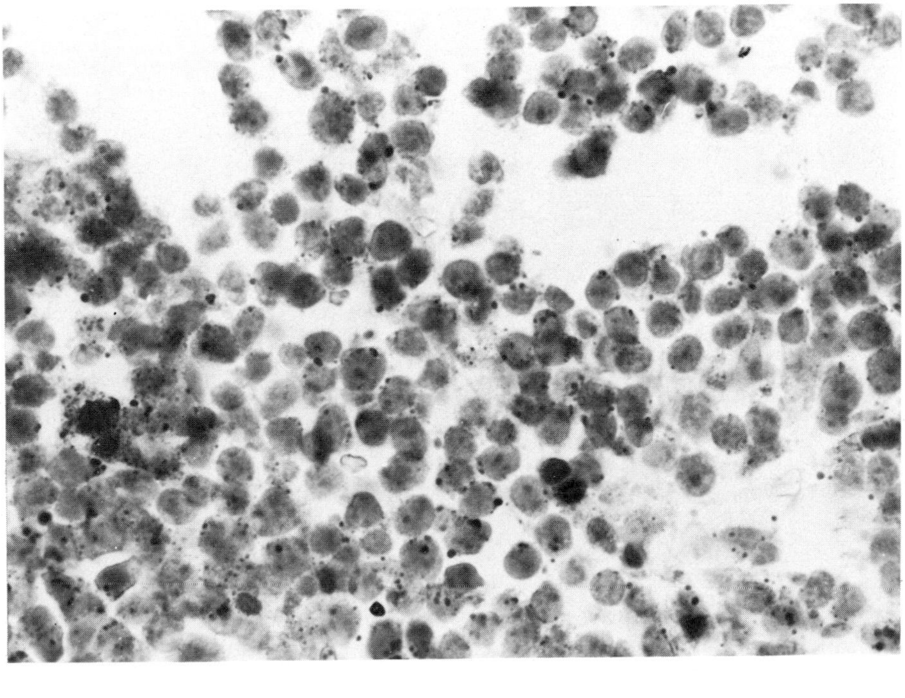

clear or foamy cytoplasm which contrasts with the darkly staining tumour cells and gives rise to the so-called 'starry sky' appearance (Fig. 8.4). Fat stains on frozen sections usually reveal a large amount of neutral lipid in these cells. They frequently contain ingested pyknotic cell remnants and occasional apparently viable tumour cells.

The diagnosis of Burkitt's lymphoma depends on the critical evaluation of the morphology of the tumour cells. Plastic sectioning techniques provide a valuable means of displaying fine cytological detail and are a most useful aid to the diagnosis of Burkitt's lymphoma. The cytological features of Burkitt's lymphoma seen in these preparations are similar to those seen in imprint preparations (Figs 8.8 and 8.9).

Electron microscopic examination (Berard *et al.*, 1969) shows rounded monomorphic nuclei although deep indentations are seen in some cases. Nuclear pockets are a characteristic but not diagnostic feature. The cytoplasm stains darkly due to the presence of large numbers of polyribosomes; only occasional short runs of rough endoplasmic reticulum are seen. Mitochondria are few and often occur at one pole of the cell. Fat droplets are seen in many cases.

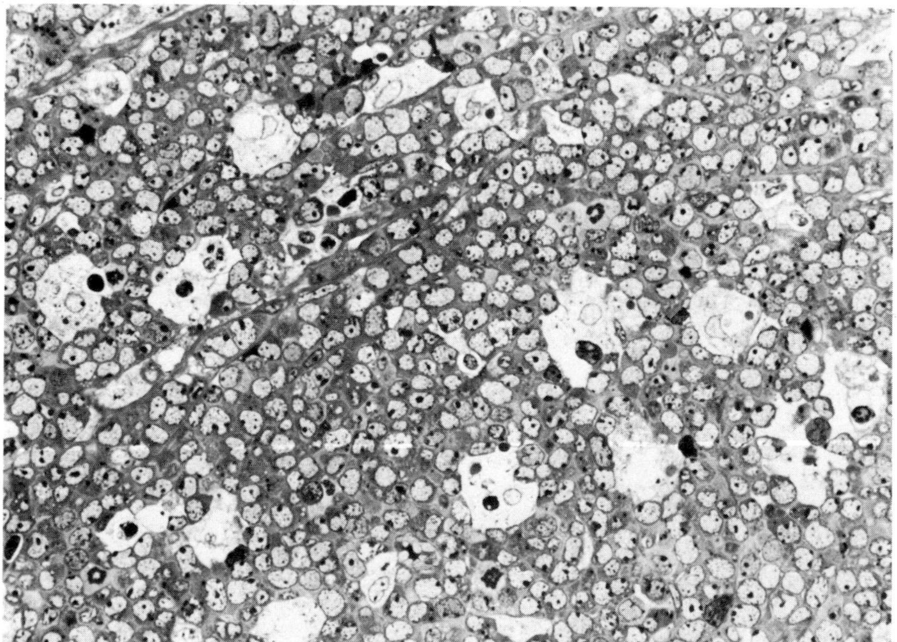

Fig. 8.8 Plastic embedded section of Burkitt's lymphoma stained with toluidine blue. Note the 'starry-sky' macrophages between the monomorphic tumour cells with their prominent nucleoli and darkly staining cytoplasm, × 300.

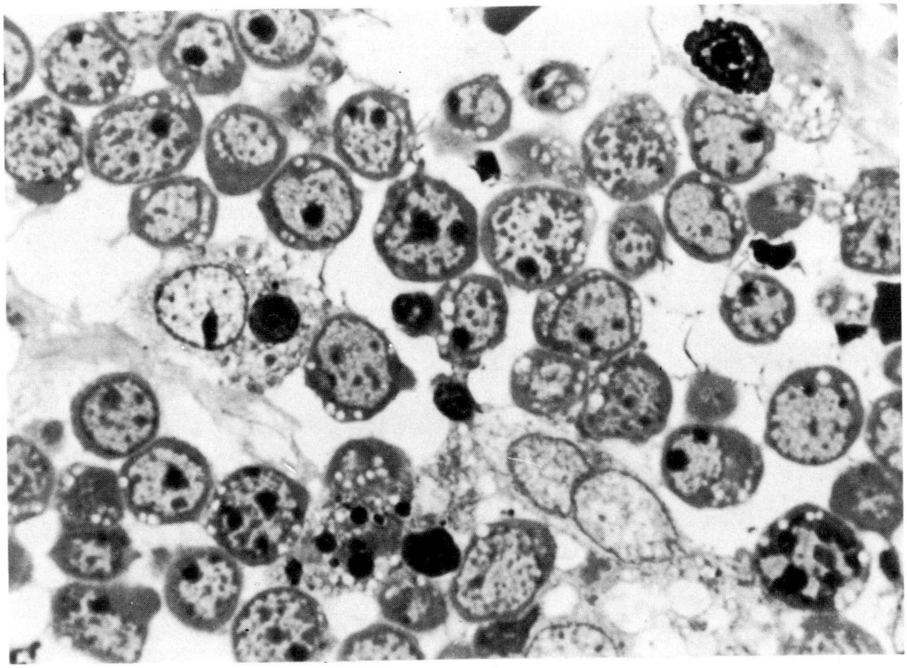

Fig. 8.9 Plastic embedded section of a poorly fixed Burkitt's lymphoma stained with toluidine blue. Note how this technique has 'rescued' the cytology of the tumour cells (compare with Fig. 8.1), × 1200.

8.2 Non-endemic Burkitt's lymphoma

Malignant lymphomas histologically indistinguishable from African cases of Burkitt's lymphoma (Figs 8.10 and 8.11) have been reported sporadically throughout the world. In some of these cases the tumours have shown a strikingly similar clinical behaviour and anatomical distribution to the African cases (Wright, 1966), although as a group significant differences are apparent.

American children with Burkitt's lymphoma diagnosed histologically have a higher incidence of lymph node, pleuropulmonary, gastrointestinal and bone marrow tumour than African cases and a lower incidence of jaw and gonadal involvement (Magrath and Ziegler, 1979). American Burkitt's lymphoma appears to be a more heterogeneous disease than African Burkitt's lymphoma (Levine *et al.*, 1982). This may reflect differences in the host response to the tumour but may be due to the difficulty in differentiating Burkitt's lymphoma from some other childhood lymphomas on histological grounds alone. Undifferentiated lymphomas with a similar morphology but showing varying degrees of

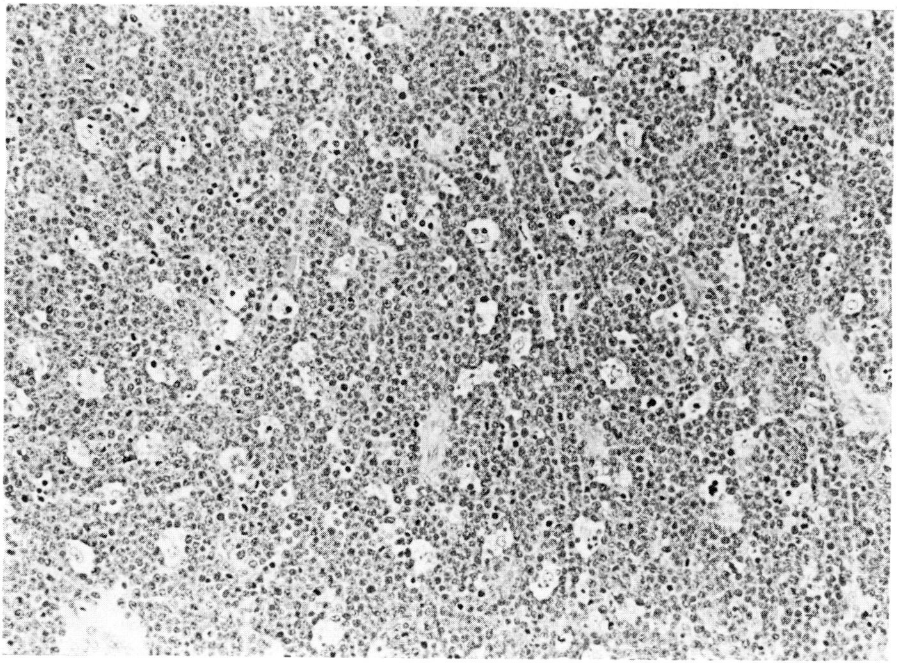

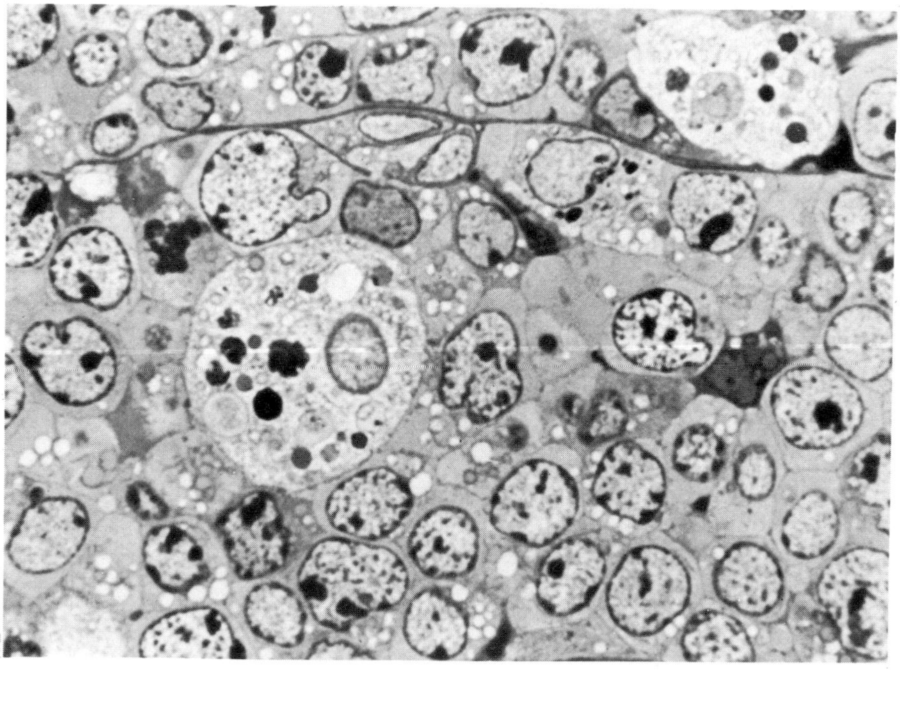

pleomorphism are separated from Burkitt's lymphoma histologically although clinically they may be indistinguishable from the non-endemic cases. Rarely follicle centre cell lymphomas occurring in childhood may resemble Burkitt's lymphoma (Wright and Isaacson, 1981).

8.3 Relationship between African and non-endemic Burkitt's lymphoma

Lukes and Collins (1975) and Mann *et al.* (1979) have proposed that Burkitt's lymphoma is of follicle centre cell origin, probably arising from a small centroblast. In support of this contention Mann *et al.* (1976) have reported American cases of Burkitt's lymphoma in which the tumour has a partly follicular structure and appears to show origin from or homing to follicle centres. It is, however, hard to imagine two more disparate tumours than African Burkitt's lymphoma and follicle centre cell lymphoma with respect to age incidence, clinical features, histological growth characteristics and anatomical distribution. If African Burkitt's lymphoma arises from a small centroblast or from a similar cell triggered to proliferate by an infectious agent such as malaria or Epstein–Barr (EB) virus, it appears frozen into a state of functional immaturity (Klein, 1979). This 'frozen' state could account for the morphological monomorphism of untreated African Burkitt's lymphoma and its failure to show other characteristics of follicle centre cell lymphomas such as differentiation towards centrocytes, cytoplasmic immunoglobulin synthesis and homing to follicle centres.

The apparent morphological identity of African and non-endemic Burkitt's lymphoma is dependent upon the quality of the biopsy material available for study and the experience of the histopathologist making the diagnosis. Tumours that appear to be typical examples of Burkitt's lymphoma in H and E stained paraffin sections may show unacceptable degrees of nuclear irregularity, probably indicative of centrocyte differentiation, in imprint preparations or plastic embedded sections. Electron microscopy may show features of centrocytic differentiation in the form of nuclear irregularity and profiles of rough endoplasmic

---

Fig. 8.10 Burkitt's lymphoma involving the ovary from an English girl. Note 'starry-sky' pattern and monomorphism of the tumour cells, an appearance identical to African Burkitt's lymphoma, × 120.

Fig. 8.11 Plastic embedded section of tumour shown in Fig. 8.10. Note 'starry-sky' phagocytes. The tumour cells are relatively monomorphic, have prominent nucleoli and darkly staining cytoplasm containing numerous lipid droplets, some of which have dissolved out to produce vacuoles. Toluidine blue, × 1200.

reticulum in tumours that at light microscopy appear to be typical examples of Burkitt's lymphoma. We have seen sections from an ovarian tumour in a 12-year-old girl that showed the typical light microscope appearances of Burkitt's lymphoma; immunohistochemical studies, however, revealed substantial cytoplasmic immunoglobulin synthesis in some of the tumour cells a feature incompatible with the diagnosis of Burkitt's lymphoma.

Magrath *et al.* (1980) have shown that the majority of American cases of Burkitt's lymphoma, in contrast to African cases, do not contain EB virus DNA and do not express receptors for C3 and EB virus. It has yet to be established with certainty whether EB virus has an aetiological role in African Burkitt's lymphoma. These studies, however, suggest that the American cases of Burkitt's lymphoma arise from a clone of cells different from the African cases that does not express, or only weakly expresses, C3 and EB virus receptors.

It would seem reasonable to propose, on the basis of the above evidence, that non-endemic Burkitt's lymphoma arises from a follicle centre cell (small centroblast) but unlike the African tumour it is not frozen into a state of immaturity and may show differentiation towards centrocytes and cytoplasmic immunoglobulin synthesis. This may account for the differences in anatomical distribution and clinical behaviour between African and non-endemic Burkitt's lymphoma. It is not yet clear whether when dealing with non-endemic cases, the separation of typical Burkitt's lymphoma from cases showing minor degrees of differentiation has any clinical or therapeutic significance. Rare cases of malignant lymphoma, centroblastic/centrocytic, sometimes with a follicular pattern, do occur in children (Frizzera and Murphy, 1979; Wright and Isaacson, 1981). These usually present as lymphadenopathy or intestinal tumours and appear to be clinically less aggressive than Burkitt's lymphoma.

8.3.1 Differential diagnosis

In the Kiel classification Burkitt's lymphoma is categorized as a lymphoblastic lymphoma. We believe, however, that Burkitt's lymphoma should be clearly separated from lymphoblastic lymphomas which are essentially bone marrow derived tumours of T- or B-cell precursors, which show marked clinical and anatomical differences from Burkitt's lymphoma (see Chapter 10) and which respond best to different treatment regimes. Histologically the separation of Burkitt's lymphoma from lymphoblastic lymphoma depends upon the positive identification of the cytological features of Burkitt's lymphoma cells as described above. Lymphoblastic lymphoma cells have a more delicate nuclear chromatin, smaller and less conspicuous nucleoli and less basophilic/pyroninophilic cytoplasm than Burkitt's lymphoma cells. The growth patterns of the two tumours are also different. Burkitt's lymphoma is usually destructive and cohesive whereas lymphoblastic lymphoma is infiltrative substituting the pre-existing cells and often leaving the underlying tissue architecture intact.

The presence of a follicular growth pattern or of cells showing features of centrocytes in a tumour that otherwise resembles Burkitt's lymphoma indicate a more differentiated follicle centre cell lymphoma and excludes a diagnosis of Burkitt's lymphoma.

References

Berard, C., O'Conor, G. T., Thomas, L. B. and Torloni, H. (1969), Histopathological definition of Burkitt's tumour. *Bull. W.H.O.* **40**, 601–7.

Burkitt, D. (1959), Sarcoma involving jaws in African children. *Br. J. Surg.*, **46**, 218–33.

Frizzera, G. and Murphy, S. B. (1979), Follicular (nodular) lymphoma in childhood: A rare clinical-pathological entity. Report of eight cases from four cancer centers. *Cancer*, **44**, 2218–35.

Klein, G. (1979), Lymphoma development in mice and humans: diversity of initiation is followed by convergent cytogenetic evolution. *Proc. Natl Acad. Sci., USA*, **76**, 2442–6.

Levine, P. H., Kamaraju, L. S., Connelly, R. R. *et al.* (1982), The American Burkitt's lymphoma Registry: Eight years' experience. *Cancer*, **49**, 1016–22.

Lukes, R. J. and Collins, R. D. (1975), New approaches to the classification of the lymphomata. *Br. J. Cancer*, **31** (Suppl. II), 1–28.

Magrath, I. T., Freeman, C. B. and Pizzo, P. (1980), Characterization of lymphoma-derived cell lines: comparison of cell lines positive and negative for Epstein–Barr virus nuclear antigen: II. Surface markers. *J. Natl Cancer Inst.*, **64**, 477–83.

Magrath, I. T. and Ziegler, J. L. (1979), Bone marrow involvement in Burkitt's lymphoma and its relationship to acute B-cell leukaemia. *Leukemia Res.*, **4**, 33–59.

Mann, R. B., Jaffe, E. S., Braylan, R. C. *et al.* (1976), Non-endemic Burkitt's lymphoma. A B-cell tumor related to germinal centers. *New Engl. J. Med.*, **295**, 685–91.

Mann, R. B., Jaffe, E. S. and Berard, C. W. (1979), Malignant lymphomas – a conceptual understanding of morphologic diversity. *Am. J. Pathol.*, **94**, 105–75.

Shepherd, J. J. and Wright, D. H. (1967), Burkitt's tumour presenting as bilateral swelling of the breast in women of child-bearing age. *Br. J. Surg.*, **54**, 776–80.

Wright, D. H. (1964), Burkitt's tumour: A post-mortem study of 50 cases. *Br. J. Surg.*, **51**, 245–51.

Wright, D. H. (1966), Burkitt's tumour in England: A comparison with childhood lymphosarcoma. *Int. J. Cancer*, **1**, 503–14.

Wright, D. H. (1970), Reed–Sternberg-like cells in recurrent Burkitt lymphomas. *Lancet*, **i**, 1052.

Wright, D. H. and Isaacson, P. (1981), Follicular center cell lymphoma of childhood: A report of three cases and a discussion if its relationship to Burkitt's lymphoma. *Cancer*, **47**, 915–25.
Wright, D. H. and Pike, P. A. (1968), Bone marrow involvement in Burkitt's tumour. *Br. J. Haematol.*, **15**, 409–18.

9 T-cell lymphomas

In Europe and North America T-cell leukaemias and lymphomas are uncommon compared with tumours of B-lymphocytes although this disparity is probably exaggerated by under-recognition. Some neoplasms of T-lymphocytes have been reasonably well defined clinically and histologically. These are T-lymphoblastic lymphoma, a tumour of precursor T-cells that is dealt with in Chapter 10, chronic lymphocytic leukaemia of T-cell type and the cutaneous T-cell lymphomas (mycosis fungoides and Sezary's syndrome). Numerous histological subtypes of node-based T-cell lymphomas have been reported in recent years. The small numbers of cases in individual series makes it difficult at the present time to determine the relationship of these subgroups to each other and to the normal maturation sequence of T-lymphocytes. Knowles and Halper (1982) have shown that tumours of the same immunological phenotype may display diverse histopathological features.

9.1 Malignant lymphoma: T-lymphocytic (T-CLL)

In Western countries approximately 2% of cases of chronic lymphocytic leukaemia are of T-lymphocyte lineage (Collins *et al.*, 1979). Brouet *et al.* (1975) reported 11 cases of CLL of T-cell origin in patients ranging from 25–78 years of age. They considered the presentation of nine of these cases to be so striking that they could be labelled as probable T-CLL before any immunological studies were performed. The main features were moderate or massive splenomegaly in five; skin lesions in three and severe neutropaenia in four cases. In all nine patients the blood and bone marrow invasion was only moderate. The neoplastic lymphocytes showed a high content of lysosomal enzymes (beta-glucuronidase and acid phosphatase) in all cases and cytoplasmic azurophil granules were prominent in six cases. Peripheral lymph node enlargement was seen in only one case.

9.1.1 *Histology and cytology*

The cytology of the tissue infiltrates in T-CLL are more pleomorphic than in B-CLL (Fig. 9.1). The neoplastic lymphocytes show irregular nuclei and blast cells with prominent central nucleoli are seen, although these do not form proliferation centres as in B-CLL (Lennert, 1981). Prominent high endothelial-lined venules are a feature of T-CLL not seen in B-CLL. Infiltrations in the spleen are characteristically periarteriolar in their distribution (Figs 9.2 and 9.3), bone marrow infiltration may be either focal or diffuse (Brouet *et al.*, 1975).

9.1.2 *Differential diagnosis*

It seems probable that T-CLL as at present recognized is a heterogeneous

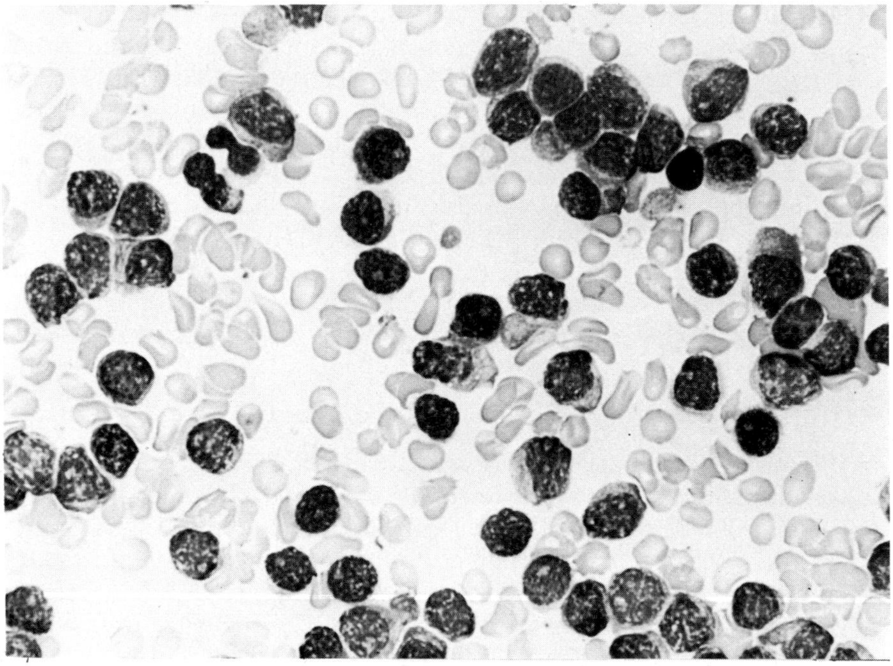

Fig. 9.1 T-CLL bone marrow smear. The tumour cells are more pleomorphic and have more blast cell features than B-CLL. Giemsa stain, × 480.

Fig. 9.2 T-CLL involving spleen. The tumour cells occupy the periarteriolar sheath, × 120.
Fig. 9.3 Higher power view of Fig. 9.2 showing pleomorphism of tumour cells, × 300.

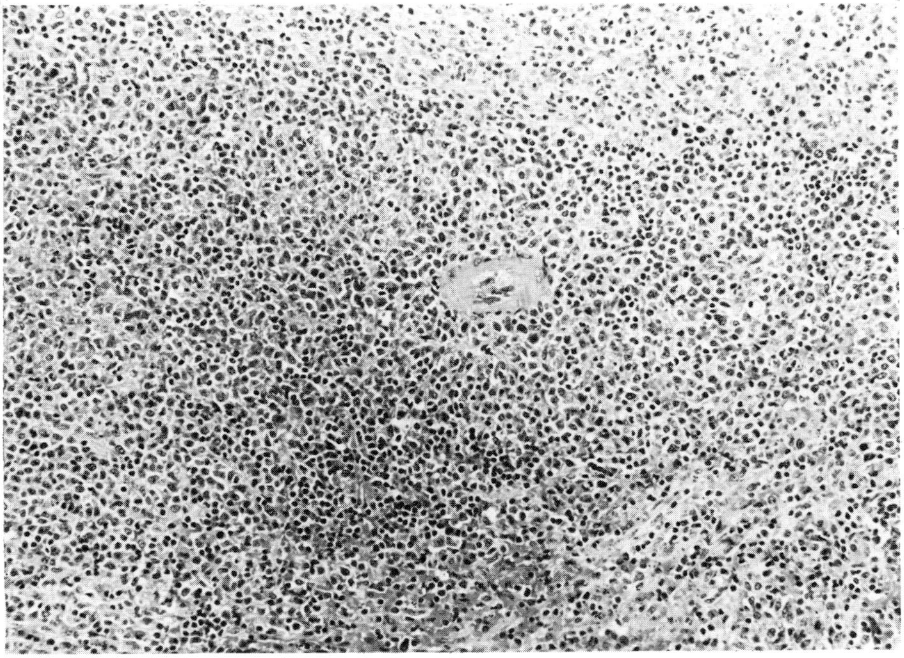

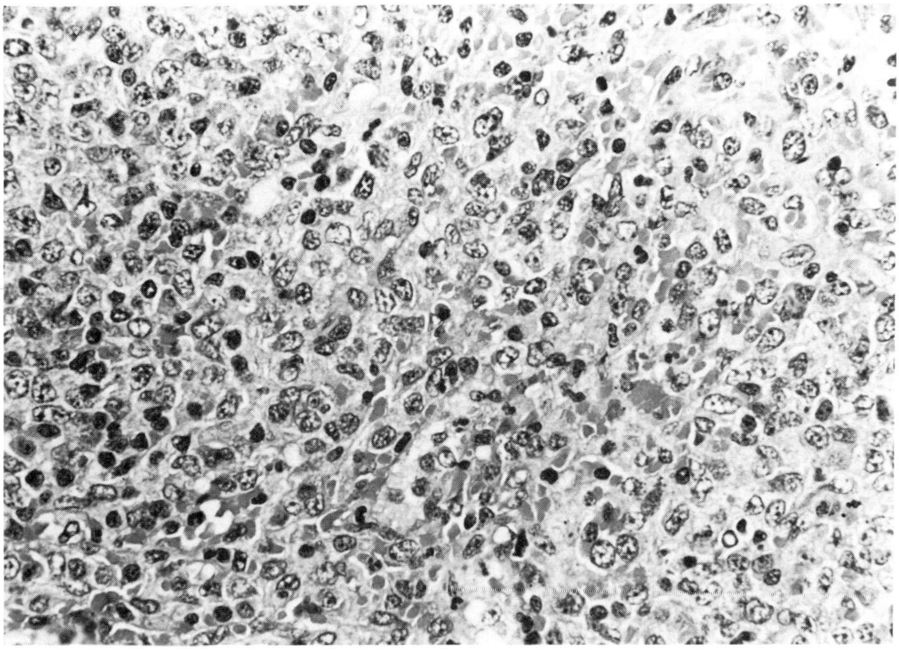

group of neoplasms representing the spillover of a number of T-cell lymphomas into the bone marrow and blood. The clinical and haematological features of T-CLL, as described above differentiate many cases from B-CLL with a moderate degree of reliability although final identification depends upon immunological marker studies. Differentiation between T-CLL with skin infiltrations and the small cell variant of Sezary's syndrome may be difficult (Watanabe *et al.*, 1981). The distinction should be made on the basis of the characteristic nuclear features of Sezary's cells and the greater epidermotropism with relative sparing of the bone marrow shown by this tumour (Lennert, 1981).

9.2 Prolymphocytic leukaemia of T-cell type

Two of the patients described by Brouet *et al.* (1975) had lymphocyte counts in their peripheral blood of 400 000 μl^{-1} and 500 000 μl^{-1} and the leukaemic cells had the morphological features of prolymphocytes. Apart from the cytological features of prolymphocytes with their prominent central nucleoli, there are no other histological differences between T–CLL and its prolymphocytic variant (Lennert, 1981).

9.3 Cutaneous T-cell lymphomas

9.3.1 Mycosis fungoides

Mycosis fungoides is a malignant lymphoma of skin-associated T-lymphocytes that exhibit epidermotropism. With evolution of the disease the skin lesions pass through premycotic, infiltrative and tumour phases; spread to lymph nodes and deeper tissues occurs late in the disease and is of bad prognostic significance. The neoplastic T-lymphocytes have irregular deeply convoluted nuclei and are referred to as cerebriform or Lutzner cells (Lutzner and Jordan, 1968; Lutzner *et al.*, 1971). They show focal positivity for acid phosphatase and acid non-specific esterase, a pattern consistent with a helper T-cell subset (Lennert, 1981). Reactivity with monoclonal antibodies to T-cell subsets (Kung *et al.*, 1981) and *in vitro* studies have confirmed this helper cell function in some cases (Lawrence *et al.*, 1978). This functional characteristic may account for the polyclonal hyperglobulinaemia sometimes associated with cutaneous T-cell lymphomas.

(a) *Histology*

Skin biopsies from patients with mycosis fungoides show a cellular infiltrate in the upper dermis. This infiltrate consists of cerebriform cells with variable numbers of reactive cells including histiocytes and eosinophils. Cerebriform cells infiltrate the epidermis either singly or in

TO SEE DR ISMAIL

NEW OF WARD 967.

Seminar

Folngia:

small groups forming the so-called Pautrier's microabscesses (Fig. 9.4), the characteristic cerebriform nuclei of these cells are best seen in plastic embedded sections (Fig. 9.5). Larger cells with multiple or polylobated nuclei, prominent nucleoli and darkly staining cytoplasm are usually present in small numbers in the infiltrate. These cells are referred to as mycosis cells and probably represent polyploid variants of the smaller cerebriform cells.

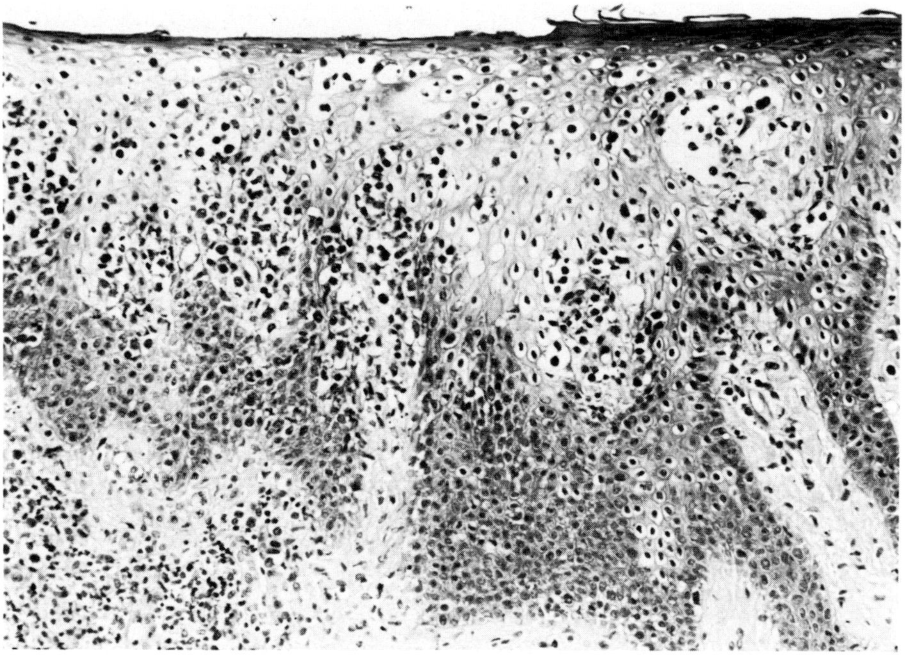

Fig. 9.4 Mycosis fungoides. The tumour cells infiltrate the papillary dermis and extend into the epidermis, × 120.

Lymphadenopathy in patients with mycosis fungoides may be due to dermatopathic lymphadenopathy and this can be difficult to distinguish histologically from lymphomatous infiltrations (Burke and Colby, 1981; Scheffer *et al.*, 1980). The infiltrate in dermatopathic lymphadenopathy consists predominantly of interdigitating reticulum cells whereas large aggregates of cerebriform cells and the presence of mycosis cells are indicative of lymphoma (Figs 9.6 and 9.7).

9.3.2 *Sezary's syndrome*

Sezary's syndrome may be regarded as a leukaemic variant of mycosis fungoides. The patients usually present with erythroderma (homme

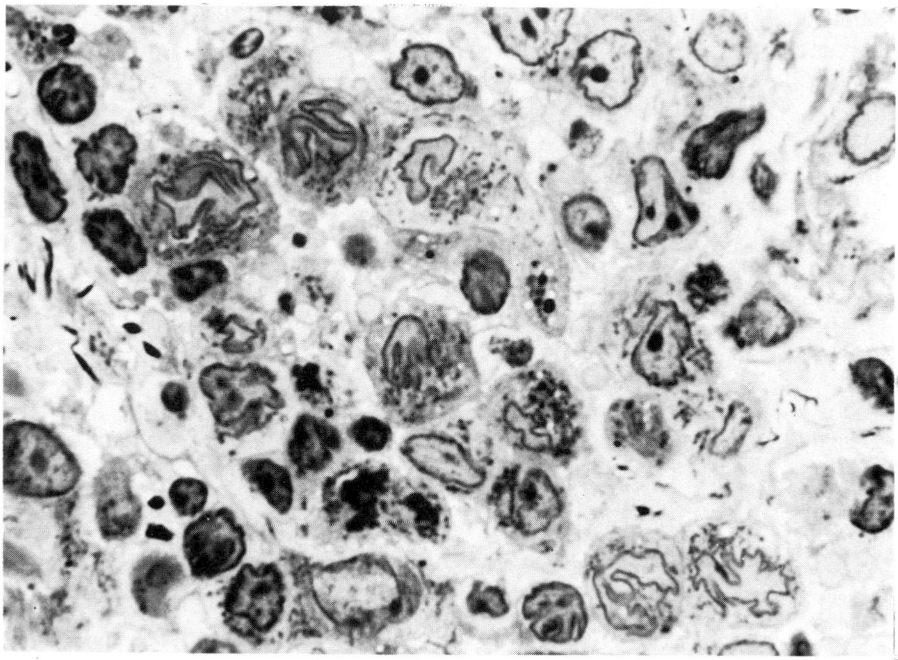

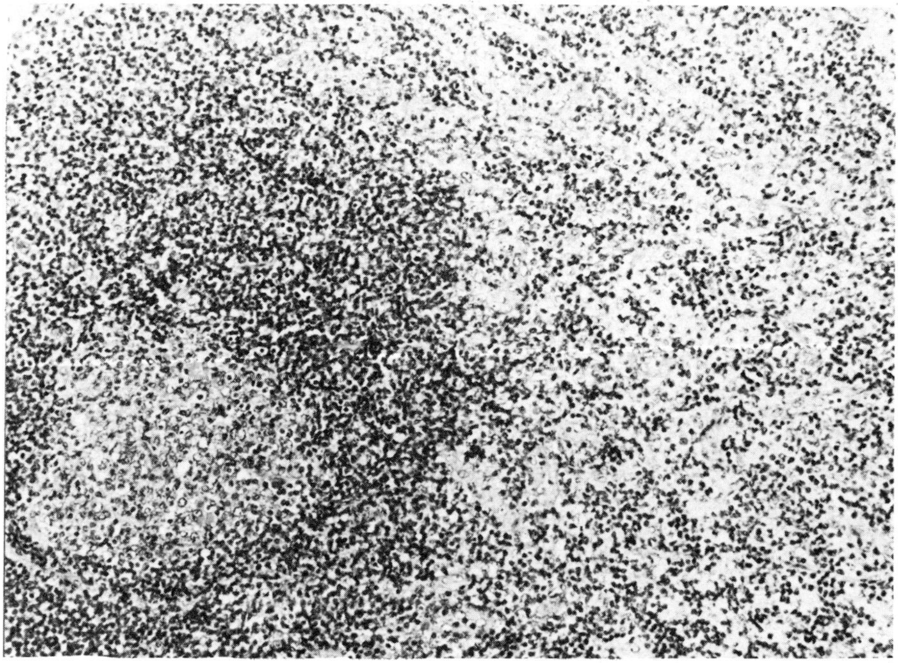

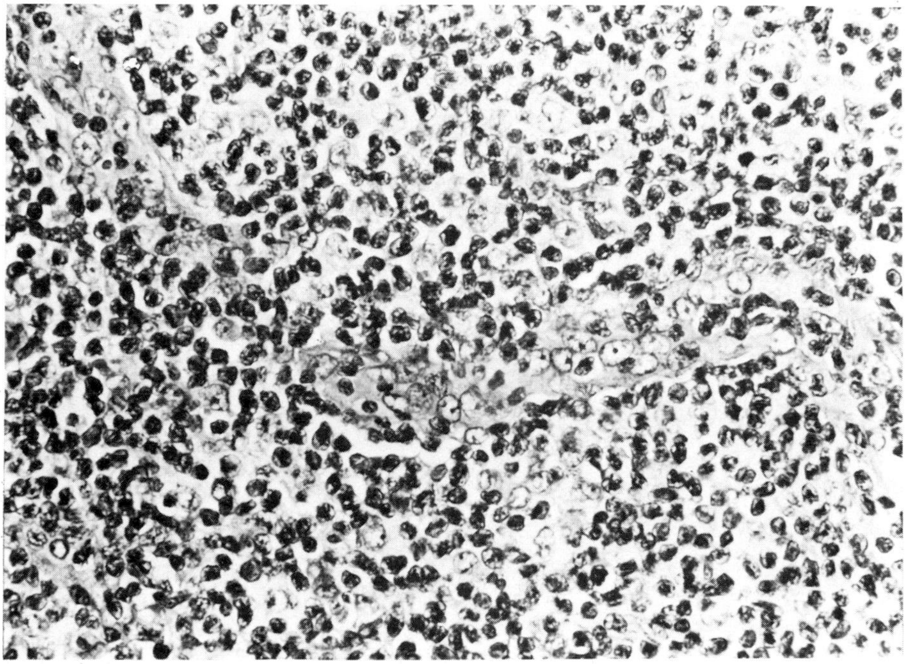

Fig. 9.7 Higher power view of Fig. 9.6 showing high endothelial lined venule surrounded by darkly staining cerebriform lymphocytes and paler blast cells, × 300.

rouge), alopecia, lymphadenopathy and a leukaemic blood picture. In contrast to other leukaemias the marrow may remain free of infiltration up to the time of death (Lennert, 1981).

(a) *Histology*

Histologically the dermal infiltrates in Sezary's syndrome are similar to those seen in the infiltrative phase of mycosis fungoides (Figs 9.8 and 9.9). Infiltration of lymph nodes occurs in the paracortex but since it is not preceded by significant dermatopathic lymphadenopathy it is generally more monomorphic than that seen in mycosis fungoides (Lennert, 1981). The infiltrate consists predominantly of Sezary cells and occasional

---

Fig. 9.5 Plastic embedded section of dermal infiltrate in mycosis fungoides showing extreme cerebriform convolutions of the nuclei of the neoplastic T-cells. Toluidine blue, × 1200.

Fig. 9.6 Lymph node section from a patient with mycosis fungoides showing expansion of the parafollicular zone by cerebriform lymphocytes. High endothelial venules are prominent in this zone, × 120.

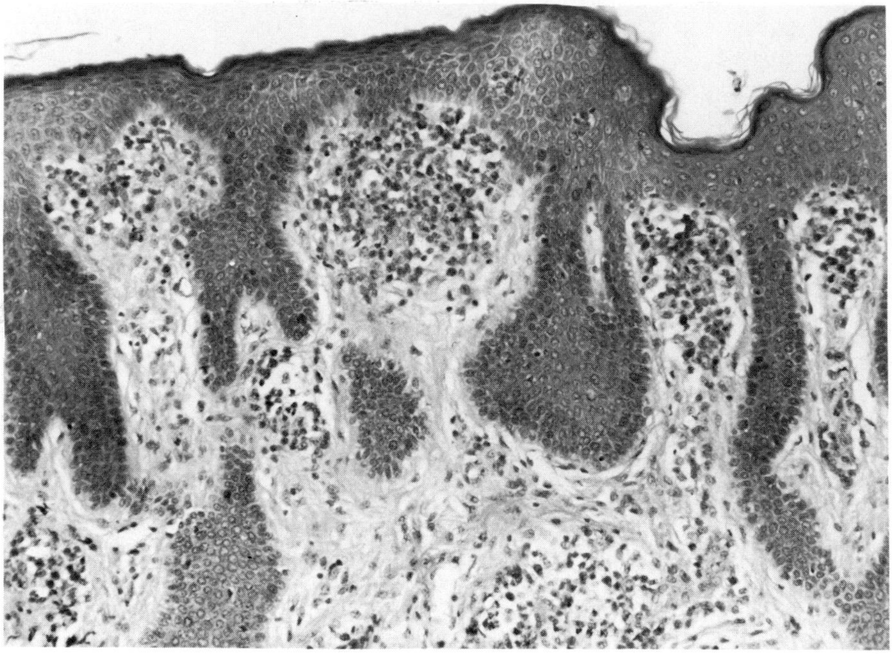

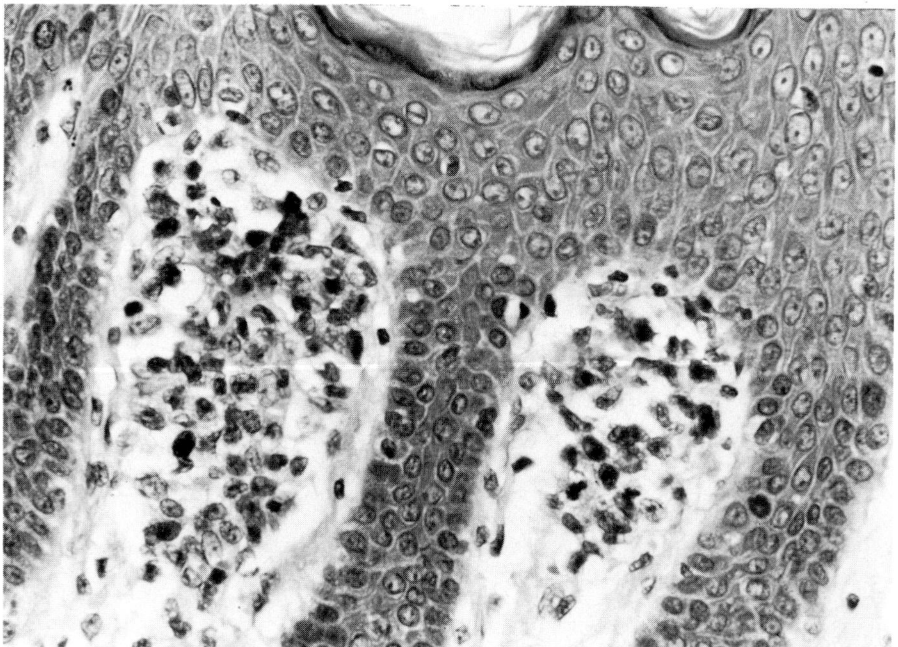

interdigitating reticulum cells (Fig. 9.10) which are best visualized in plastic embedded sections (Fig. 9.11). High endothelial lined venules are prominent (Fig. 9.12).

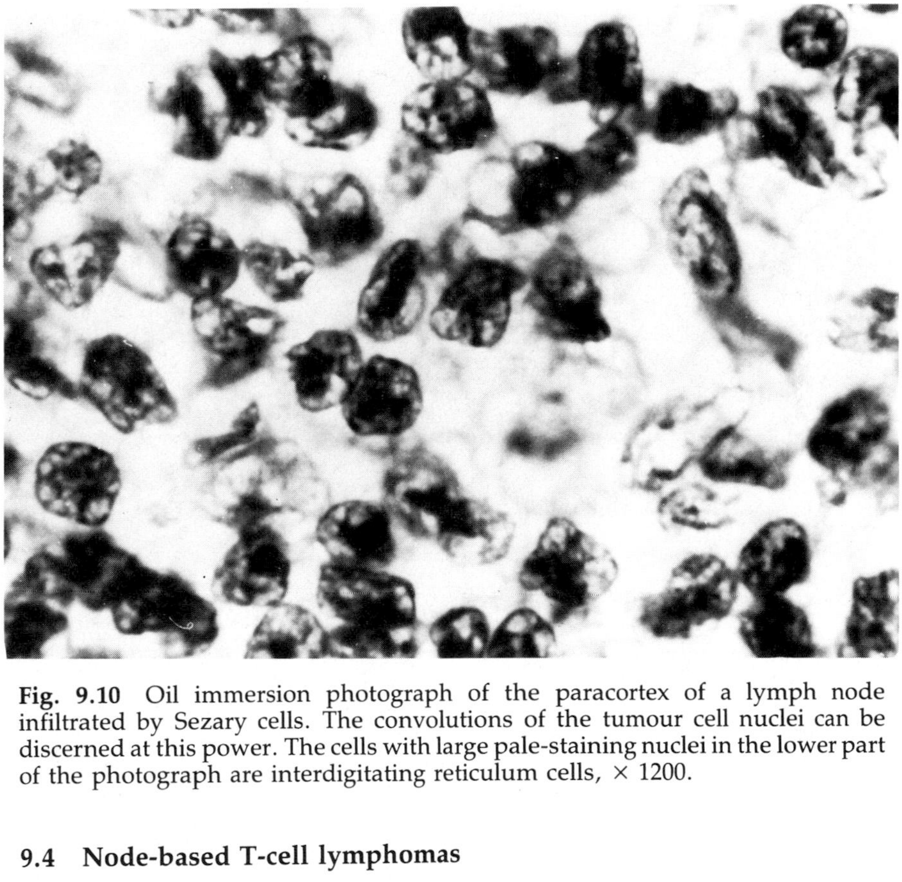

Fig. 9.10 Oil immersion photograph of the paracortex of a lymph node infiltrated by Sezary cells. The convolutions of the tumour cell nuclei can be discerned at this power. The cells with large pale-staining nuclei in the lower part of the photograph are interdigitating reticulum cells, × 1200.

9.4 Node-based T-cell lymphomas

In this group we describe lymphomas of T-cell type that present primarily with lymphadenopathy. Several authors have reported small series of node-based T-cell lymphomas and the full spectrum of clinical behaviour and morphology within each group and between groups is not, as yet, entirely clear. Larger series have been reported from Japan (Watanabe *et al.*, 1979; 1981) where T-cell tumours account for 40% of non-Hodgkin's

---

Fig. 9.8 Skin biopsy from a patient with Sezary's syndrome. Sezary cells infiltrate the papillary dermis, × 120.
Fig. 9.9 Higher power view of Fig. 9.8 showing irregularity of the tumour cell nuclei, × 300.

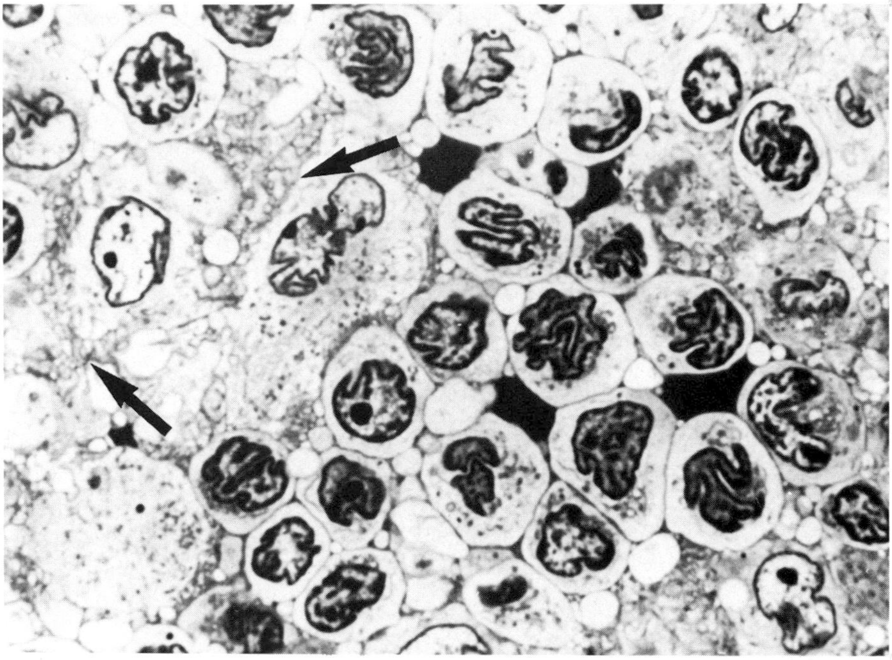

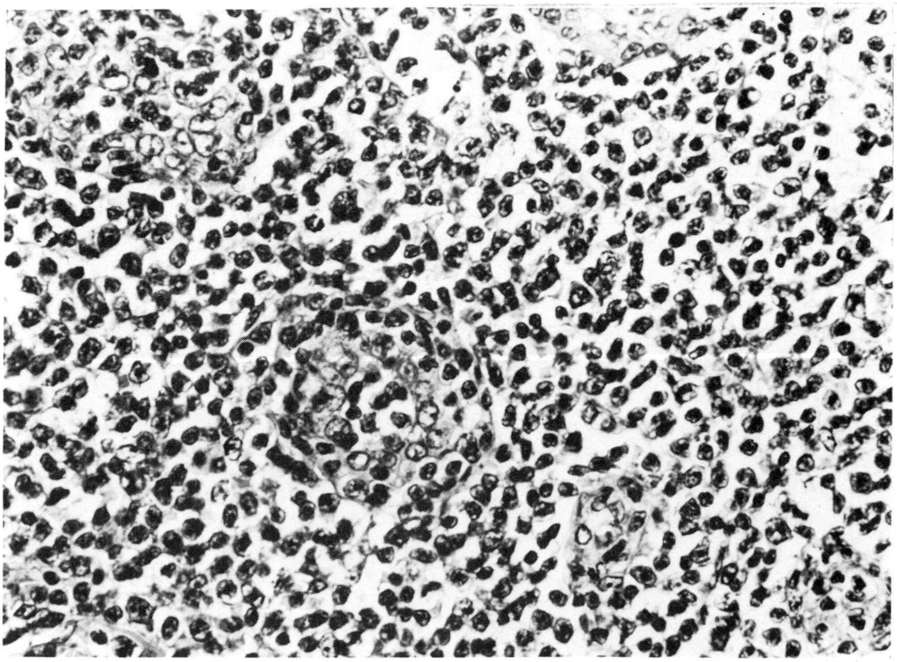

lymphomas. The relationship between the Japanese cases and those seen in Europe and North America has yet to be firmly established.

The node-based T-cell lymphoma was designated T-zone lymphoma by Lennert (1981) because the tumour contains all the components of the T-zones of lymphoid tissue and is, in a sense, analagous to follicular lymphoma which contains all the components of the follicle centre. As the disease progresses large blast cells replace all other elements and the tumour becomes a T-immunoblastic lymphoma. T-zone lymphoma is now considered to be the same entity as the peripheral T-cell lymphoma described by Waldron *et al.* (1977) and to show considerable overlap with the T-immunoblastic sarcoma of Lukes *et al.* (1978) and the T-cell lymphoma of pleomorphic type (Watanabe *et al.*, 1979; 1981).

The proliferation of high endothelial venules, epithelioid cells and plasma cells and, in some instances, the prominence of reactive follicle centres in peripheral T-cell lymphomas may be related to lymphokine production by the neoplastic T-cells. These neoplastic T-cells vary in shape and size and may assume giant cell forms resembling Reed–Sternberg cells. For this reason we have used the term 'T-cell lymphoma of pleomorphic type' to describe these tumours. However, the same term has been used by Watanbe *et al.* (1981) to describe a type of lymphoma that shows differences from the tumour that we designate pleomorphic T-cell lymphoma. The Japanese cases are not accompanied by infiltrates of eosinophils and epithelioid cells, nor the proliferation of high endothelial-lined venules. One-third of the patients have hypercalcaemia and they show a remarkable geographical distribution in Japan. Catovsky *et al.* (1982) reported six cases of T-cell lymphoma-leukaemia in blacks from the West Indies. Five of these patients had hypercalcaemia. Histologically these cases showed replacement of the lymph node architecture by small to medium lymphocytes with convoluted nuclei often exhibiting bizarre forms. This morphology corresponds to that described by Watanabe *et al.* (1981) for Japanese cases of pleomorphic T-cell lymphoma. Hypercalcaemia associated with T-cell lymphomas appears to be due to the production of osteoclast-activating factors by the tumour cells (Grossman *et al.*, 1981).

Fig. 9.11 Plastic embedded section of the same lymph node shown in Fig. 9.10. In this preparation the characteristic cerebriform nuclei of the Sezary cells are clearly visible. A group of interdigitating reticulum cells are seen to the left of the photograph. Their interdigitating cell membranes are clearly visible (arrows). Toluidine blue, × 1200.

Fig. 9.12 Involved lymph node from a patient with Sezary's syndrome. Note prominent high endothelial venules showing an active traffic of lymphoid cells, × 300.

Watanabe *et al.* (1980) also described a T-cell lymphoma with hyperglobulinaemia that histologically resembles angioimmunoblastic lymphadenopathy. This might represent a distinct entity but could be part of the spectrum of T-cell lymphoma, polymorphic type in which there is unusually marked stimulation of immunoglobulin production and of high endothelial venules.

The Japanese workers have described two types of monomorphic T-cell lymphoma (Watanabe *et al.*, 1979; 1981). One of these composed of medium-sized cells, may resemble malignant lymphoma centrocytic histologically and is frequently associated with skin lesions. The other is a large cell lymphoma which probably shows some overlap with the T-immunoblastic lymphoma of Lukes *et al.* (1978). Progression from polymorphic T-cell lymphoma to monomorphic large cell lymphoma has been described (Leong *et al.*, 1981), and Knowles and Halper (1982) reported two patients who showed progression from small cell cutaneous T-cell lymphomas to large pleomorphic and T-immunoblastic lymphomas.

Pinkus *et al.* (1979) described four cases of large T-cell lymphoma with clover-leaf or mulberry-like nuclei. In a retrospective study Weinberg and Pinkus (1981) subsequently reported ten cases of multilobated lymphoma identified by morphological criteria only. These cases had a predilection for skin, soft tissues and bone and had a good prognosis compared with other large cell lymphomas.

Malignant lymphomas with a high content of epithelioid cells (lymphoepithelioid lymphoma, Lennert's lymphoma) include T-cell lymphomas (Lennert, 1981). The infiltration of the tumour by epithelioid histiocytes in these cases is presumably related to the production of lymphokines by the neoplastic T-cells. The precise characterization of this type of T-cell lymphoma and its relationship to the other types requires further study.

Two cases of a unique T-cell lymphoma designated erythrophagocytic T-γ lymphoma with clinical and pathological features resembling malignant histiocytosis have been described by Kadin *et al.* (1981). The patients presented with hepatosplenomegaly and minimal lymphadenopathy, showed a poor response to chemotherapy and died after a short illness. The tumour cells formed rosettes with sheep red cells, reacted with monoclonal antibodies to T-cell antigens and bore receptors for the Fc components of IgG. They were non-specific esterase negative but showed phagocytosis of autologous red cells best seen in methacrylate-embedded sections. Kadin *et al.* (1981) postulate that this tumour arises from the population of T-γ lymphocytes normally resident in the spleen.

For the general pathologist this apparent profusion of subtypes of T-cell lymphoma is, no doubt, daunting, particularly in view of the small proportion of T-cell lymphomas in relation to other lymphomas seen in most practices. Nevertheless, T-cell lymphomas have a number of characteristic histological features that may alert the pathologist to their nature and stimulate him to seek further advice or further immunological marker studies. These features are set out in Table 9.1.

Table 9.1 Histopathological features of T-cell lymphomas

Many subtypes show:
Epidermotropism
Proliferation in paracortical region of lymph nodes or periarterial region of spleen
Irregular nuclear outline of tumour cells (cerebriform, squiggly, multilobated)
Large numbers of blood vessels lined by plump endothelial cells – often showing pronounced lymphocyte traffic
Epithelioid cells in sheets or clusters. Occasional giant cells
Variable eosinophil infiltrates

9.5 T-cell lymphoma: pleomorphic type (Lennert's T-zone lymphoma)

This lymphoma occurs over a wide age range but has a maximum incidence in the seventh decade. Clinically the patients usually present with lymphadenopathy which may rapidly become widespread. Hepatosplenomegaly and involvement of the lungs and pleura are common. Atypical cells are often present in the peripheral blood and may provide a convenient source of cells for immunological marker studies.

9.5.1 Histology

The tumour is first seen in the paracortical areas of the lymph node. Follicle centres may appear numerous and hyperplastic at this stage, possibly because they are being stimulated by the neoplastic T-cells (Fig. 9.13). As the disease progresses the follicles are displaced by neoplastic T-cells. The tumour cells usually show a range of sizes and appearances. The smallest cells have dark chromatin and nuclei that may be rounded but that are frequently very irregular. Interspersed amongst these are larger cells with rounded open vesicular nuclei with 2–4 prominent nucleoli. The cytoplasm is abundant and pale staining. All gradations between the large and small cells may be present (Figs 9.14 and 9.15). As the disease progresses blast cells come to dominate the picture.

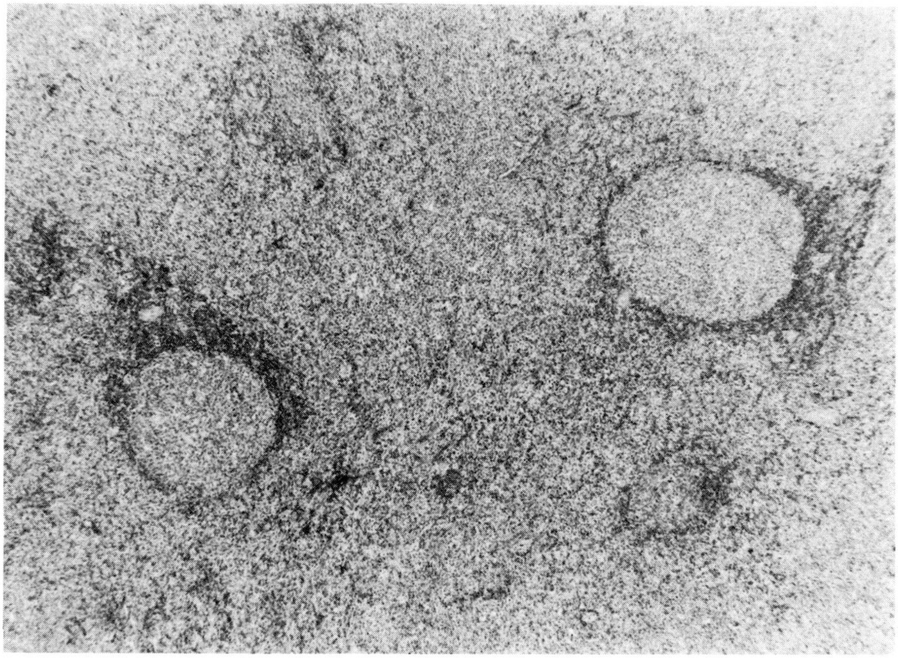

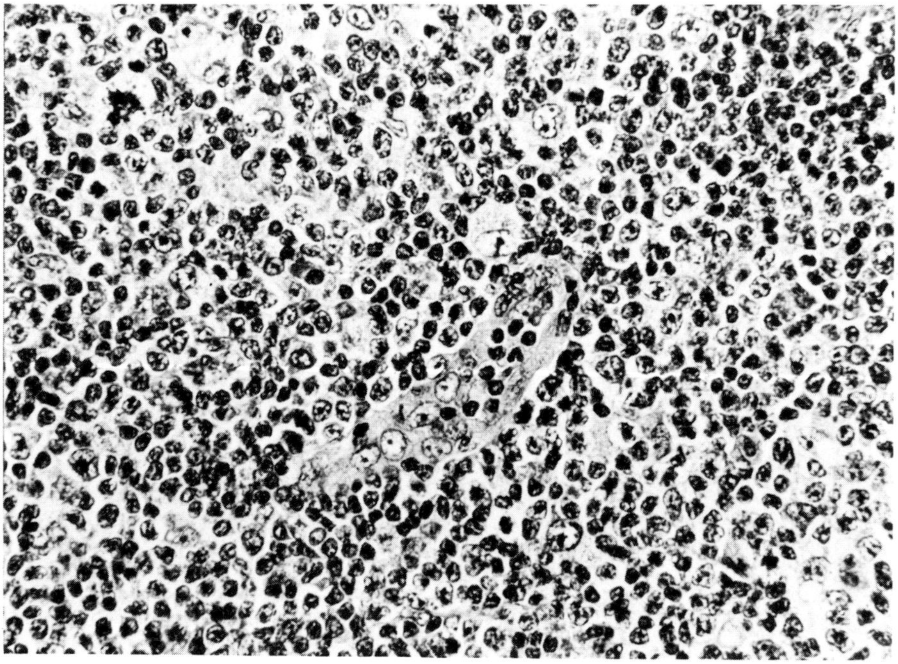

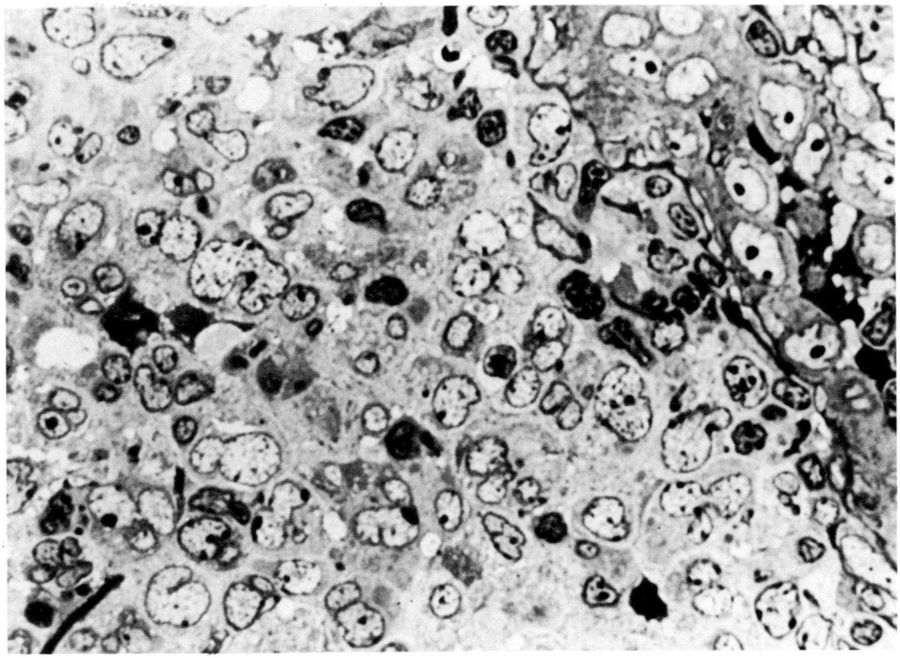

Fig. 9.15 Plastic embedded section of pleomorphic T-cell lymphoma. There is a high endothelial venule to the right of the photograph. Note the marked pleomorphism of the tumour cell nuclei. Toluidine blue, × 480.

Pleomorphic polylobated blast cells are not uncommon and may superficially resemble Reed–Sternberg cells (Fig. 9.16).

Blood vessels lined by plump endothelial cells are usually abundantly distributed between the tumour cells (Figs 9.14 and 9.15). Numerous small lymphoid cells are present in the walls of these vessels and may, to some extent, obscure them. The vessels may be highlighted by the PAS or the reticulin stain. Epithelioid cells and/or eosinophils may be present in the tumours in variable numbers. Plasma cells are sometimes present and may be numerous often appearing in clusters or islands.

9.5.2 Differential diagnosis

In our experience T-cell lymphoma of pleomorphic type is most

---

Fig. 9.13 Pleomorphic T-cell lymphoma (T-zone lymphoma) of lymph node. Prominent reactive lymphoid follicles are surrounded by lymphoma tissue, × 30.
Fig. 9.14 Pleomorphic T-cell lymphoma showing a prominent high endothelial lined venule surrounded by lymphoma cells showing a range of morphologies from small lymphocytes to large blast cells, × 300.

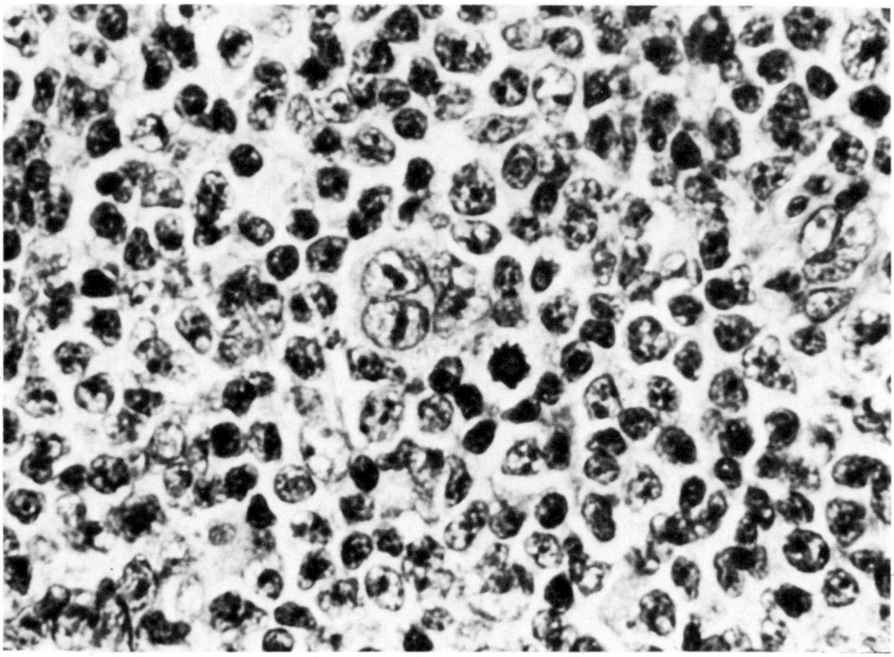

Fig. 9.16 Multinucleated 'Reed–Sternberg-like' cell in a pleomorphic T-cell lymphoma. The surrounding cells range from small lymphocytes to blast cells and would be inconsistent with any subtype of Hodgkin's disease, × 480.

frequently misdiagnosed as Hodgkin's disease. The pleomorphic giant cell forms of the T-blasts superficially resemble Reed–Sternberg cells and this impression may be reinforced by the presence of eosinophils and epithelioid cells. However, the background infiltrates of T-blasts and intermediate cells is not compatible with any sub-type of Hodgkin's disease.

The irregularity of the smaller T-cells may suggest centrocytes and lead to a diagnosis of centroblastic/centrocytic lymphoma. The blast cells do not, however, have the characteristic nuclear morphology of centroblasts and lack the cytoplasmic basophilia/pyroninophilia of these cells. Follicle centre cell lymphomas never occupy the paracortex in the presence of reactive follicles.

The differentiation between pleomorphic T-cell lymphoma with hypergammaglobulinaemia and angioimmunoblastic lymphadenopathy may be difficult. Plasma blasts and plasma cells are usually much more abundant in angioimmunoblastic lymphadenopathy and more widely dispersed throughout the lymph node. T-cell lymphomas rarely show the complex arborizing pattern of blood vessels that is characteristic of angioimmunoblastic lymphadenopathy. The presence of collections of blasts cells and polymorphism should always raise suspicions of lymphoma in such cases.

9.6 T-cell lymphoma: monomorphic, medium-sized cell type

9.6.1 Histology

The cells that comprise these lymphomas are medium sized and usually have markedly convoluted or irregular nuclei. Larger cells have more vesicular and less irregular nuclei with one or two eosinophilic nucleoli, mitotic figures are usually plentiful. High endothelial blood vessels showing an active traffic of lymphocytes may be prominent (Figs 9.17 and 9.18).

9.6.2 Differential diagnosis

The separation of this tumour from follicle centre cell lymphoma centrocytic or centroblastic/centrocytic diffuse can be difficult on

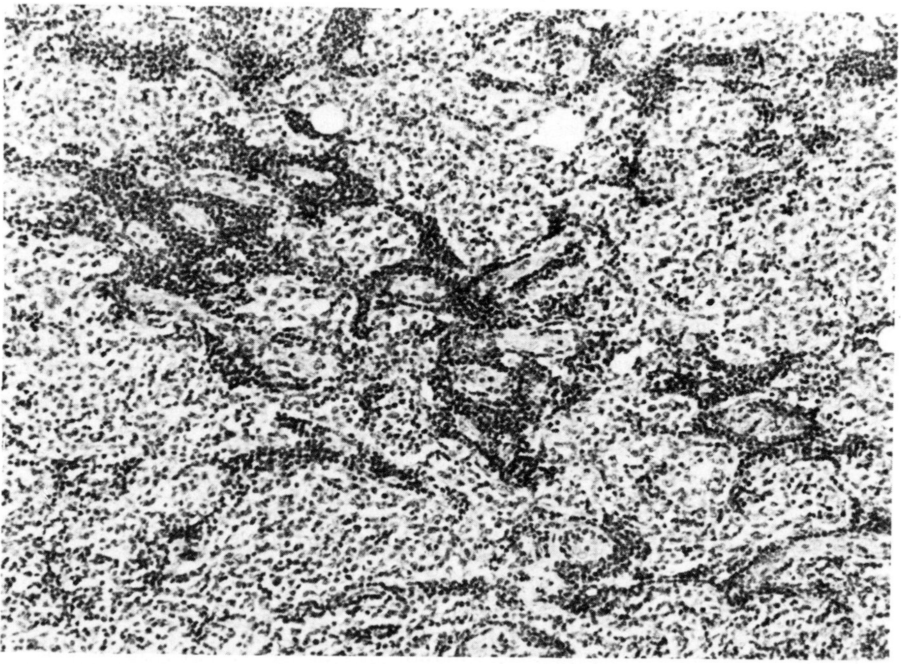

Fig. 9.17 T-cell lymphoma monomorphic medium-sized cell type. Note the prominent high endothelial vessels showing active lymphocyte traffic, × 120.

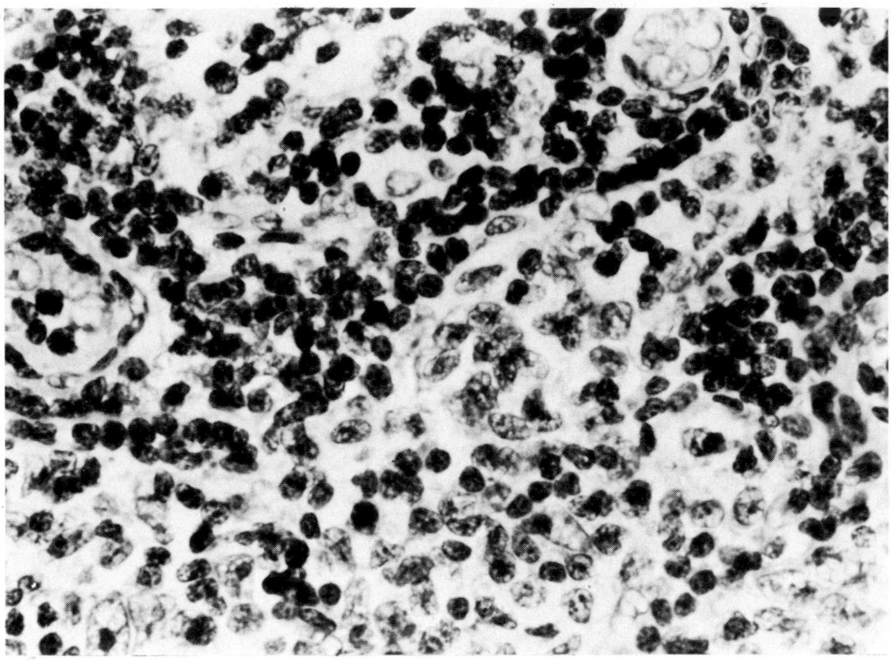

Fig. 9.18 Higher power view of the lymphoma illustrated in Fig. 9.17. Note the resemblance of the tumour cells to centrocytes, × 480.

histological features alone. The presence of high endothelial blood vessels is highly suggestive of a T-cell lymphoma but marker studies will be required to confirm the diagnosis.

9.7 T-cell lymphoma: monomorphic, large cell type

9.7.1 Histology

This tumour is composed of large blast cells with basophilic/pyronino-philic cytoplasm and nuclei that have a relatively regular or rounded outline in paraffin sections (Fig. 9.19) although greater degrees of pleomorphism may be seen in plastic embedded sections. Cytological preparations (Fig. 9.20) show blast cells with prominent nucleoli and

---

Fig. 9.19 T-cell lymphoma, monomorphic large cell type. The tumour cells have rounded nuclei, prominent nucleoli and dark-staining cytoplasm. Serpiginous T-lymphocytes can be seen between the blast cells, × 480.

Fig. 9.20 Cytocentrifuge preparation of tumour cells from lymphoma illustrated in Fig. 9.19 showing E-rosettes. The tumour cells have deeply staining basophilic cytoplasm with a pale area adjacent to the nuclear hof. Giemsa, × 1200.

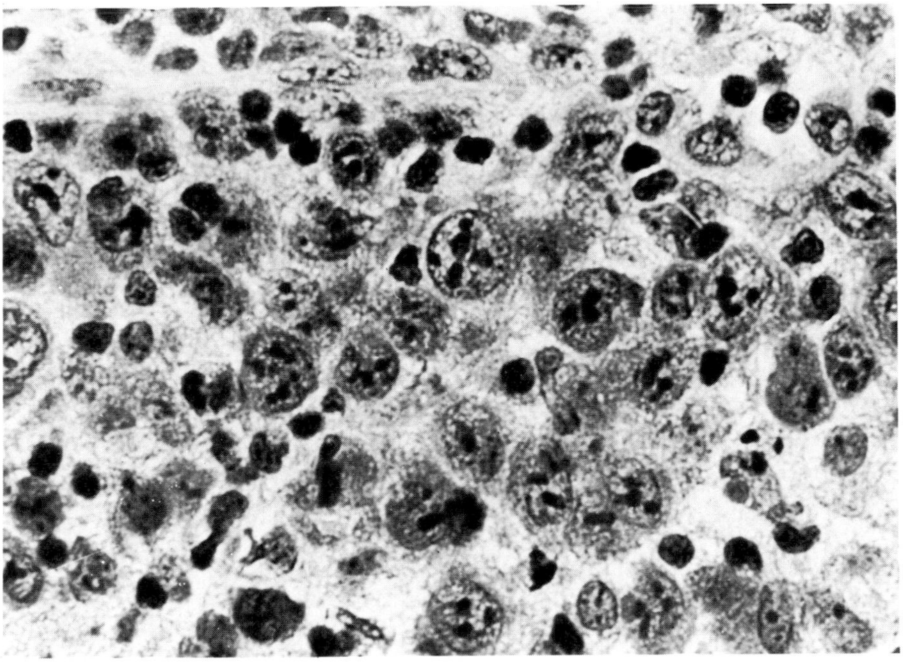

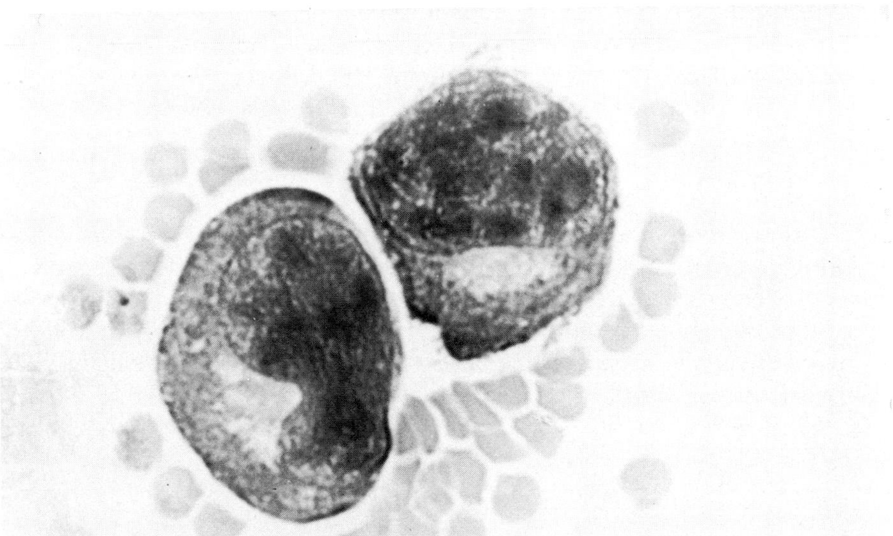

deeply basophilic cytoplasm. The nuclear chromatin is granular or clumped and from 2–4 prominent nucleoli are seen. Small irregular serpiginous T-lymphocytes are seen in clusters between the large cells, often in association with high endothelial venules.

9.7.2 *Differential diagnosis*

This tumour is most likely to be confused with centroblastic or immunoblastic lymphoma. A clue to its identity is provided by the presence of high endothelial venules and scattered small serpiginous T-lymphocytes. Final identification depends upon the use of immunological methods.

9.8 T-cell lymphoma of multilobated type

9.8.1 *Histology*

The characteristic feature of this large cell lymphoma is the extreme multilobation of the tumour cell nuclei giving them a clover leaf or mulberry appearance in histological sections (Fig. 9.21). This feature is best visualized in plastic embedded sections (Fig. 9.22). The tumour cells are relatively monomorphic and are not accompanied by the same proliferation of blood vessels, eosinophils and epithelioid histiocytes that is seen in many other T-cell lymphomas. The neoplastic T-cells have very finely dispersed nuclear chromatin, small inconspicuous nucleoli and a broad rim of pale or water clear cytoplasm.

9.8.2 *Differential diagnosis*

This tumour is most likely to be mistaken for a centroblastic or centroblastic/centrocytic lymphoma. Large follicle centre cells can show polylobated nuclei and this feature alone should not be used to diagnose the T-cell lymphoma of multilobated type. Follicle centre cell lymphomas have relatively coarse nuclear chromatin, large eosinophilic nuclei and pyroninophilic cytoplasm in contrast to the fine chromatin, small

---

Fig. 9.21 Multilobated T-cell lymphoma. Note mulberry-like configuration of many of the tumour cell nuclei, × 480.

Fig. 9.22 Plastic embedded section of tumour shown in Fig. 9.21 showing the multilobated tumour cell nuclei and their abundant pale-staining cytoplasm. Toluidine blue, × 1200.

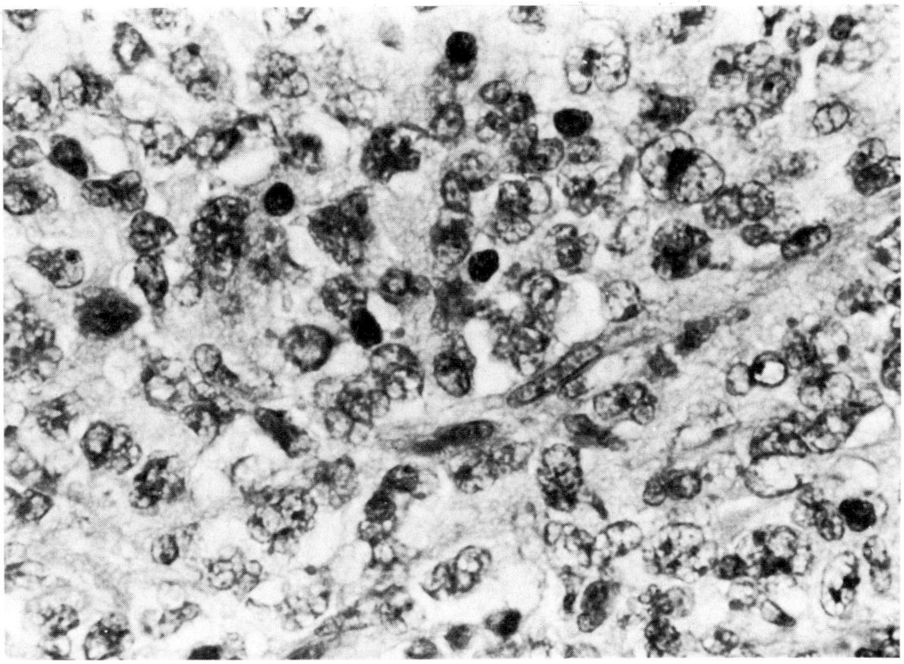

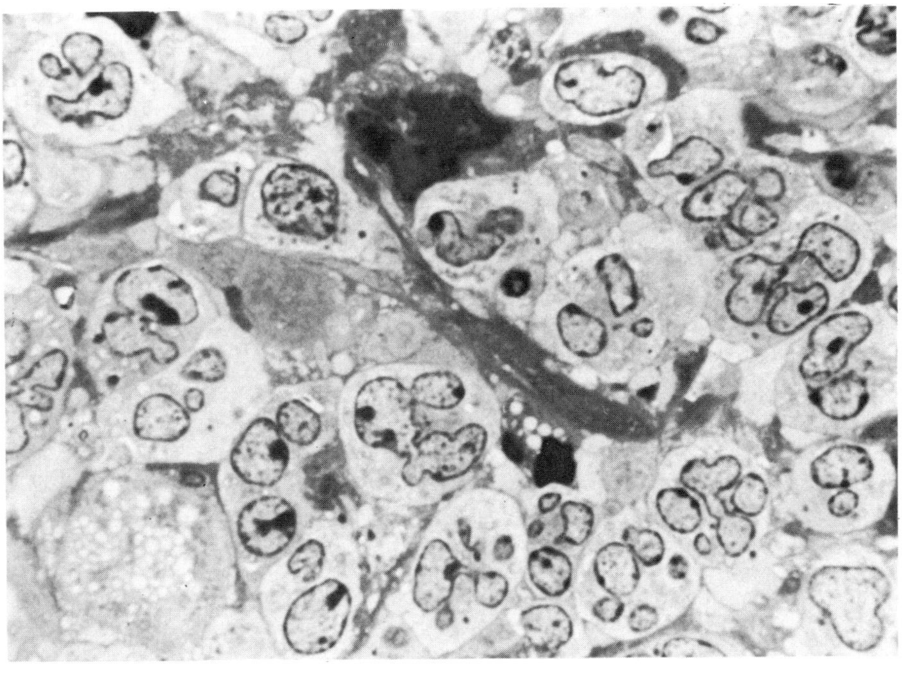

inconspicuous nucleoli and water clear cytoplasm of the multilobated T-cells.

9.9 Malignant lymphoma with a high content of epithelioid cells (Lennert's lymphoma)

Lennert and Mestdagh (1968) described a malignant lymphoma with a high content of epithelioid cells since when there has been considerable debate as to the nature of this tumour. These tumours were originally thought to be a form of Hodgkin's disease but because of the absence of typical Reed–Sternberg cells and the unusual progression of some of these cases, Lennert *et al.* (1975) recommended the term 'lymphoepithelioid lymphoma'. Dorfman (1975) and Lukes and Tindle (1975) adopted the term 'Lennert's lymphoma' for this tumour. Unfortunately this designation implies a specific entity whereas it is apparent that intense epithelioid cell infiltration may occur in a number of lymphomas of differing histogenetic type (Kim *et al.*, 1980). It is important, therefore, to attempt to identify the underlying lymphoma. This identification will be based on the morphological and functional characteristics of the lymphoid cells intervening between the clusters and sheets of epithelioid cells.

Many malignant lymphomas with a high content of epithelioid cells appear to be of the T-cell lineage. If the term 'Lennert's lymphoma' is to be used it is our opinion that it should be restricted to this epithelioid cell-rich lymphoma of T-cell type. It is not yet clear whether the tumour is part of the spectrum of pleomorphic T-cell lymphoma or a separate entity.

9.9.1 Histology

The epithelioid cells may appear as loose clusters or form almost confluent sheets (Figs 9.23 and 9.24). In lymph nodes showing early involvement the epithelioid cells are found predominantly in the paracortex. The neoplastic T-cells show a range of appearances between small, irregular serpiginous T-cells and T-immunoblasts (Fig. 9.25). Pleomorphic T-immunoblasts may show some resemblance to Reed–Sternberg cells (Fig. 9.26). Other characteristics of T-cell lymphomas may

---

Fig. 9.23 T-cell lymphoma with a high content of epithelioid cells. Low power view shows loss of nodel architecture and loose aggregates of epithelioid cells, × 30.

Fig. 9.24 Higher power view of Fig. 9.23. High endothelial venules are visible amongst the lymphoid cells between the epithelioid cell aggregates (arrows), × 120.

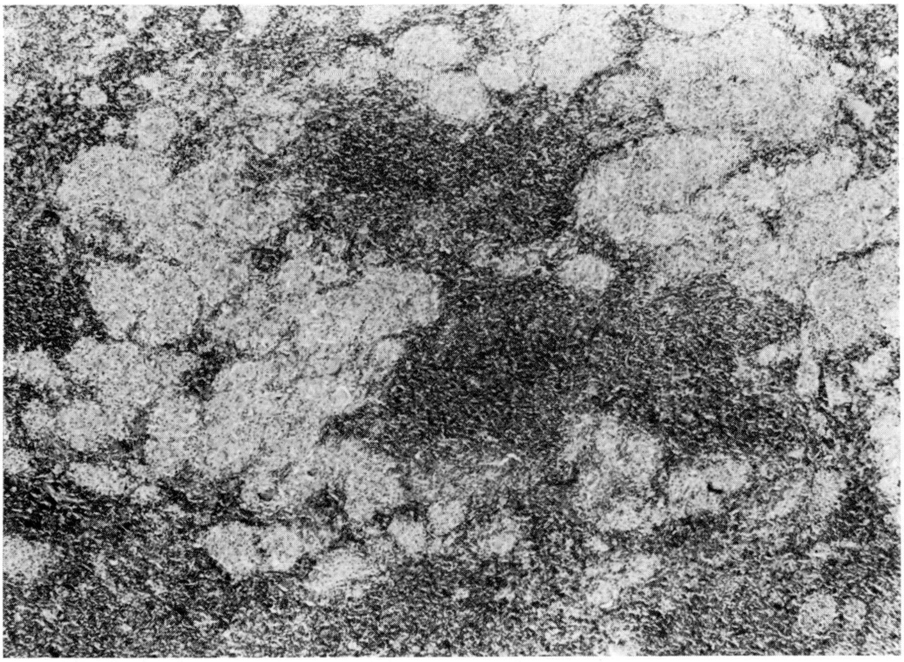

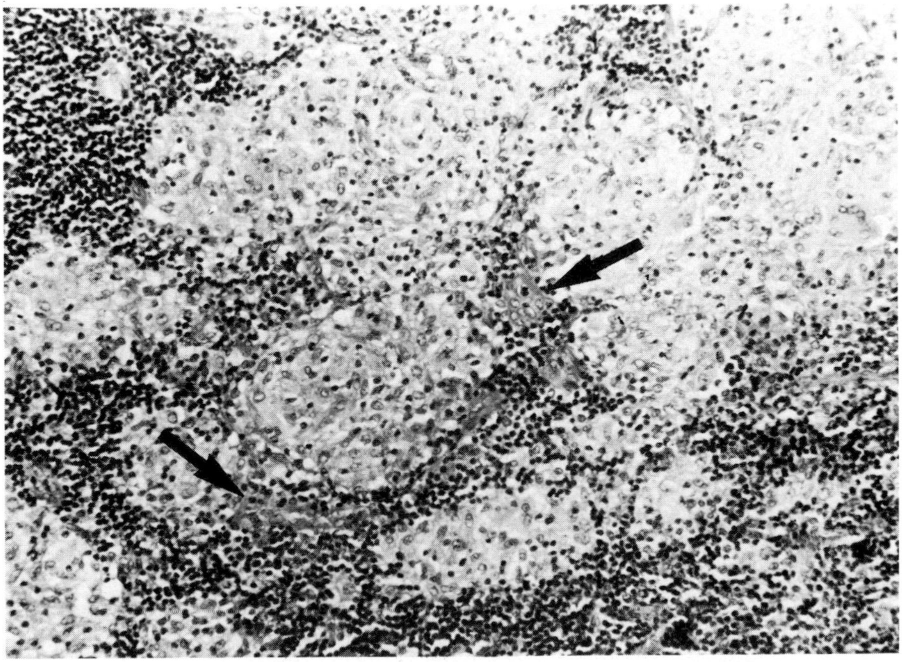

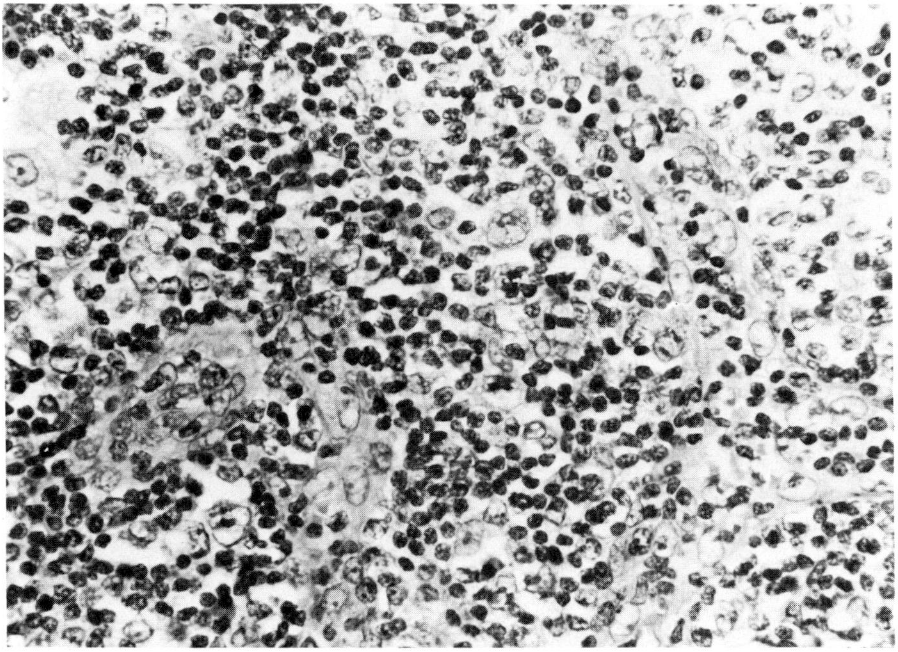

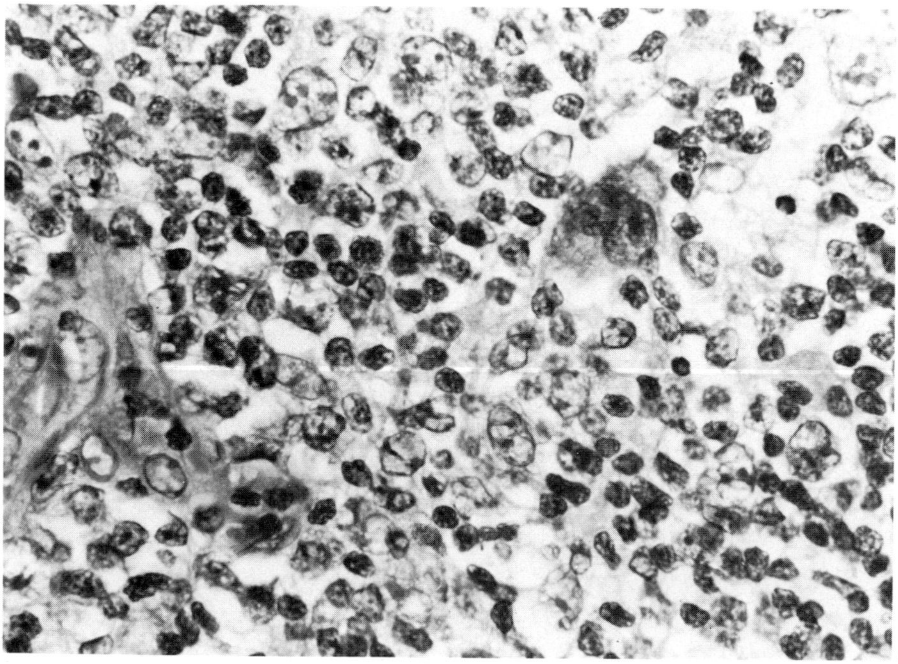

be present such as high endothelial venules and eosinophils. Focal collections of plasma cells may also be prominent particularly in sections stained by methyl green pyronin.

9.9.2 *Differential diagnosis*

When confronted with a lymph node containing large numbers of epithelioid cells, an attempt should be made to identify the underlying tumour or other pathology. In some cases this will be Hodgkin's disease in which case characteristic Reed–Sternberg cells in an appropriate cellular setting should be seen. Lymphoplasmacytic/cytoid and follicle centre cell lymphomas sometimes contain an intense infiltrate of epithelioid cells. Immunohistochemistry and marker studies will often help in the identification of these cases. Large numbers of epithelioid cells have been reported in some cases of angioimmunoblastic lymphadenopathy. In view of the difficulty that may be experienced in separating angioimmunoblastic lymphadenopathy from T-cell lymphomas it is possible that some of the reported cases with a high content of epithelioid cells have, in fact, been T-cell lymphomas.

Epithelioid cells that are part of a granulomatous process must be differentiated from those occurring in association with malignant lymphomas. The granulomas in sarcoidosis are usually much better defined than the loose collections of epithelioid cells seen in malignant lymphoma. The presence of areas of necrosis should raise suspicions of infection with acid-fast bacilli, fungi or other organisms. In toxoplasmosis the lymph node shows reactive hyperplasia and the epithelioid cell clusters surround and often invade germinal centres (see Chapter 2).

References

Brouet, J. C., Flandrin, G., Sasportes, M. *et al.* (1975), Chronic lymphocytic leukaemia of T-cell origin. Immunological and clinical evaluation in 11 patients. *Lancet*, **ii**, 890–3.

Burke, J. S. and Colby, T. V. (1981), Dermatopathic lymphadenopathy. Comparison of cases associated and unassociated with mycosis fungoides. *Am. J. Surg. Pathol.*, **5**, 343–52.

Catovsky, D., Greaves, M. F., Rose, M. *et al.* (1982), Adult T-cell lymphoma-leukaemia in blacks from the West Indies. *Lancet*, **i**, 639–43.

Fig. 9.25 Higher power view of Fig. 9.24 showing high endothelial venules and mixed lymphoid population, × 300.

Fig. 9.26 Binucleate cells in the tumour illustrated in Fig. 9.23. Note that the accompanying population of lymphoid cells ranging from small lymphocytes to blast cells is inappropriate for any subtype of Hodgkin's disease, × 480.

Collins, R. D., Waldron, J. A. and Glick, A. D. (1979), Results of multiparameter studies of T-cell lymphoid neoplasms. *Am. J. Clin. Pathol.*, **72**, 699–707.

Dorfman, R. (1975), Lymphadenopathy. Letter to the Editor. *Human Pathol.*, **6**, 264.

Grossman, B., Schechter, G. P., Horton, J. E. *et al.* (1981), Hypercalcemia associated with T-cell lymphoma-leukemia. *Am. J. Clin. Pathol.*, **75**, 149–55.

Kadin, M. E., Kamoun, M. and Lamberg, J. (1981), Erythrophagocytic Tγ lymphoma. A clinicopathologic entity resembling malignant histiocytosis. *New Engl. J. Med.*, **304**, 648–53.

Kim, H., Nathwani, B. N. and Rappaport, H. (1980), So-called 'Lennert's lymphoma'. Is it a clinicopathological entity? *Cancer*, **45**, 1379–99.

Knowles, D. M. II. and Halper, J. P. (1982), Human T-cell malignancies. Correlative clinical, histopathologic, immunologic and cytochemical analysis of 23 cases. *Am. J. Pathol.*, **106**, 187–203.

Kung, P. C., Berger, C. L., Goldstein, G. *et al.* (1981), Cutaneous T-cell lymphoma: characterization by monoclonal antibodies. *Blood*, **57**, 261–6.

Lawrence, E. C., Broder, S., Jaffe, E. S. *et al.* (1978), Evolution of a lymphoma with helper T-cell characteristics in Sezary's syndrome. *Blood*, **52**, 481–92.

Lennert, K. (1981), *Histopathology of Non-Hodgkin's Lymphomas (Based on the Kiel Classification)*, Springer-Verlag, Berlin.

Lennert, K. and Mestdagh, J. (1968), Lymphogranulomatosen mit konstant hohem Epitheloidzellgehalt. (Hodgkin's disease with constantly high content of epithelioid cells). *Virchow Arch. (Pathol. Anat.)*, **344**, 1–20.

Lennert, K., Stein, H. and Kaiserling, E. (1975), Cytological and functional criteria for the classification of malignant lymphomata. *Br. J. Cancer*, **31** (Suppl. II), 29–43.

Leong, A. S.-Y., Dale, B. M., Liew, S.-H. *et al.* (1981), Node based T-cell lymphoma. The clinical immunological and morphological spectrum. *Pathology*, **13**, 79–95.

Lukes, R. J., Parker, J. W., Taylor, C. R. *et al.* (1978), Immunological approach to non-Hodgkin's lymphomas and related leukemias. Analysis of the results of multiparameter studies of 425 cases. *Semin. Haematol.*, **15**, 322–51.

Lukes, R. J. and Tindle, B. H. (1975), Immunoblastic lymphadenopathy. A hyperimmune entity resembling Hodgkin's disease. *New Engl. J. Med.*, **292**, 1–8.

Lutzner, M. A., Hobbs, J. W. and Horvath, P. (1971), Ultrastructure of abnormal cells in Sezary's syndrome, mycosis fungoides and parapsoriasis en plaque. *Arch. Dermatol.*, **103**, 375–86.

Lutzner, M. A. and Jordan, H. W. (1968), The ultrastructure of an abnormal cell in Sezary's syndrome. *Blood*, **31**, 719–26.

Pinkus, G. S., Said, J. W. and Hargreaves, H. (1979), Malignant lymphoma, T-cell type. A distinct morphologic variant with large multilobated nuclei, with a report of four cases. *Am. J. Clin. Pathol.*, **72**, 540–50.

Scheffer, E., Meijer, C. J. L. M. and Van Vloten, W. A. (1980), Dermatopathic lymphadenopathy and lymph node involvement in mycosis fungoides. *Cancer*, **45**, 137–48.

Waldron, J. A., Leech, J. H., Glick, A. D. *et al.* (1977), Malignant lymphoma of peripheral T-lymphocyte origin. Immunologic pathologic and clinical features in six patients. *Cancer*, **40**, 1604–17.

Watanabe, S., Nakajima, T., Schimosata, Y. *et al.* (1979), T-cell malignancies: Subclassification and interrelationship. *Jpn. J. Clin. Oncol.*, **9** (Suppl.), 423–42.

Watanabe, S., Shimosato, Y., Shimoyama, M. *et al.* (1980), Adult T-cell lymphoma with hypergammaglobulinemia. *Cancer*, **46**, 2472–83.

Watanabe, S., Shimosato, Y. and Shimoyama, M. (1981), Lymphoma and leukemia of T-lymphocytes in *Pathology Annual* 1981, Part 2 (eds S. C. Sommers and P. P. Rosen), Appleton-Century Crofts, New York, pp. 155–203.

Weinberg, D. S. and Pinkus, G. (1981), Non-Hodgkin's lymphoma of large multilobated cell type. A clinicopathologic study of ten cases. *Am. J. Clin. Pathol.*, **76**, 190–6.

10 Malignant lymphoma of B- and T-cell precursors

10.1 Lymphoblastic lymphomas

Lymphoblastic lymphoma occurs at all ages (Nathwani *et al.*, 1981; Streuli *et al.*, 1981) but is most frequently seen in childhood and adolescence. In Europe and North America it is the commonest non-Hodgkin's lymphoma of the paediatric age group. A high proportion of patients with lymphoblastic lymphoma, particularly in the younger age groups have, or subsequently develop, lymphoblastic leukaemia. The use of marker studies, specific antibodies and cytochemistry has identified four subtypes of acute lymphoblastic leukaemia (ALL), (Greaves, 1981) (Table 10.1). Lymphoblastic lymphoma and leukaemia share immunological and clinical features and may be regarded as different stages of

Table 10.1 (Modified from Greaves, 1981)

Type	M : F	WBC> $100 \times 10^9\ l^{-1}$ (%)	Hb> $8\ g\ dl^{-1}$ (%)	Mediastinal mass
C-ALL	1.3 : 1	8.7	38	0/274
Null	1.5 : 1	12.3	34.8	0/68
T-ALL	4.6 : 1	23.5	68.6	33/63
B-ALL	4 : 0	0	–	0/4

C-ALL Common acute lymphoblastic leukaemia. Tumour cells have no recognizable T- or B-cell surface markers but bear the common acute lymphoblastic leukaemia antigen (C-ALL).
Null-ALL Same as C-ALL but tumour cells do not bear C-ALL antigen.
T-ALL T-cell acute lymphoblastic leukaemia. Tumour cells form E-rosettes and have focal positivity for acid phosphatase. Surface marker and cytochemical reactions indicate that the majority of these tumours arise at the prothymocyte stage of differentiation (Stein *et al.*, 1976; Lennert, 1981).
B-ALL B-cell acute lymphoblastic leukaemia. Tumour cells have membrane immunoglobulin.

progression of the same neoplasm (Crist *et al.*, 1981). However although the most prevalent subtypes of lymphoblastic leukaemia are of the common or null-cell phenotype, the T-cell or B-cell phenotypes are more frequently associated with tumour masses and are, therefore, more likely to be seen by histopathologists. The anatomical distribution of the tumour gives a clue to its phenotype. Most abdominal tumours are of B-cell type and mediastinal tumours of T-cell type whereas those presenting as peripheral lymphadenopathy are usually of null-cell or T-cell type (Crist *et al.*, 1981).

The phenotype of most cases of C-ALL and null-ALL identified by the use of monoclonal antibodies indicates that these arise from a B-cell precursor in bone marrow (Greaves, 1981; Vogler *et al.*, 1981). The tumour cells may express or lose the common ALL antigen during the course of the disease. These two leukaemias have similar clinical and haematological features and may be regarded as a single tumour entity.

The tumour cells of B-ALL have features of Burkitt's lymphoma cells (Bennett *et al.*, 1976), and these cases are sometimes referred to as Burkitt's cell leukaemia. B-ALL is usually associated with extramedullary tumour masses, particularly in the gastrointestinal tract. Greaves (1981) is of the opinion that B-ALL is not a primary bone marrow-derived leukaemia but is a rapidly disseminated lymphoma. It would appear that most, if not all cases of B-ALL represent involvement of the bone marrow with spillover into the blood from a Burkitt's or Burkitt's-like lymphoma. These tumours appear to arise from a functionally more mature cell than those that give rise to lymphoblastic lymphoma (Bernard *et al.*, 1979) and should not be classified with them.

Lymphoblastic lymphoma of T-cell type occurs at all ages but the majority of cases are seen in the first two decades of life. It has a higher male-to-female ratio than other lymphoblastic lymphomas. The tumour commonly presents as lymphadenopathy or as a mediastinal (thymic) mass. Barcos and Lukes (1975) proposed the term 'malignant lymphoma of convoluted lymphocytes' for this neoplasm, and it is designated as 'lymphoblastic lymphoma of convoluted cell type' in the Kiel classification. Nathwani *et al.* (1976), however, investigated 30 cases of lymphoblastic lymphoma and could find no clinical or anatomical differences between those with and those without nuclear convolutions. Similarly Pangalis *et al.* (1979) in a study of 101 patients with acute lymphoblastic leukaemia found no correlation between nuclear convolutions and clinical parameters. In neither of these studies were immunological and cytochemical data presented. Our own experience, and that of other workers (Bernard *et al.*, 1979; Lennert, 1981; Navas Palacios *et al.*, 1981) is that some T-cell lymphoblastic lymphomas do not have convoluted nuclei. It would not seem appropriate, therefore, to designate this tumour convoluted cell lymphoma although deep nuclear convolutions when present, are usually indicative of a T-cell neoplasm.

10.1.1 Histology and cytology

The cytology of lymphoblastic lymphoma/leukaemia may be studied in blood and bone marrow smears, malignant effusions or touch preparations of biopsies. The morphology of the cells varies slightly in specimens from these different sources. The tumour cells have rounded or oval nuclei and convolutions, when present, appear in these preparations as lines or folds across the nucleus. Nucleoli number from 2–5 and the nuclear chromatin is fine and evenly dispersed (Fig. 10.1). A moderately basophilic rim of cytoplasm sometimes contains small vacuoles corresponding to dissolved neutral fat droplets.

Lymphoblastic lymphomas infiltrate tissues in a characteristic fashion displacing resident cells without destroying the underlying tissue structure (Figs 10.2 and 10.3). Thus, in the lymph nodes the reticulin stain will often show preservation of the pattern of the sinusoids which have become filled out and obscured by lymphoma cells (Fig. 10.4). The tumour cells characteristically infiltrate between connective tissue fibres in an indian-file fashion, this being particularly well seen in the capsule of the lymph node and around blood vessels (Figs 10.5 and 10.6). Lymphoblastic lymphoma cells have rounded, oval, or convoluted nuclei (Figs 10.7–10.10). The nuclear chromatin is fine and evenly dispersed with from 2–5 small eosinophilic nucleoli. The cytoplasm is not well defined and is only moderately basophilic/pyroninophilic. Plastic embedded tissues sectioned at 1 μm are particularly valuable for studying the cytological features of lymphoblastic lymphomas and nuclear convolutions are best demonstrated in these preparations (Fig. 10.10). Mitotic figures are frequent and in many cases numerous pyknotic nuclei and nuclear fragments indicate a high rate of cell death (Fig. 10.11). In such cases the presence of reactive histiocytes that have phagocytosed cell debris may give a starry-sky pattern. Preferential invasion of the paracortex of the lymph node with sparing of the follicles is a morphological feature suggestive of T-lymphoblastic lymphoma (Figs 10.12 and 10.13). In many cases confirmation of the phenotype can be obtained by performing immunological marker studies and cytochemistry on the tumour cells present in bone marrow or blood. Focal positivity

---

Fig. 10.1 Cytology of lymphoblastic lymphoma-leukaemia, (a) showing tumour cells in a bone marrow smear, (b) in an imprint preparation from a lymph node biopsy. Giemsa, × 1200.

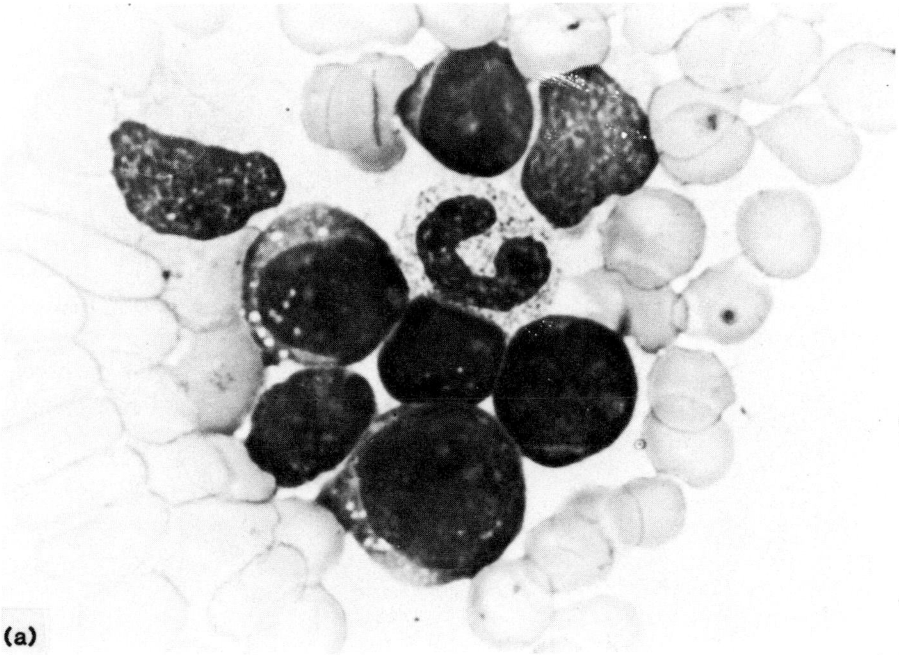
(a)

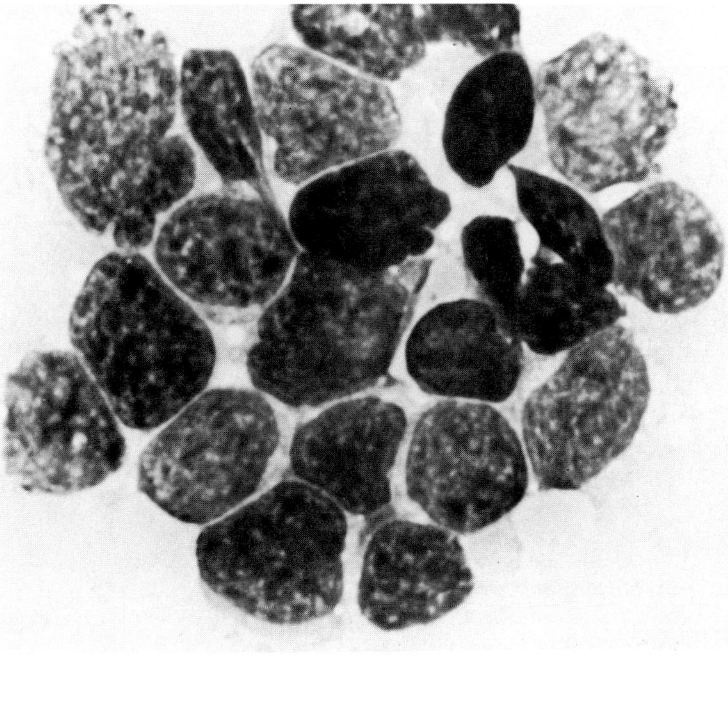
(b)

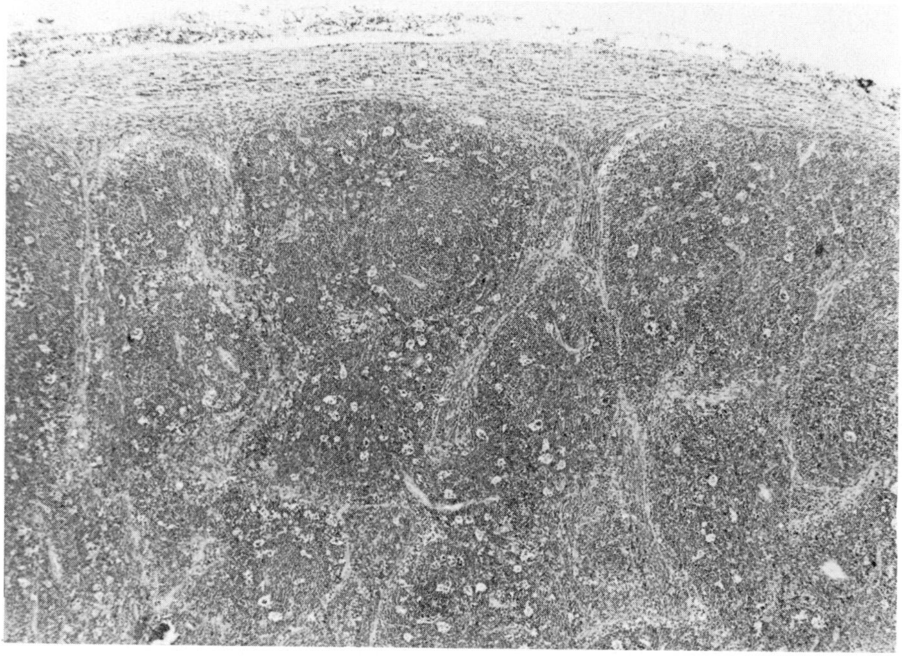

Fig. 10.2 Lymphoblastic lymphoma. Low power view of lymph node biopsy. The lymph node is diffusely infiltrated by lymphoma cells but the pre-existing structure can still be discerned, × 30.

for acid phosphatase (Fig. 10.14) appears to be a particularly reliable cytochemical method for identifying T-lymphoblasts and may be particularly useful when insufficient cells are available for rosetting techniques (Savage *et al.*, 1981).

In relapse, lymphoblastic leukaemia/lymphoma commonly infiltrates the meninges and the gonads. Some centres undertake testicular biopsy at the end of treatment to exlude occult disease. Whereas it is usually easy to recognize frank tumour infiltration (Fig. 10.15), it can be difficult to identify small numbers of neoplastic cells. Immunohistochemical staining of frozen sections for terminal transferase, an enzyme present in leukaemic lymphoblasts, may assist in this identification (Greaves, 1981).

Fig. 10.3 Lymphoblastic lymphoma showing preserved lymph node sinusoids filled out with lymphoma cells, × 300.
Fig. 10.4 Reticulin stain of lymphoblastic lymphoma showing preservation of much of the pre-existing lymph node structure, × 30.

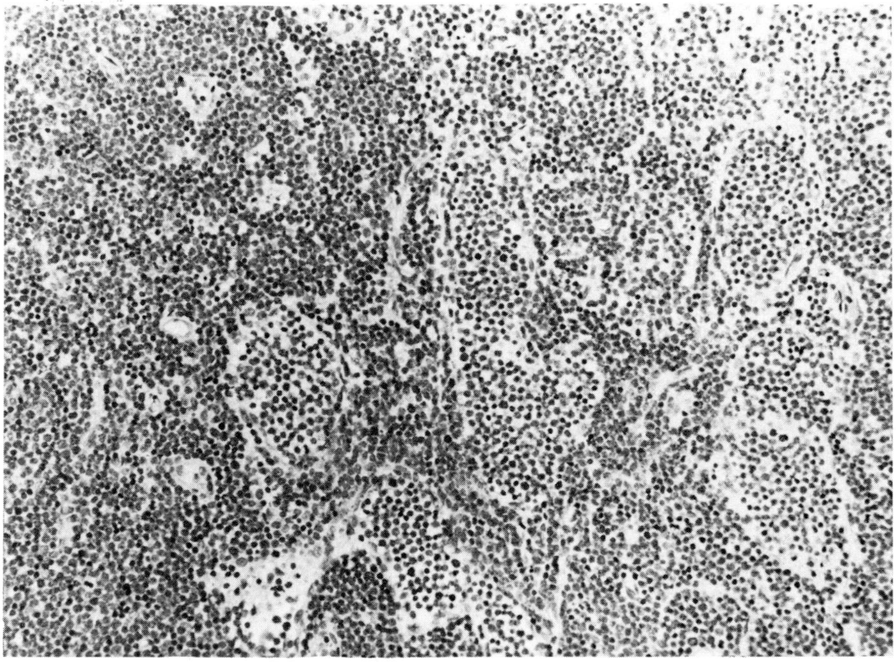

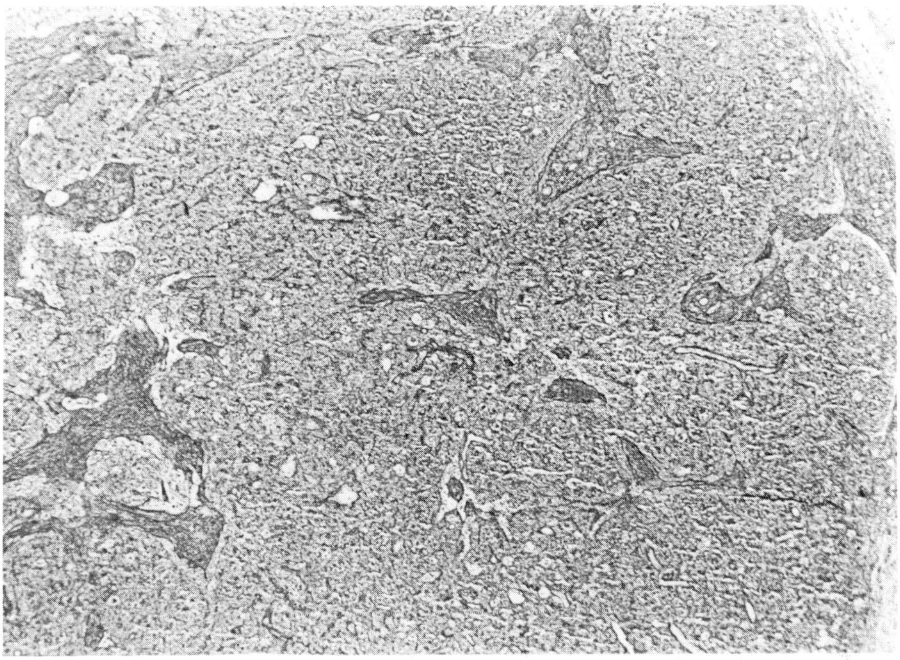

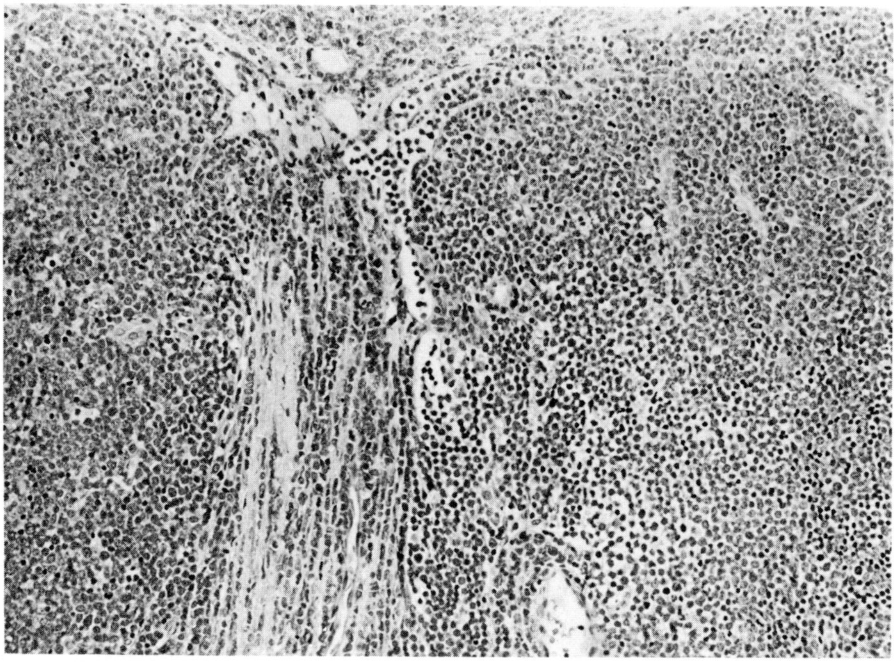

Fig. 10.5 Section of lymphoblastic lymphoma showing indian-file infiltration of a fibrous trabeculum. The adjacent sinus is loosely filled with lymphoma cells, × 120.

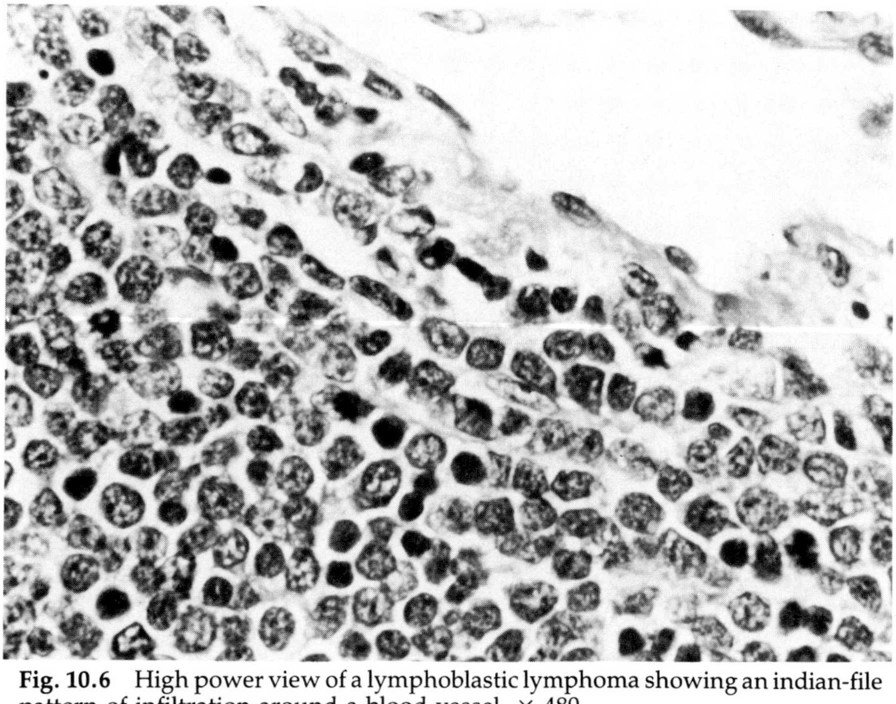

Fig. 10.6 High power view of a lymphoblastic lymphoma showing an indian-file pattern of infiltration around a blood vessel, × 480.

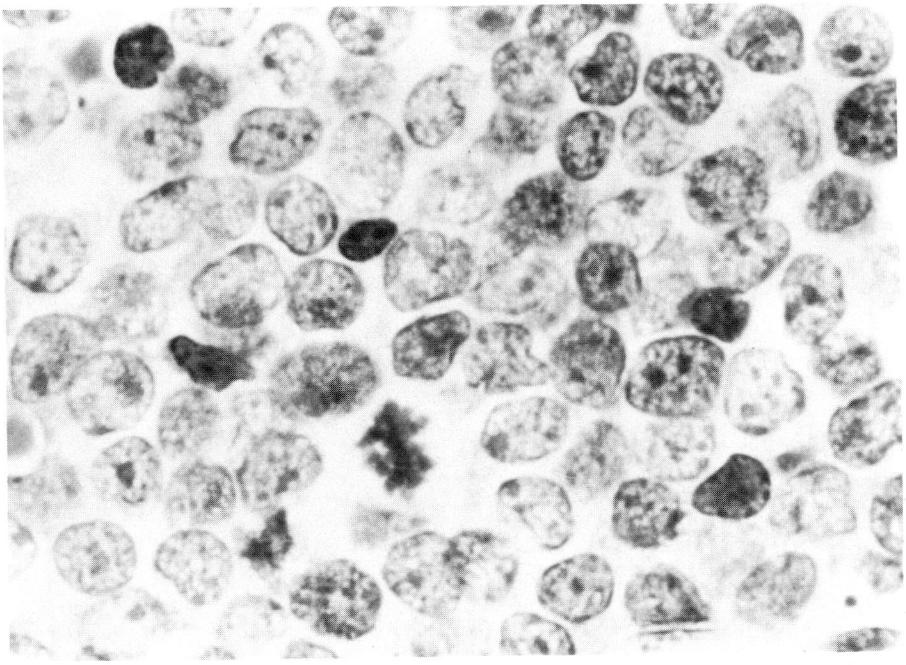

Fig. 10.7 Lymphoblastic lymphoma, high power view, showing delicate nuclear chromatin structure, small nucleoli and poorly defined cytoplasm. Few cells show nuclear convolutions, × 1200.

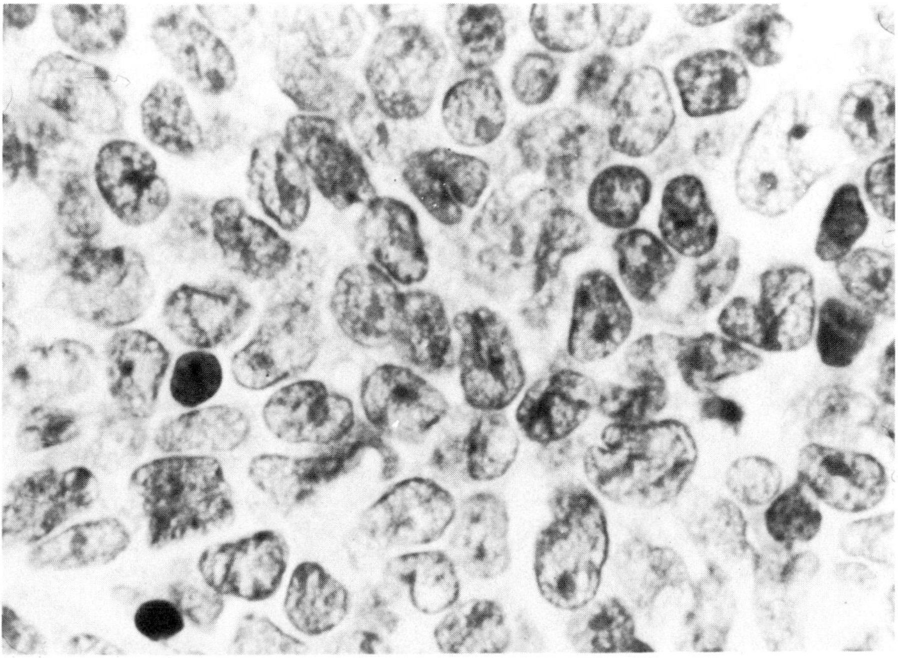

Fig. 10.8 High power photograph of a lymphoblastic lymphoma. Most of the cells in this tumour show nuclear convolutions, × 1200.

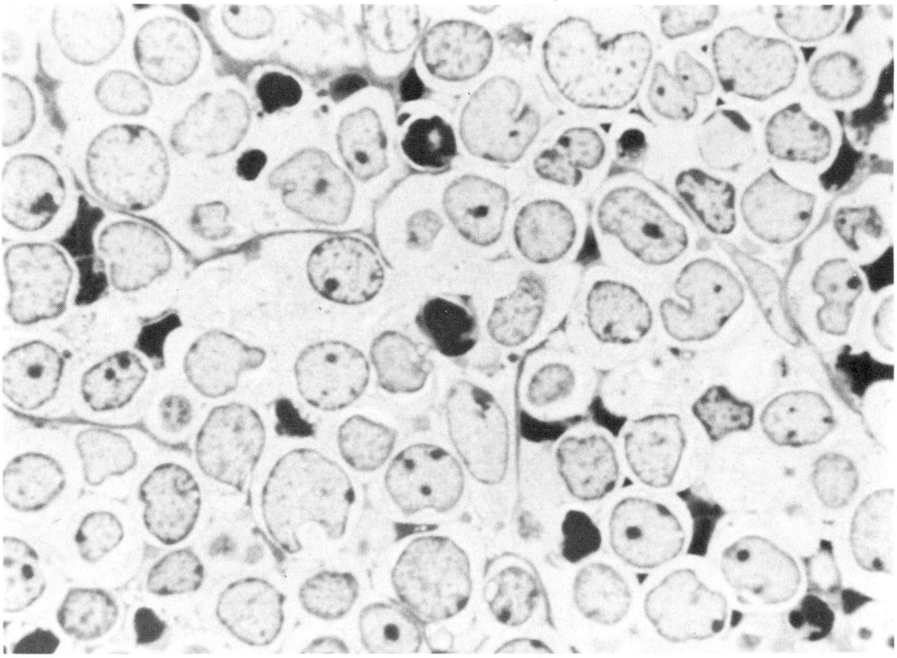

Fig. 10.9 Plastic embedded section of lymphoblastic lymphoma. Nuclear clefts are infrequent. Note the fine nuclear chromatin, small nucleoli and pale-staining cytoplasm. Toluidine blue, × 1200.

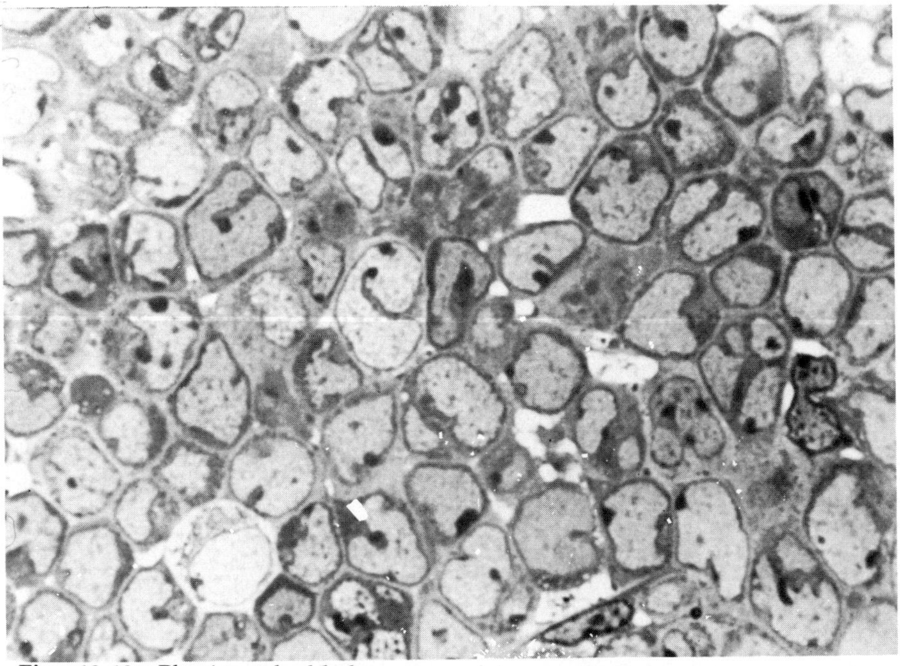

Fig. 10.10 Plastic embedded section of lymphoblastic lymphoma showing prominent nuclear convolutions. Toluidine blue, × 1200.

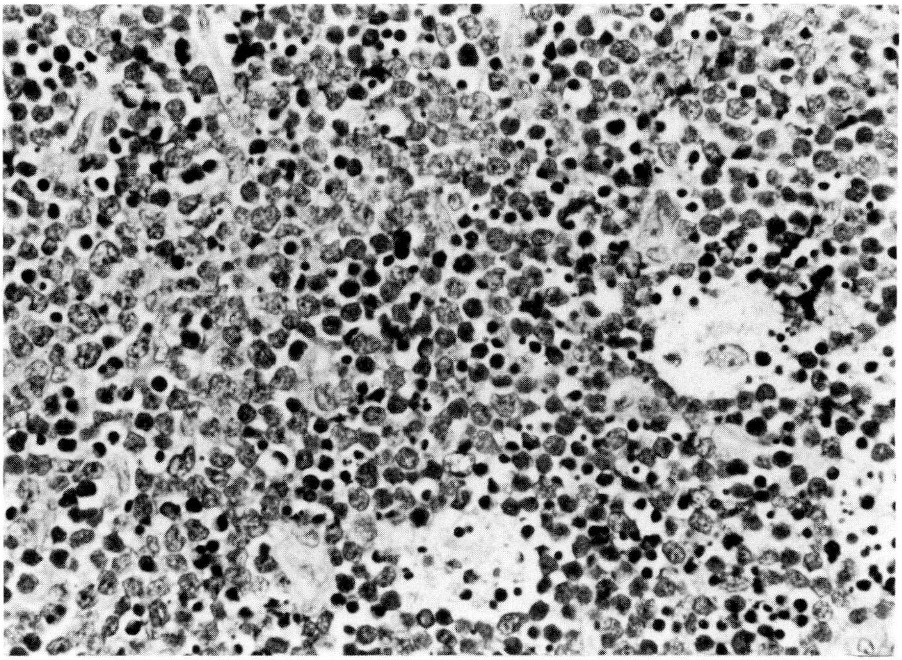

Fig. 10.11 Lymphoblastic lymphoma showing numerous pyknotic nuclei. Foamy macrophages containing ingested cell debris are seen lower right, × 400.

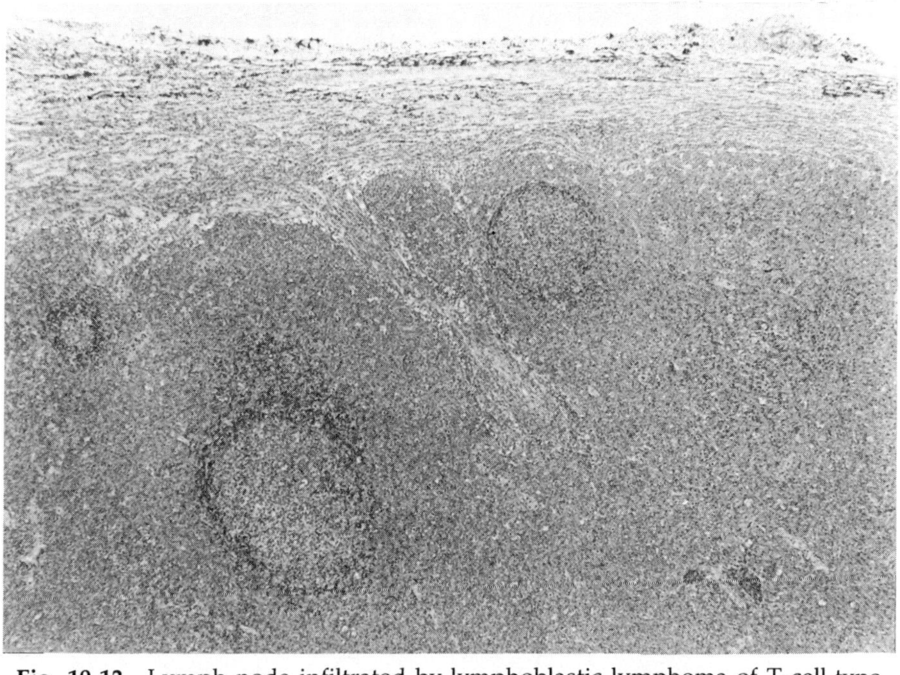

Fig. 10.12 Lymph node infiltrated by lymphoblastic lymphoma of T-cell type showing preservation of reactive follicles, × 25.

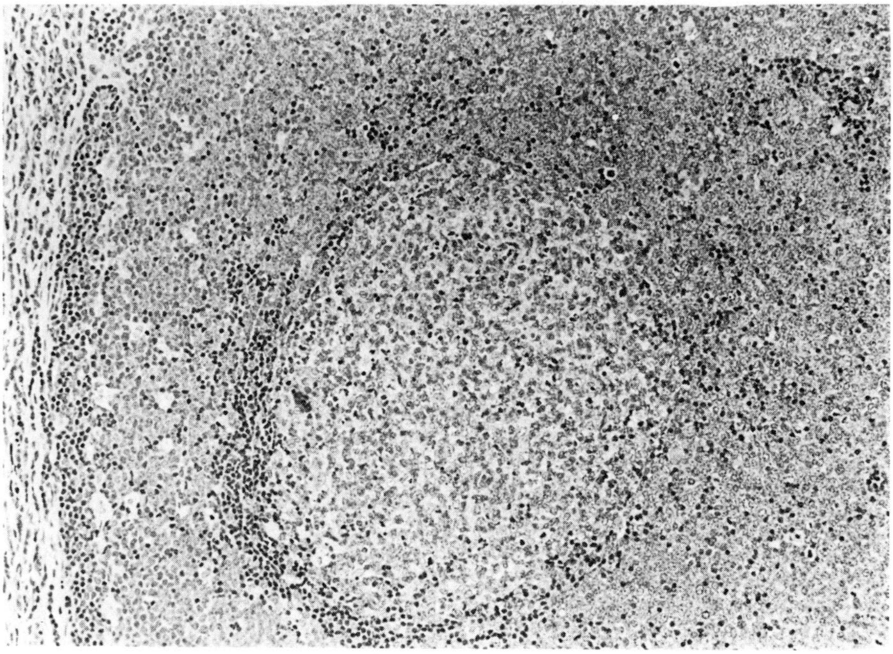

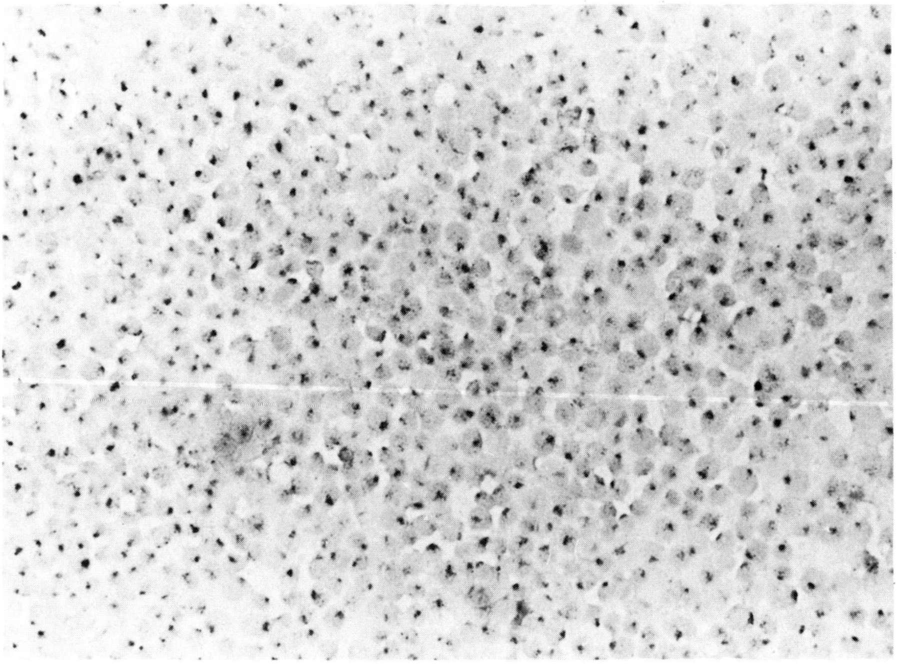

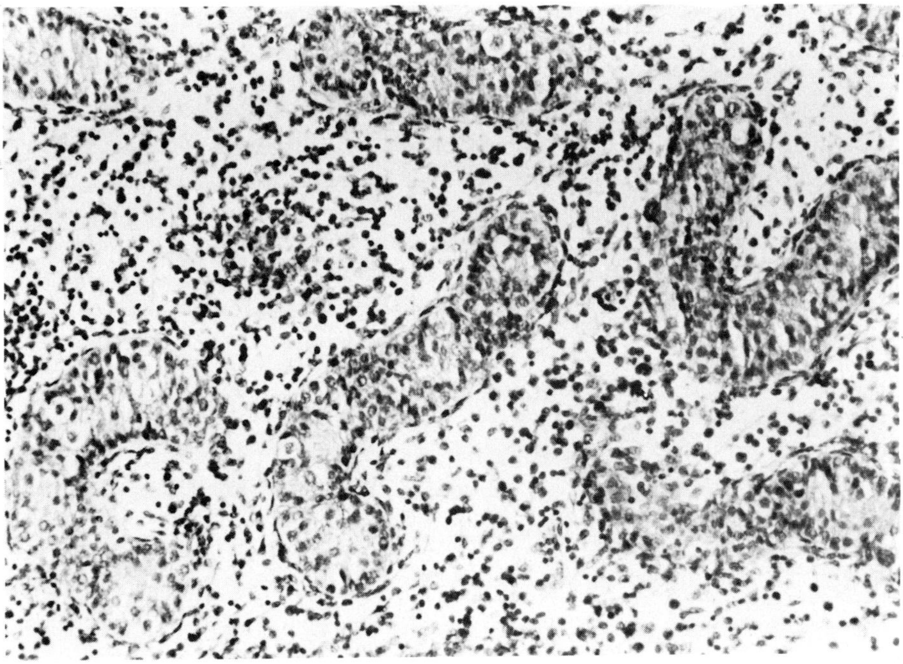

Fig. 10.15 Testicular biopsy from a boy with treated lymphoblastic leukaemia. Note infiltration of lymphoblasts between the seminiferous tubules, × 120.

10.1.2 Differential diagnosis

Lymphoblastic lymphoma usually presents a characteristic histological appearance with its cytological monomorphism, fine nuclear chromatin and infiltrative growth pattern. Lymphocytic and prolymphocytic lymphomas may exhibit similar growth patterns but are cytologically distinct although this distinction can be blurred by poor fixation. Lennert (1978) drew attention to the histological similarity between malignant lymphoma centrocytic and lymphoblastic lymphoma in some preparations. These two lymphomas can usually be distinguished by the smoother nuclear chromatin of the cells of lymphoblastic lymphoma and their higher mitotic rate. The growth pattern of malignant lymphoma centrocytic is destructive and it has a coarse reticulin pattern in contrast to

---

Fig. 10.13 Higher power view of Fig. 10.12 showing infiltration of the parafollicular area by a T-lymphoblastic lymphoma, × 120.
Fig. 10.14 Imprint preparation of T-lymphoblastic lymphoma stained for acid phosphatase. Note dot-positive staining of tumour cells, × 300.

the infiltrative growth pattern with preservation of the pre-existing reticulin structure exhibited by lymphoblastic lymphomas.

We believe that lymphoblastic lymphoma should be differentiated from Burkitt's lymphoma since they are histogenetically and clinically distinct and respond best to different treatment regimes (Ziegler, 1977). Burkitt's lymphoma cells have coarser nuclear chromatin, larger and more prominent nucleoli and better defined and more intensely basophilic/pyroninophilic cytoplasm than the cells of lymphoblastic lymphoma. Both tumours exhibit a high mitotic rate and may show a 'starry-sky' pattern. Burkitt's lymphoma has destructive growth characteristics in contrast to the infiltrative pattern of lymphoblastic lymphoma.

References

Barcos, M. P. and Lukes, R. J. (1975), Malignant lymphoma of convoluted lymphocytes: A new entity of possible T-cell type. In *Conflicts in Childhood Cancer. An Evaluation of Current Management*. Vol. 4 (eds L. F. Sinks and J. O. Godden), Alan R. Liss, New York, pp. 147–78.

Bennett, J. M., Catovsky, D., Daniel, M. T. *et al.* (1976), Proposals for the classification of the acute lymphomas. *Br. J. Haematol.*, **33**, 451–8.

Bernard, A., Boumsell, L., Bayle, C. *et al.* (1979), Subsets of malignant lymphomas in children related to the cell phenotype. *Blood*, **54**, 1058–68.

Crist, W. M., Kelly, D. R., Ragab, A. H. *et al.* (1981), Predictive ability of Lukes–Collins classification for immunological phenotypes of childhood non-Hodgkin lymphoma: An institutional series and literature review. *Cancer*, **48**, 2070–5.

Greaves, M. F. (1981), Analysis of the clinical and biological significance of lymphoid phenotypes in acute leukemia. *Cancer Res.*, **41**, 4752–66.

Lennert, K. (1978), Malignant lymphomas other than Hodgkin's disease. In *Handbuch der Speziellen Pathologischen Anatomie und Histologie*, Springer-Verlag, Berlin.

Lennert, K. (1981), *Histopathology of Non-Hodgkin's Lymphomas (Based on the Kiel Classification)*, Springer-Verlag, Berlin.

Nathwani, B. N., Diamond, L. W., Winberg, C. D. *et al.* (1981), Lymphoblastic lymphoma: A clinicopathological study of 95 patients. *Cancer*, **48**, 2347–57.

Nathwani, B. N., Kim, H. and Rappaport, H. (1976), Malignant lymphoma, lymphoblastic. *Cancer*, **38**, 964–83.

Navas Palacios, J. J., Valdes, M. D., Montalban Pallares, M. A. *et al.* (1981), Lymphoblastic lymphoma/leukemia of T-cell origin: Ultrastructural, cytochemical, and immunological features of ten cases. *Cancer*, **48**, 1982–91.

Pangalis, G. A., Nathwani, B. N., Rappaport, H. and Rosen, R. B. (1979), Acute lymphoblastic leukemia. The significance of nuclear convolutions. *Cancer*, **43**, 551–7.

Savage, R. A., Valenzuela, R. and Hoffman, G. C. (1981), Acid phosphatase staining pattern as an indicator of T-cell acute leukemia. *Am. J. Clin. Pathol.*, **76**, 760–4.

Stein, H., Peterson, N., Gaedick, F. G. *et al.* (1976), Lymphoblastic lymphoma of convoluted or acid phosphatase type. A tumour of T-precursor cells. *Int. J. Cancer*, **17**, 292–5.

Streuli, R. A., Kaneko, Y., Variakojis, D. *et al*. (1981), Lymphoblastic lymphoma in adults. *Cancer*, **47**, 2510–16.

Vogler, B. L., Crist, W. M., Sarrif, A. M. *et al*. (1981), An analysis of clinical and laboratory features of acute lymphocytic leukemias with emphasis in 35 children with pre-B leukemia. *Blood*, **58**, 135–40.

Ziegler, J. L. (1977), Treatment of 54 American patients with Burkitt's lymphoma are similar to the African experience. *New Engl. J. Med.*, **297**, 75–80.

11 Malignant lymphomas of the monocyte/macrophage system (histiocytic lymphomas)

Using morphological criteria alone Jaffe *et al.* (1982) were able to predict the correct phenotype in only 61% of diffuse large cell lymphomas. These tumours previously designated as reticulum cell sarcomas, were termed histiocytic lymphomas in the Rappaport classification in the belief that they were derived from cells of the monocyte/macrophage system (Rappaport, 1966). Immunological and cytochemical marker studies (Table 11.1) have shown that the majority of these tumours are, in fact, of B-cell origin and that true histiocytic lymphomas are uncommon. Lukes *et al.* (1978) found only one histiocytic lymphoma amongst 425 cases

Table 11.1 Marker studies in diffuse large cell lymphomas

Authors	Number of patients	B-cell	T-cell	Histiocytic	Undefined
Bloomfield *et al.*, 1977	10	7	–	–	3
Bronet *et al.*, 1976	9	2	2	1	4
Davey *et al.*, 1976	7	5	1	–	1
Epstein *et al.*, 1978	10	6	–	2	2
Filippa *et al.*, 1978	13	10	2	1	–
Jaffe *et al.*, 1982	27	15	9	1	2
Li and Harrison, 1978	79	74	1	4	–
Said *et al.*, 1979	14	10	4	–	–
Total	169	129	19	9	12
%	100	76	11	5	7

submitted to multiparameter analysis and the category 'histiocytic lymphoma' does not appear at all in the Kiel classification.

Variations in the incidence of histiocytic lymphoma between different studies may relate to differences in the criteria used for the identification of these tumours. Large cell lymphomas are often difficult to disperse for marker studies and the presence of many non-neoplastic cells may mask the reaction of the tumour cells. Fluoride-sensitive alpha-naphthyl-acetate esterase activity and staining for acid phosphatase are good markers for most cells of the monocyte/macrophage system. The staining intensity of these enzymes in malignant histiocytes is, however, often weak and may be obscured by the intense staining of non-neoplastic histiocytes that are abundant in many lymphomas. Kim *et al.* (1982) have recently described a cytochemical technique utilizing 2-naphthyl thiol acetate as a substrate at both the light microscope and ultrastructural level that may prove useful for the identification of malignant histiocytes.

Workers employing immunohistochemical techniques often use the presence of lysozyme as a marker to identify tumours of histiocytic origin. Although initially thought to be a dependable marker for histiocytes (Taylor, 1978; Isaacson *et al.*, 1979) we have since found it to be unreliable, possibly because although synthesized by cells of the monocyte/ macrophage system it is rapidly exported from the cell and therefore not present in readily detectable quantities. We have found granular, paranuclear aggregations of alpha-1-antitrypsin to be the most consistent marker of histiocytes (Isaacson *et al.*, 1981). This antigen is best detected in trypsinized sections of formalin-fixed tissues. It cannot be reliably demonstrated in tissues fixed in mercurial solutions which are widely used as fixatives for lymphoid tissues.

The wide morphological and functional diversity of cells of the monocyte/macrophage system may present problems in identifying the neoplastic counterparts of these cells. Dendritic reticulum cells and interdigitating reticulum cells, for example, although considered part of the monocytic/macrophage system, have different cytochemical profiles from tissue macrophages (Lennert, 1978). Neoplasms of these specialized histiocytes have recently been reported (Feltkamp *et al.*, 1981; Valk *et al.*, 1982).

At the present time it is difficult to determine the true incidence of histiocytic lymphomas. Table 11.1 shows that, taking a number of series together, 5% of 169 large cell lymphomas were positively identified as histiocytic but that 7% remained undefined by the markers used. In view of the lack of entirely satisfactory monocyte/macrophage markers it is likely that some of this undefined group are histiocytic lymphomas.

The spectrum of histiocytic malignancies, those of specialized histiocytes apart, includes histiocytic lymphoma (HL), malignant histiocytosis

(MH) and malignant histiocytosis of the intestine (MHI). Cases of HL present with solid tumours and are clinically indistinguishable from other malignant lymphomas, while in MH the formation of solid tumours is infrequent. In MHI solid tumours of the intestine are often present but the pattern of dissemination in other organs is identical to MH.

11.1 Histiocytic lymphomas

In view of the confusion surrounding the identification of histiocytic lymphomas, it is difficult to establish a clear-cut clinicopathological description of these tumours. They occur at all ages and their presentation with lymphadenopathy or extranodal tumours may be indistinguishable from that of other malignant lymphomas (Valk *et al.*, 1981). Cases may later show dissemination to the bone marrow and at this stage they may resemble malignant histiocytosis. The distinction between malignant histiocytosis and histiocytic lymphoma is thus not always clear-cut.

11.1.1 Histology

In its early stages histiocytic lymphoma fills out the sinuses of the node and spreads into the paracortex isolating the B-cell areas (Fig. 11.1). Histiocytic lymphoma shows a range of appearances. At one end of the spectrum the tumour cells have pleomorphic nuclei, often with clumped heterochromatin and one or more prominent nucleoli. Giant forms may be frequent (Fig. 11.2). Tumour cells may have relatively abundant cytoplasm that is poorly defined, often vacuolated and weakly pyroninophilic (Fig. 11.3). In plastic embedded sections the cytoplasm is usually seen more clearly (Fig. 11.4). At the other end of the spectrum histioblastic forms have much more regular, rounded vesicular nuclei with usually a single prominent eosinophilic nucleolus that is usually situated at the centre of radiating nuclear folds or close to indentations in the nucleus (Figs 11.5 and 11.6). The cytoplasm of these cells is less abundant and more strongly pryoninophilic than that of the more pleomorphic forms.

Fig. 11.1 Histiocytic lymphoma showing intrasinusoidal pattern of infiltration, × 40.
Fig. 11.2 Histiocytic lymphoma showing pleomorphism of tumour cells with giant cell forms. Note numerous benign histiocytes between tumour cells, × 400.

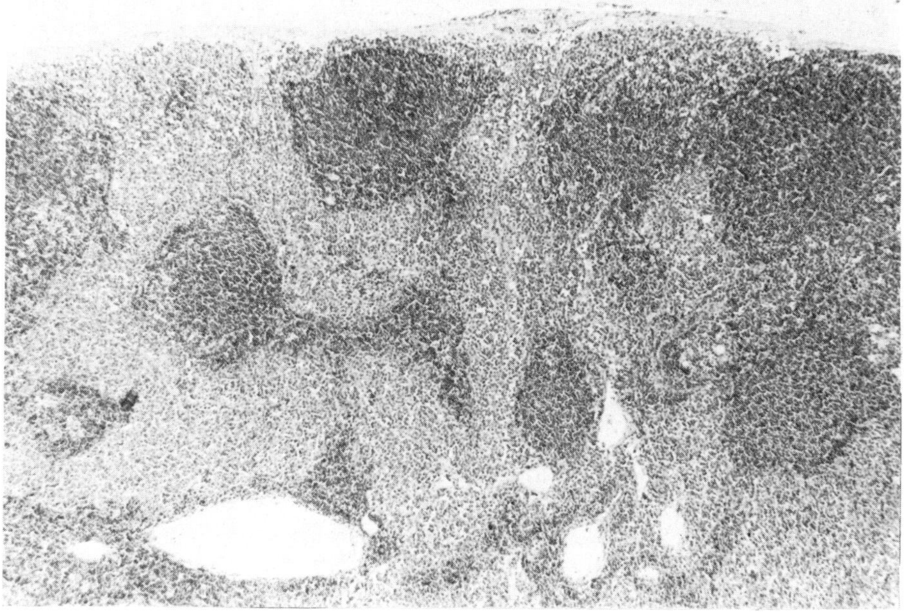

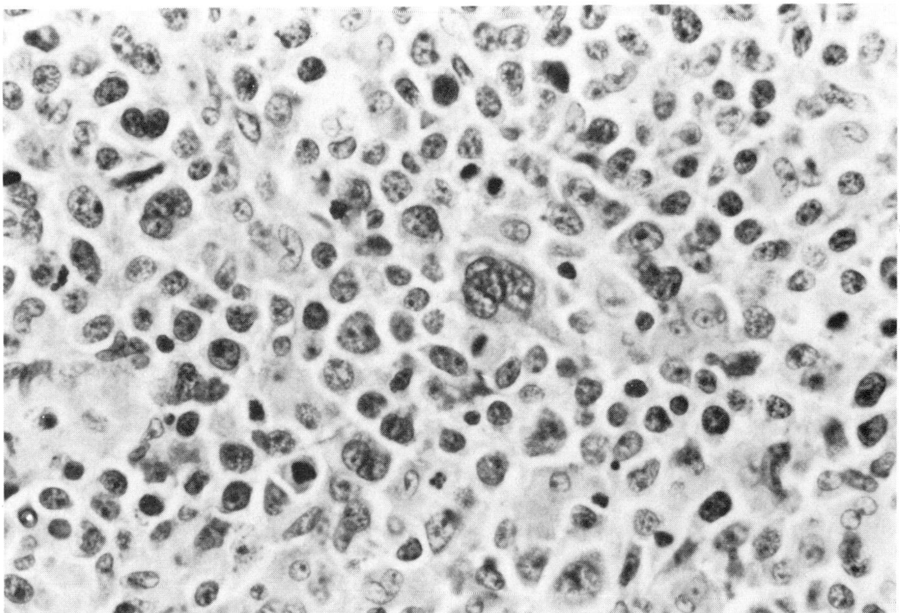

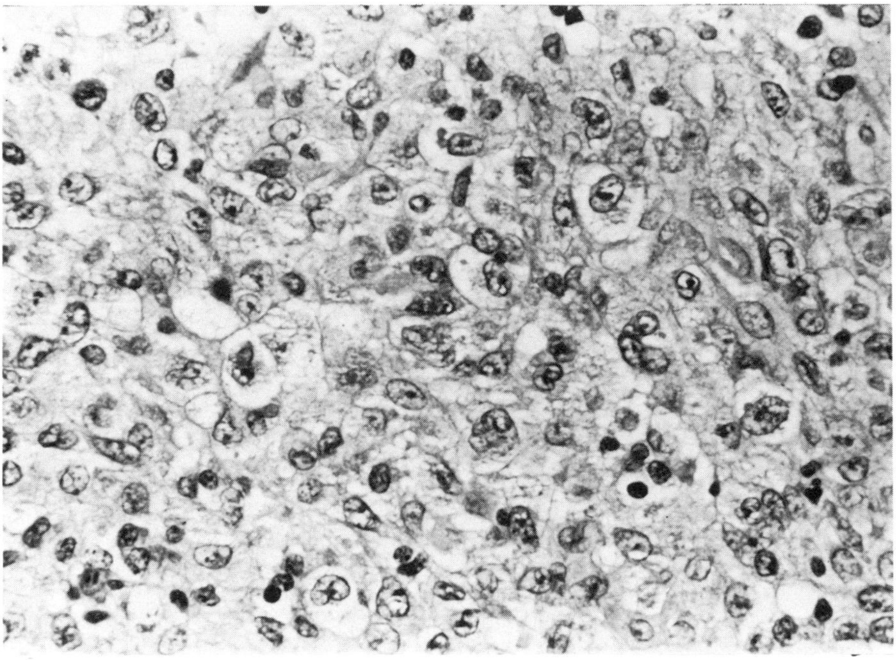

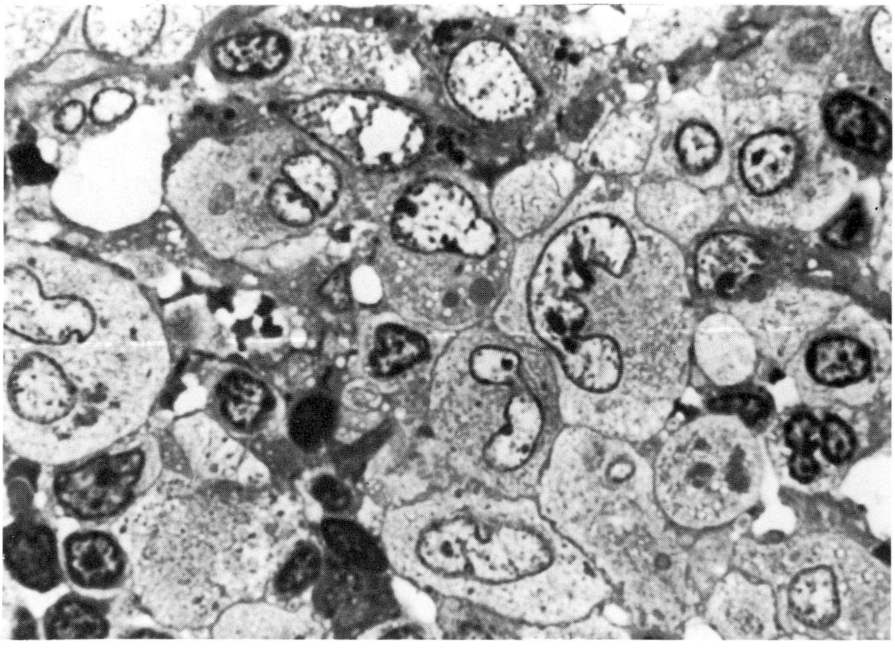

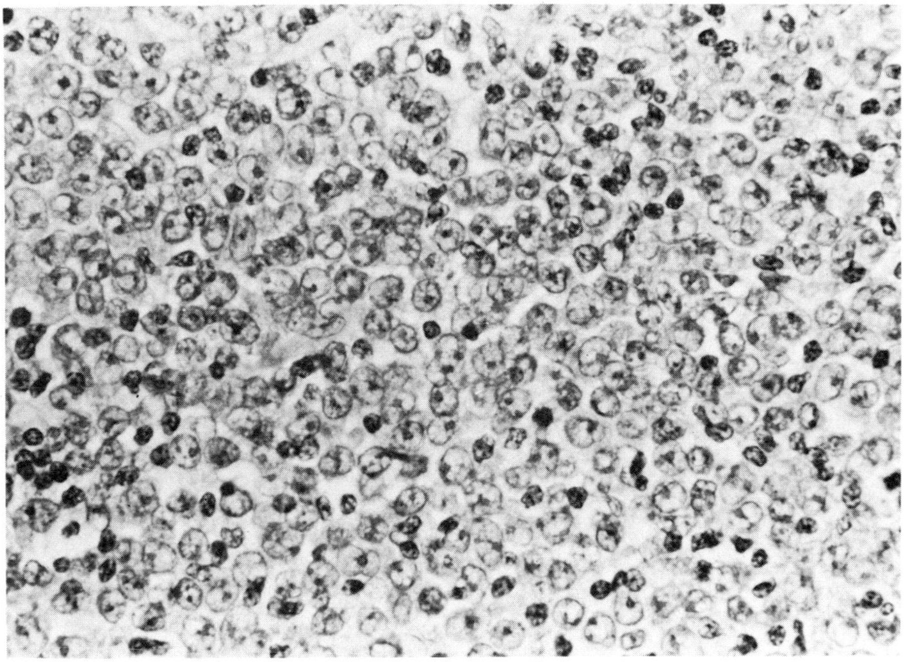

Fig. 11.5 Undifferentiated (histioblastic) histiocytic lymphoma. The tumour cells have rounded nuclei, delicate nuclear chromatin and a single prominent nucleolus, × 400.

11.1.2 *Differential diagnosis*

We have experienced considerable difficulty in separating histiocytic lymphoma from other non-Hodgkin's lymphomas on morphological features alone and differentiation from metastatic carcinoma may prove difficult. The histological features described above are characteristic of histiocytic lymphoma but need to be supplemented by special techniques such as cytochemistry or immunohistochemistry before a definite diagnosis is possible. Histioblastic forms of histiocytic lymphoma tend to be misdiagnosed as immunoblastic sarcomas. They do not show evidence of monoclonal immunoglobulin synthesis and unlike immunoblasts they contain paranuclear alpha-1-antitrypsin granules (Fig. 11.7). Phagocy-

---

Fig. 11.3 Section of histiocytic lymphoma showing abundant pale-staining cytoplasm of tumour cells, × 400.

Fig. 11.4 Plastic embedded section of histiocytic lymphoma. The nuclear pleomorphism and abundant cytoplasm is well illustrated in this preparation. Toluidine blue stain, × 1200.

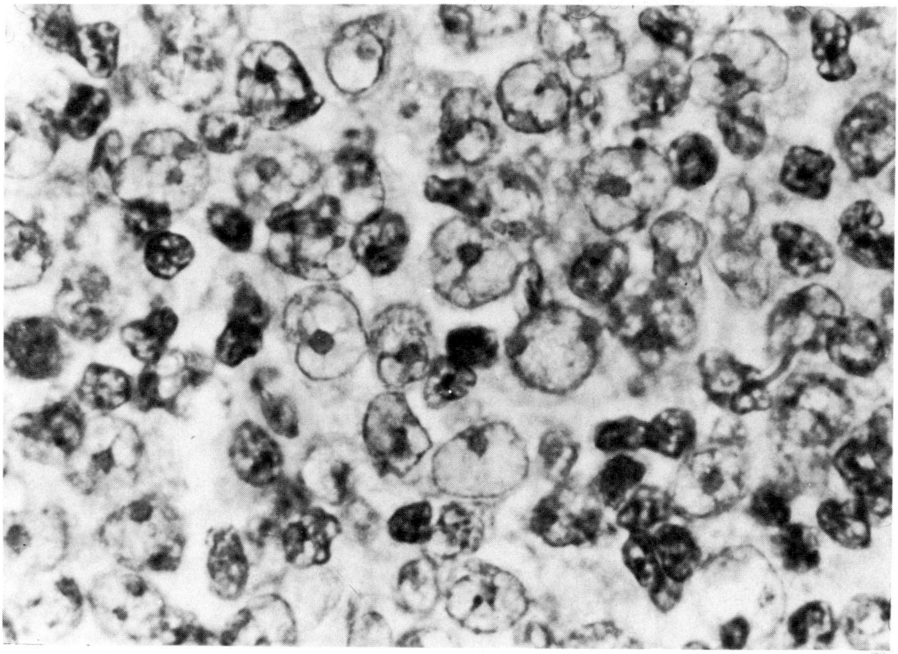

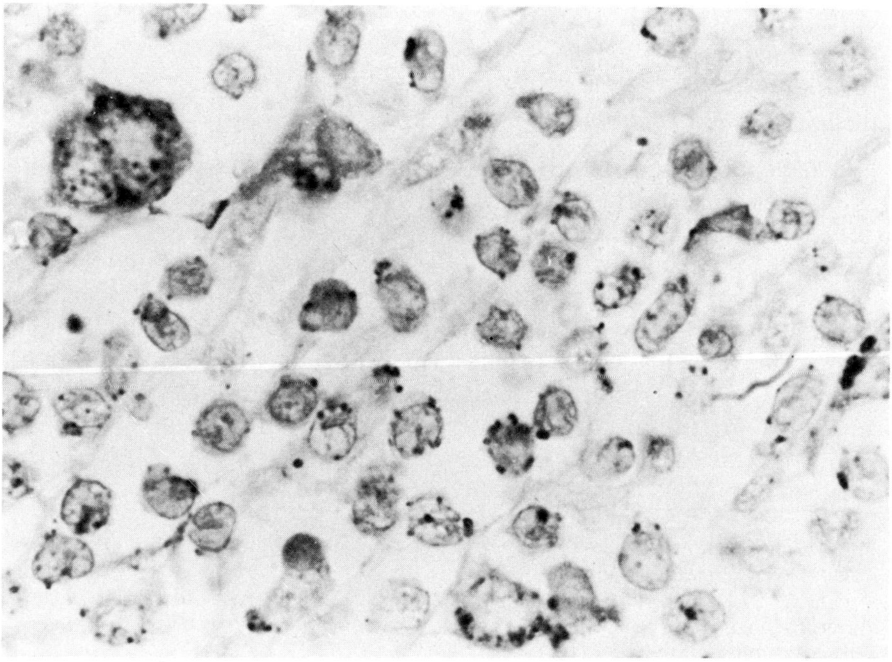

tosis of cell debris or red cells by tumour cells has been cited as a feature of malignant histiocytes (Valk *et al.*, 1981) but we have found that this is uncommon although benign phagocytic histiocytes may be a prominent component of many histiocytic lymphomas.

Histiocytic lymphomas are frequently infiltrated by eosinophils and sometimes plasma cells. This feature together with the findings of multinucleated tumour cells in many cases may suggest a diagnosis of Hodgkin's disease. However, the tumour giant cells rarely resemble classic Reed–Sternberg cells and the background infiltrate is not usually appropriate for any of the histological subtypes of Hodgkin's disease.

11.2 Malignant histiocytosis

11.2.1 Histiocytic medullary reticulosis (HMR)

Scott and Robb-Smith (1939) described ten patients with fever, wasting and generalized lymphadenopathy associated with splenic and hepatic enlargement and in the final stages jaundice, purpura and anaemia with profound leukopenia. They designated this condition histiocytic medullary reticulosis. Rappaport (1966) introduced the term malignant histiocytosis for a systemic, progressive proliferation of abnormal histiocytes. In recent years the term malignant histiocytosis has become widely accepted as a synonym for HMR. Malignant histiocytosis affects all age groups. Patients usually present with fever, anaemia, lymphadenopathy and hepatosplenomegaly (Warnke *et al.*, 1975). Malignant histiocytosis is essentially a malignancy of bone marrow histiocytes but usually shows dissemination to the sinuses of the lymph nodes, liver and spleen at the time of presentation. Patients may, however, present with apparent localized lymphadenopathy or extranodal tumour masses (Warnke *et al.*, 1975).

11.2.2 Histology

Lymph node sections, at least in the early stages of the disease, show an intrasinusoidal proliferation of atypical histiocytes (Fig. 11.8). The nodal architecture may become totally obliterated in the later stages of the

---

Fig. 11.6 Higher power view of the tumour shown in Fig. 11.5. Note that the nucleolus often appears to be attached to folds of nuclear chromatin, × 1000.
Fig. 11.7 Histiocytic lymphoma stained by the immunoperoxidase technique to show alpha-1-antitrypsin. Note paranuclear granules of alpha-1-antitrypsin activity, × 1000.

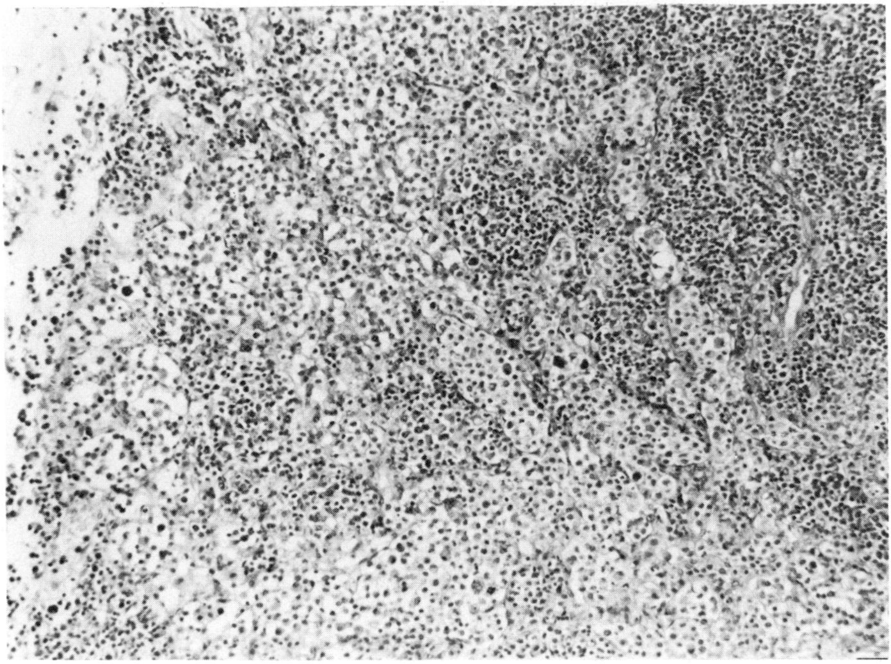

Fig. 11.8 Lymph node involved by malignant histiocytosis. The sinusoids are infiltrated by malignant histiocytes some of which have hyperchromatic nuclei, × 100.

disease. Multinucleated cells occur in approximately two-thirds of the cases and these may resemble Reed–Sternberg cells (Warnke *et al.*, 1975). Erythrophagocytosis which has been stressed as a feature of this disease is not always seen and when present may be in reactive rather than in neoplastic histiocytes. Necrosis is a prominent feature of many cases of malignant histiocytosis. This may be related to vascular invasion which is also a feature of the tumour. Infiltration of the spleen, liver and bone marrow is diffuse without the formation of tumour masses (Figs 11.9–11.11). Bone marrow infiltration is more reliably detected in smear preparations than in trephine biopsies (Fig. 11.12). Infiltration of the liver is predominantly sinusoidal although aggregates of tumour cells are also frequently seen in the portal tracts.

Fig. 11.9 Section of spleen from a patient with malignant histiocytosis. Note the scattered hyperchromatic tumour cells in the remnants of a lymphoid follicle and in the sinusoids, × 100.

Fig. 11.10 Malignant histiocytosis involving the liver. Note intrasinusoidal infiltration by pleomorphic tumour cells, × 100.

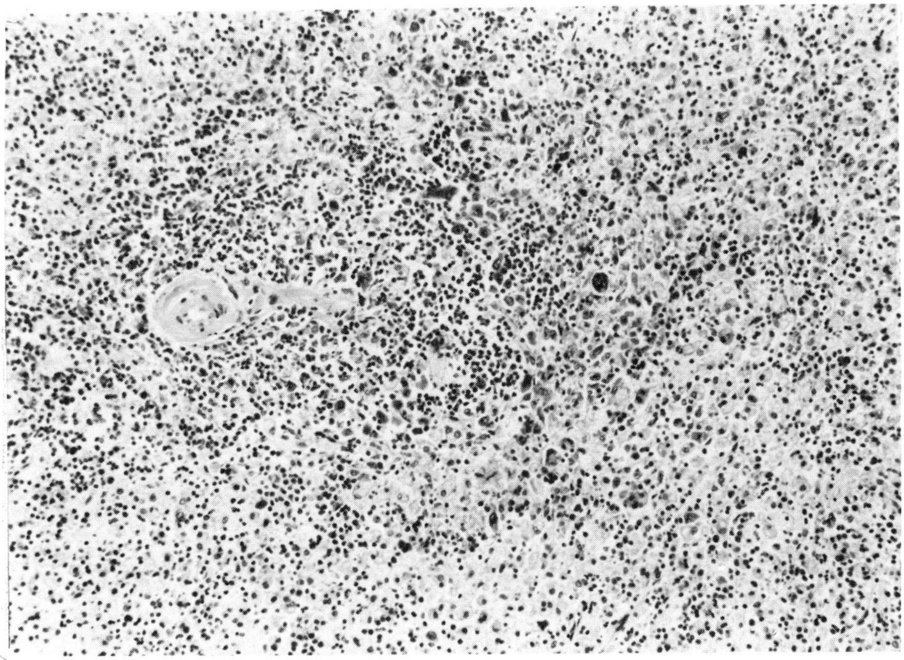

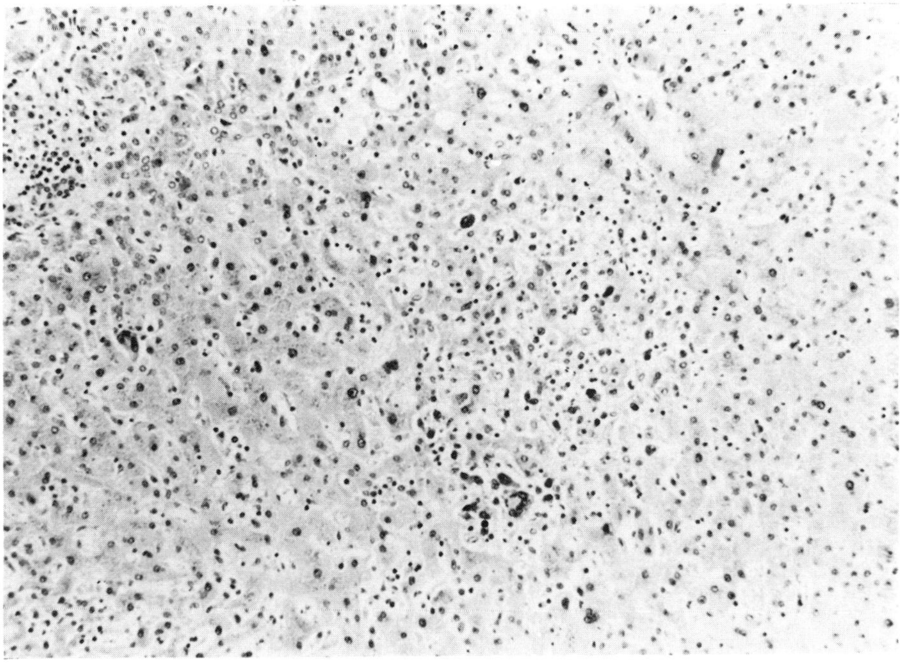

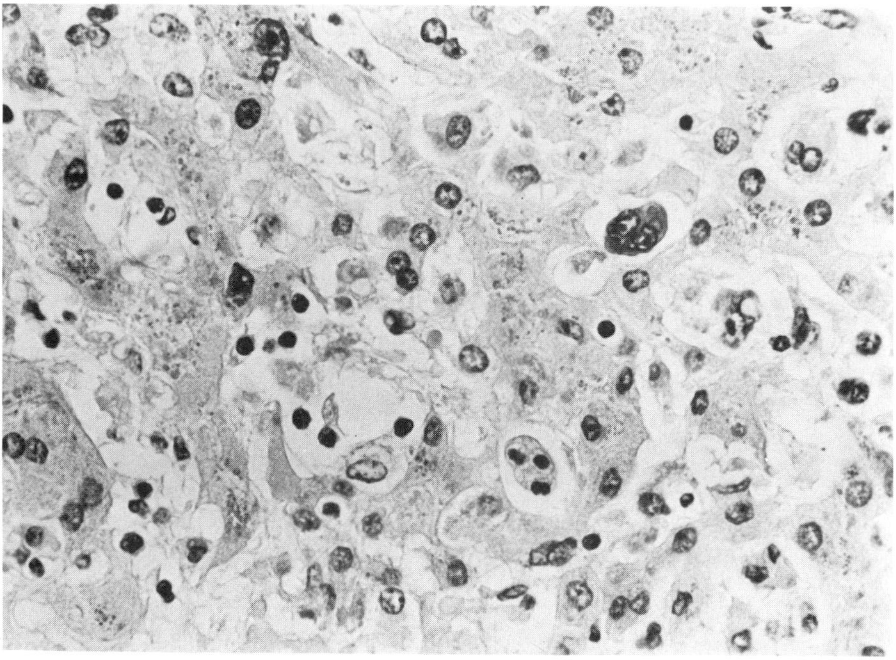

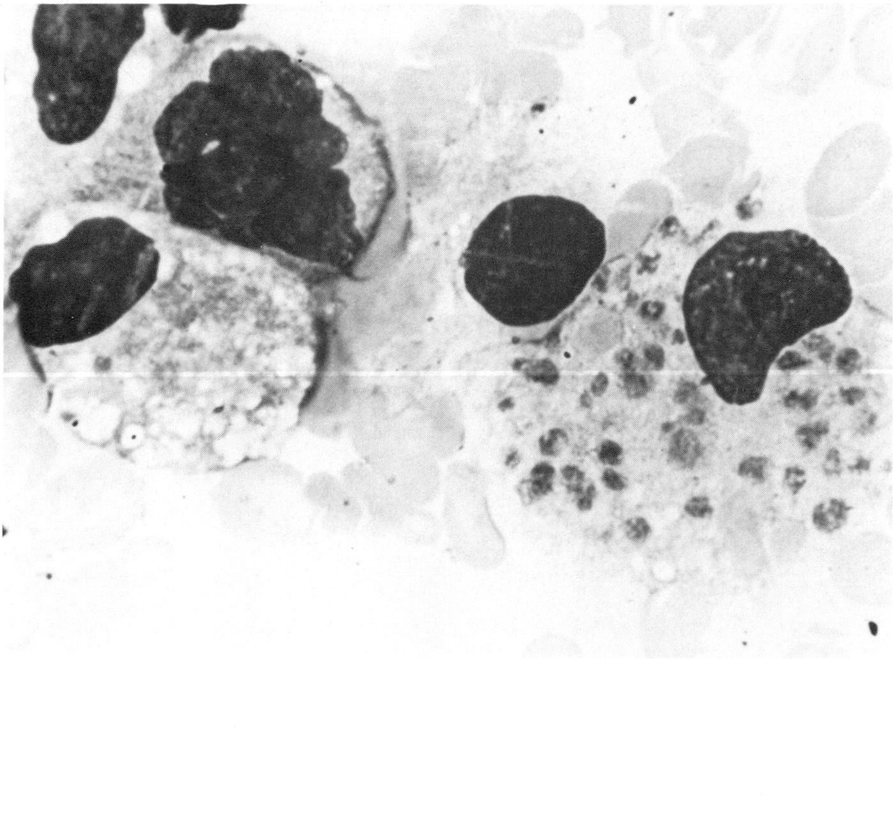

11.2.3 Differential diagnosis

The diffuse intrasinusoidal pattern of infiltration differentiates malignant histiocytosis from histiocytic lymphoma. However, occasional cases of malignant histiocytosis present with solid tumour masses (Warnke *et al.*, 1975) and in lymph node biopsies malignant histiocytes may totally obliterate the nodal architecture. In such cases the clinical follow-up information and subsequent biopsies of other organs or tissues may be necessary to make the differentiation. Large cell lymphomas may rarely infiltrate the lymph nodes in a sinusoidal pattern (Osborne *et al.*, 1980) and must be differentiated from malignant histiocytosis on the basis of the tumour cell morphology, cytochemistry or immunohistochemistry.

Perhaps of greater importance is the differentiation of malignant histiocytosis from benign, haemophagocytic syndromes associated with immunodeficiency and virus infections (Risdall *et al.*, 1979). Rappaport (1966) noted the proliferating histiocytes in malignant histiocytosis may appear relatively benign. However, Risdall *et al.* (1979) and McKenna *et al.* (1981) have stressed the need to identify morphologically atypical histiocytes before making a diagnosis of malignant histiocytosis. Kadin (1981) and Kadin *et al.* (1981) have described a malignant lymphoma of T-cells bearing Fcγ receptors and associated clinically with hepatosplenomegaly in which both the tumour cells and benign histiocytes exhibit erythrophagocytosis. The presence of T-cell leukaemia in many of these patients would appear to differentiate this condition from MH.

Monocytic leukaemia like malignant histiocytosis is a bone marrow-derived malignancy of the monocyte/macrophage system. It differs from malignant histiocytosis in that the tumour cells are more regular and monocytoid in their morphology. Diffuse bone marrow infiltration with a leukaemic blood picture is usually present in monocytic leukaemia whereas in malignant histiocytosis the bone marrow infiltration may be sparse and peripheral blood involvement is either absent or very scanty.

11.3 Malignant histiocytosis of the intestine

The association of coeliac disease and malignant lymphoma has been recognized for many years but the lymphoma that develops in these patients had not been well categorized until Isaacson and Wright (1978)

Fig. 11.11 Higher power view of Fig. 11.10. Note the proliferation of benign histiocytes as well as the tumour cells, × 400.

Fig. 11.12 Bone marrow smear from a patient with malignant histiocytosis. Two histiocytes show ingested platelets and lipid. The most atypical histiocyte shows little evidence of phagocytosis. Giemsa, × 1200.

identified the tumour cells in this condition as malignant histiocytes. Because the tumour disseminates in a diffuse fashion throughout the sinusoids of the lymph nodes, liver, spleen and bone marrow they designated it as malignant histiocytosis of the intestine. This tumour is described in Chapter 13.

References

Bloomfield, C. D., Kelsey, J. H. and Brunning, R. D. (1977), Prognostic signficance of lymphocytic surface markers and histology in adult non-Hodgkin's lymphoma. *Cancer Treat. Rep.*, **61**, 963–70.

Brouet, J. C., Preud'homme, J. L., Flandrin, G. *et al.* (1976), Membrane markers in 'histiocytic' lymphomas (reticulum cell sarcomas). *J. Natl Cancer Inst.*, **56**, 631–3.

Epstein, A. C., Levy, R., Kim, H. *et al.* (1978), Biology of the human malignant lymphomas. IV. Functional characterization of ten diffuse histiocytic lymphoma cell lines. *Cancer*, **42**, 2379–91.

Feltkamp, C. A., Van Heerde, P., Feltkamp-Vroom, T. H. and Koudstaal, J. (1981), Malignant tumor arising from interdigitating cells: light microscopical ultrastructural, immuno and enzyme histochemical characteristics. *Virchows Arch. A. (Pathol. Anat.)*, **393**, 183–92.

Filippa, D. A., Lieberman, P. H., Erlandson, R. A. *et al.* (1978), A study of malignant lymphomas using light and ultramicroscopic cytochemical and immunologic technics. Correlation with clinical features. *Am. J. Med.*, **64**, 258–68.

Isaacson, P. and Wright, D. H. (1978), Intestinal lymphoma associated with malabsorption. *Lancet*, **i**, 67–70.

Isaacson, P., Wright, D. H., Judd, M. A. and Mepham, B. L. (1979), Primary gastrointestinal lymphomas: a classification of 66 cases. *Cancer*, **43**, 1805–19.

Isaacson, P., Jones, D. B., Millward-Sadler, G. H. *et al.* (1981), Alpha-1-antitrypsin in human macrophages. *J. Clin. Pathol.*, **34**, 982–90.

Jaffe, E. S., Strauchen, J. A. and Berard, C. W. (1982), Predictability of immunologic phenotype by morphologic criteria in diffuse aggressive non-Hodgkin's lymphomas. *Am. J. Clin. Pathol.*, **77**, 46–9.

Kadin, M. E. (1981), T Gamma cells: A missing link between malignant histiocytosis and T-cell leukemia-lymphoma. *Human Pathol.*, **12**, 771–2.

Kadin, M. E., Kamonn, M. and Lamberg, J. (1981), Erythrophagocytic Tγ lymphoma. A clinicopathologic entity resembling malignant histiocytosis. *New Engl. J. Med.*, **304**, 648–53.

Kim, H., Pangalis, G. A., Payne, B. C. *et al.* (1982), Ultrastructural identification of neoplastic histiocytes–monocytes. An application of a newly developed cytochemical technique. *Am. J. Pathol.*, **106**, 204–23.

Lennert, K. (1978), Malignant lymphomas other than Hodgkin's disease in *Handbuch der Speziellen Pathologischen Anatomie und Histologie*, Springer-Verlag, Berlin.

Li, C. Y. and Harrison, E. G. (1978), Histochemical and immunohistochemical study of diffuse large cell lymphomas. *Am. J. Clin. Pathol.*, **70**, 721–32.

Lukes, R. J., Parker, J. W., Taylor, C. R. *et al.* (1978), Immunological approach to non-Hodgkin's lymphomas and related leukemias. Analysis of the results of multiparameter studies of 425 cases. *Semin. Hematol.*, **15**, 322–51.

McKenna, R. W., Risdall, R. J. and Brunning, R. D. (1981), Virus associated hemophagocytic syndrome. *Human Pathol.*, **12**, 395–8.

Osborne, B. M., Butler, J. J. and Mackay, B. (1980), Sinusoidal large cell ('histiocytic') lymphoma. *Cancer*, **46**, 2484–91.

Rappaport, H. (1966), *Tumors of the Hematopoietic system. Atlas of Tumor Pathology (Sect. 3, Fasc. 8)*, Armed Forces Institute of Pathology, Washington, D.C.

Risdall, R. J., McKenna, R. W., Nesbit, M. E. *et al.* (1979), Virus associated hemophagocytic syndrome: A benign histiocytic proliferation distinct from malignant histiocytosis. *Cancer*, **44**, 993–1002.

Said, J. W., Hargreaves, H. K. and Pinkus, G. S. (1979), Non-Hodgkin's lymphomas: An ultrastructural study correlating morphology with immunologic cell type. *Cancer*, **44**, 504–28.

Scott, R. B. and Robb-Smith, A. H. T. (1939), Histiocytic medullary reticulosis. *Lancet*, **ii**, 194–8.

Taylor, C. R. (1978), Immunoperoxidase techniques: Theoretical and practical aspects. *Arch. Pathol. Lab. Med.*, **102**, 113–21.

Warnke, R. A., Kim, H. and Dorfman, R. F. (1975), Malignant histiocytosis (histiocyte medullary reticulosis). I. Clinico-pathologic study of 29 cases. *Cancer*, **35**, 215–30.

Valk, P. van Der, Te Velde, J., Jansen, J. *et al.* (1981), Malignant lymphoma of true histiocytic origin: histiocytic sarcoma. A morphological, ultrastructural, immunological, cytochemical and clinical study of 10 cases. *Virchows Arch. A. (Pathol. Anat.)*, **391**, 249–65.

Valk, P. van Der, Ruiter, D. J., Ottolander, G. J. *et al.* (1982), Dendritic reticulum cell sarcoma? Four cases of a lymphoma probably derived from dendritic reticulum cells of the follicular compartment. *Histopathology*, **6**, 269–87.

12 Miscellaneous

12.1 Hairy cell leukaemia (leukaemic reticuloendotheliosis)

The cell of origin of hairy cell leukaemia has not yet been identified and this histogenetic uncertainty has resulted in the inclusion of a number of heterogeneous conditions in reported series of hairy cell leukaemia (Palutke *et al.*, 1981). The cells are characterized by the presence of cytoplasmic tartrate-resistant acid phosphatase and at the ultrastructural level by ribosomal lamellae, although these features are not entirely specific (Palutke *et al.*, 1981). Most patients present with pancytopenia and many have splenomegaly. Peripheral lymphadenopathy is not a feature of hairy cell leukaemia. Histopathologists are most likely therefore to see this condition in bone marrow trephine, liver biopsies and spleens removed either for diagnostic or therapeutic purposes. Hairy cell leukaemia is classed as a low grade neoplasm and many patients survive for ten years or more. Death is usually due to intercurrent infection whether or not the patient has had a splenectomy (Stewart and Bodey, 1981).

12.1.1 Histology

The cells of hairy cell leukaemia are very monomorphic in tissue sections. They have oval, often slightly indented, nuclei with fine uniformly dispersed chromatin and inconspicuous nucleoli. The cytoplasm stains weakly and is poorly defined but is more abundant than that of small lymphocytes, so the nuclei appear more widely dispersed than in other lymphocytic malignancies. Hairy cells infiltrate tissues in a very characteristic fashion. They appear to attach to the walls of sinusoids in the bone marrow, liver (Fig. 12.1) and spleen (Figs 12.2 and 12.3) and to damage the sinusoidal lining cells. The resulting sinusoidal ectasia gives rise to characteristic pseudo-angiomatous formations in the bone marrow and liver and to blood lakes in the spleen (Nanba *et al.*, 1977). Infiltration

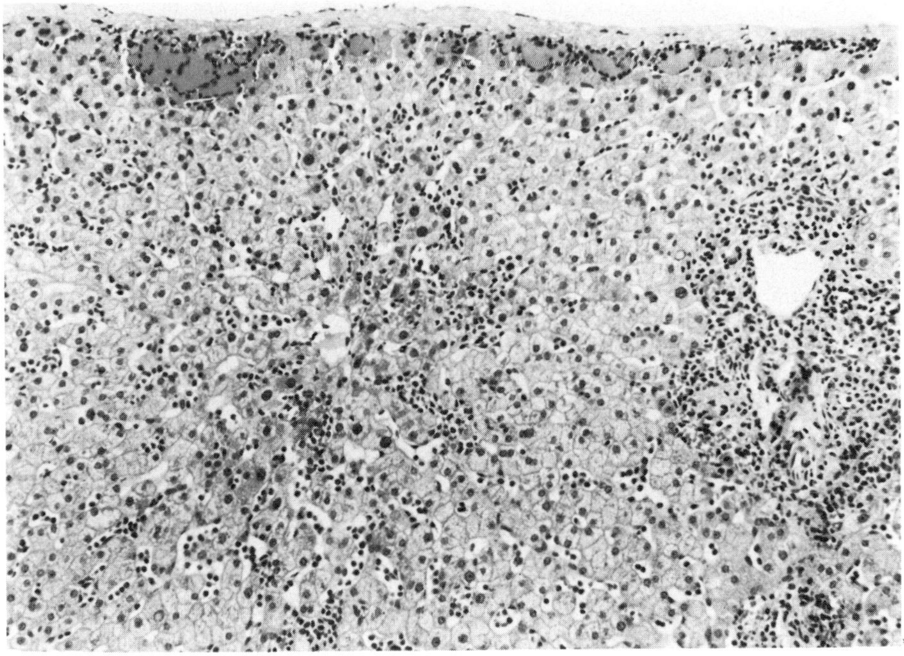

Fig. 12.1 Section of liver from a patient with hairy cell leukaemia. The leukaemic cells infiltrate sinusoids and portal areas. Note dilated blood-filled sinusoids lined by hairy cells, × 120.

of lymph nodes begins in the sinusoids and extends in the perifollicular compartment leaving the follicles isolated in a sea of hairy cells (Fig. 12.4).

12.2 Granulocytic sarcoma (chloroma)

Chloromas were so-called because the presence of myeloperoxidase in the tumour cells imparts a green colour to the neoplasm. This colour, which fades rapidly on exposure to oxygen, is not a constant feature and the term 'granulocytic sarcoma' introduced by Rappaport (1966) is now much more widely used. The tumour occurs over a wide age range from infancy to old age. The tissues most commonly involved are bone periosteum, soft tissue, lymph node and skin. The tumours are a manifestation of granulocytic leukaemia although they may present before other features of leukaemia are apparent. In a series of 50 patients studied by Neiman *et al.* (1981) 15 had no evidence of leukaemia at the time of biopsy, 13 of these 15 patients developed acute granulocytic leukaemia over a period of 1–49 months (mean 10.5 months). Tumours occurring in patients with known leukaemia were usually associated with blast crises.

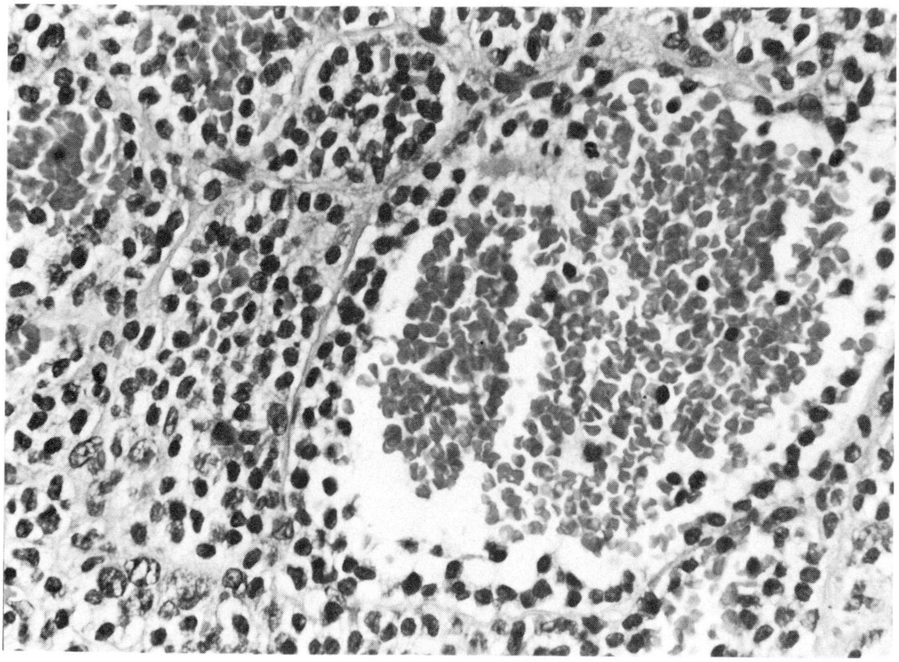

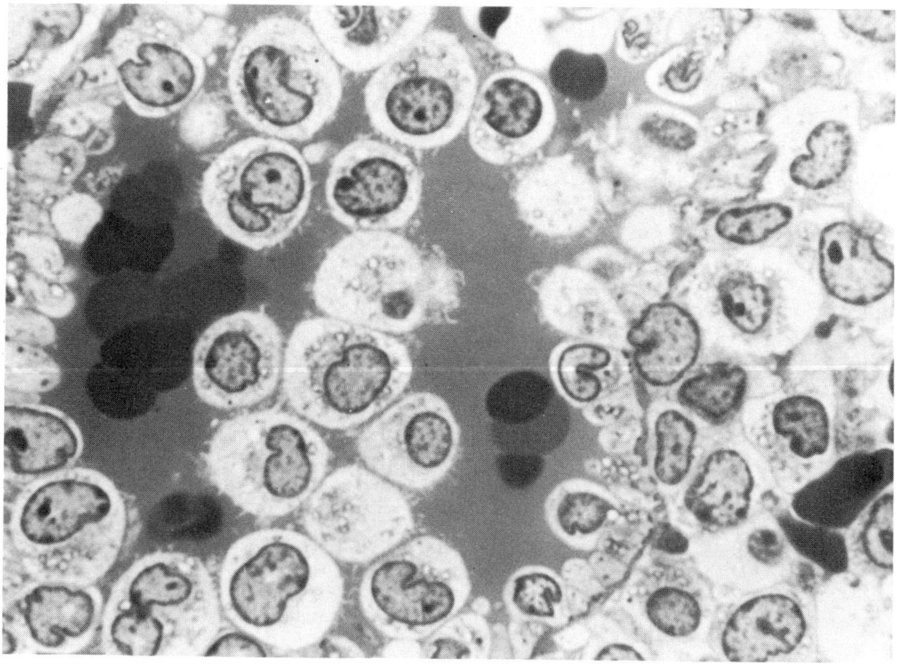

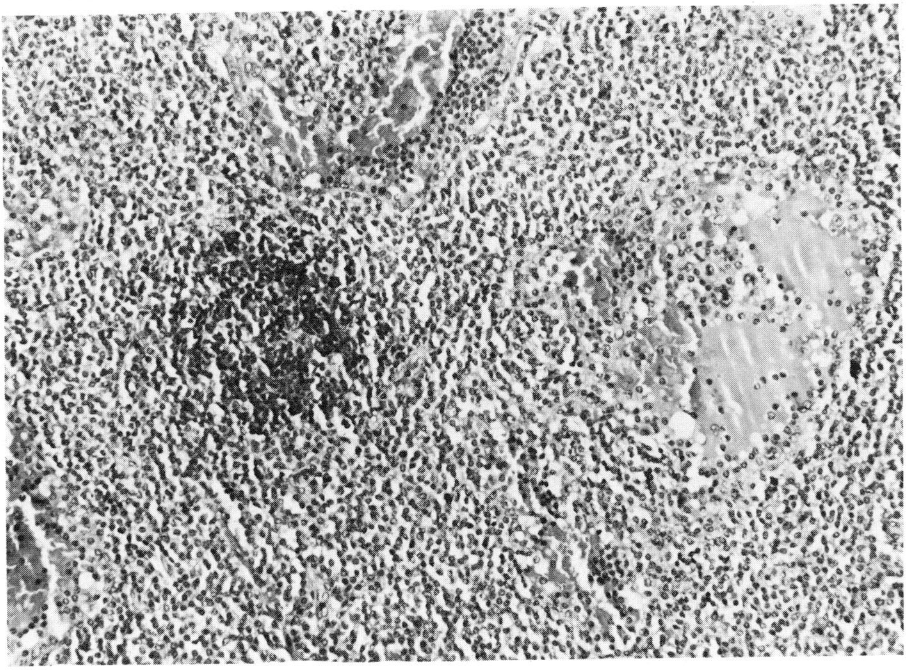

Fig. 12.4 Section of splenic hilar lymph node from a patient with hairy cell leukaemia. An island of residual lymphocytes can be seen surrounded by larger paler-staining hairy cells. Note dilated sinuses lined by hairy cells, × 120.

12.2.1 Histology

Granulocytic sarcoma shows a range of appearances from undifferentiated blast cell tumours to well-differentiated tumours containing many granulated cells. The undifferentiated tumours may closely resemble malignant lymphoma, particularly of the lymphoblastic type. The presence of occasional granulated cells, of which eosinophil myelocytes are usually the most conspicuous, is a good pointer to the identity of this tumour (Fig. 12.5), although pathologists should always maintain a high index of suspicion when dealing with undifferentiated lymphomas. The naphthyl ASD chloroacetate esterase stain (Leder, 1964) is widely used to

---

Fig. 12.2 Hairy cell leukaemia of spleen. Note sinusoid distended by blood and lined by hairy cells, × 300.
Fig. 12.3 Plastic embedded section of spleen from patient with hairy cell leukaemia. Hairy cells can be seen within a sinusoid, attached to its wall and apparently migrating through into the adjacent tissues. Toluidine blue, × 1200.

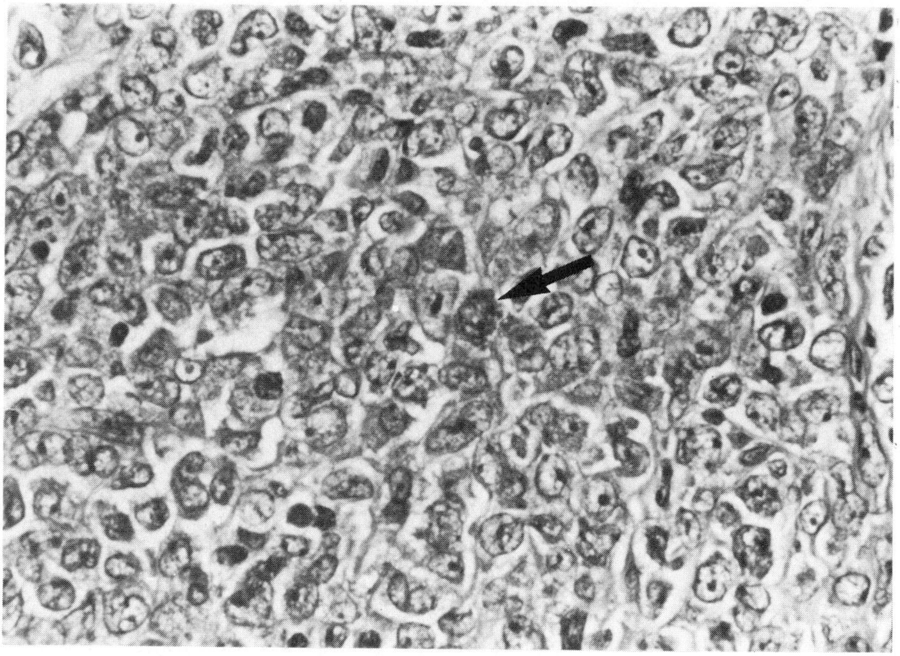

Fig. 12.5 Granulocytic sarcoma. A single eosinophil myelocyte is seen amongst the tumour cells (arrow), × 480.

identify granulocytic sarcoma. However, in some tumours only a very small minority of cells may stain and these must be carefully distinguished from non-neoplastic polymorphs infiltrating the tumour. Neiman *et al.* (1981) found that immunohistochemical staining for lysozyme is a more reliable marker for the diagnosis of granulocytic sarcoma. Our own experience supports this observation (Figs 12.6 and 12.7). In addition we have found alpha-1-antitrypsin to be a good marker for these tumours.

12.2.2 *Differential diagnosis*

A small proportion of patients with granulocytic leukaemia enter a blast crisis in which the tumour cells express the phenotype of lymphoblastic

---

Fig. 12.6 Section of lymph node from a patient with granulocytic leukaemia of several years duration. The appearances are consistent with either granulocytic sarcoma or lymphoblastic transformation, × 300.

Fig. 12.7 The same tumour as shown in Fig. 12.6 stained by the immunoperoxidase technique for lysozyme. A high proportion of the tumour cells are positive indicating their granulocytic lineage, × 300.

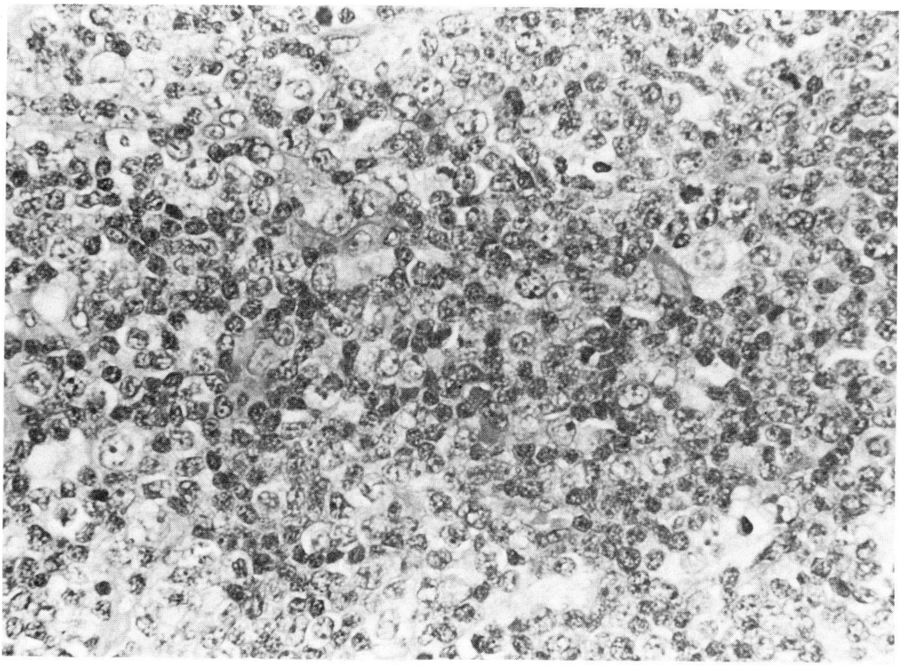

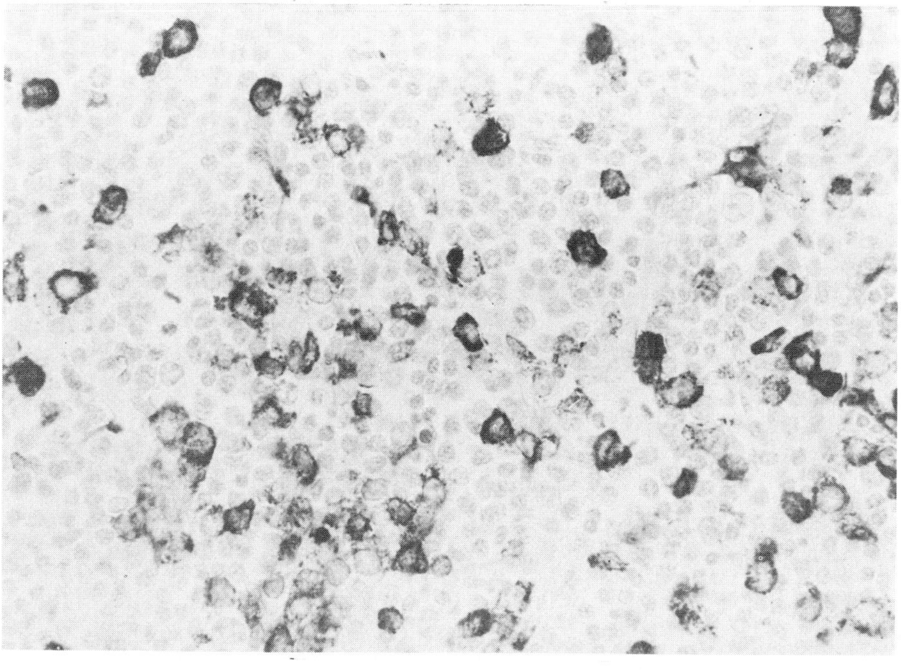

leukaemia (Janossy *et al.*, 1976). These patients may develop lymphadenopathy in which the histological appearances are similar to those of lymphoblastic lymphoma. Cytochemical and immunological profiles are necessary to distinguish these cases from undifferentiated granulocytic sarcoma.

12.3 Systemic mastocytosis (malignant mastocytosis)

Cutaneous mastocytosis associated with diffuse or localized mast cell infiltrations usually presents clinically with urticaria pigmentosa. Systemic mastocytosis is an uncommon but probably underdiagnosed manifestation of mast cell disease. It is not always associated with urticaria pigmentosa and such cases are particularly likely to escape diagnosis. Urticaria pigmentosa developing in adult life is more likely to be associated with disseminated mastocytosis than the childhood form (Webb *et al.*, 1982). Patients with systemic mastocytosis commonly present with gastrointestinal symptoms possibly related to the production of histamine by the mast cells. Approximately half the patients have hepatosplenomegaly and lymphadenopathy (Webb *et al.*, 1982) and widespread osteopenia with fractures is common (Fallon *et al.*, 1981). In a study of 43 cases (25 from the literature and 16 of their own) Lennert and Parwaresch (1979) reported the development of leukaemia in 16 cases. In six this was mast cell, in five granulocytic and five monocytic leukaemia. They cite the latter cases as supporting a common origin of mast cells and monocytes.

12.3.1 Histology

Mast cell proliferations are often accompanied by large numbers of eosinophils. Abdominal lymph nodes are more frequently involved than peripheral lymph nodes. They show infiltration of the perifollicular areas with mast cells and eosinophils. Total replacement of the follicles may give the proliferation a nodular appearance. Infiltrates of the spleen occur along the fibrous trabeculae which become thickened and prominent. The liver infiltrates are portal in distribution. Involvement of the bone marrow is usually paratrabecular. In skin biopsies mast cells are typically polygonal in shape with abundant and rather clear cytoplasm (Figs 12.8 and 12.9). In other tissues they often appear more like histiocytes and

---

Fig. 12.8 Skin biopsy from a patient with systemic mastocytosis. The dense infiltrate of mast cells extends to the epidermis, × 120.

Fig. 12.9 Higher power view of Fig. 12.8. Note the resemblance of some of the spindle-shaped cells to epithelioid cells, × 300.

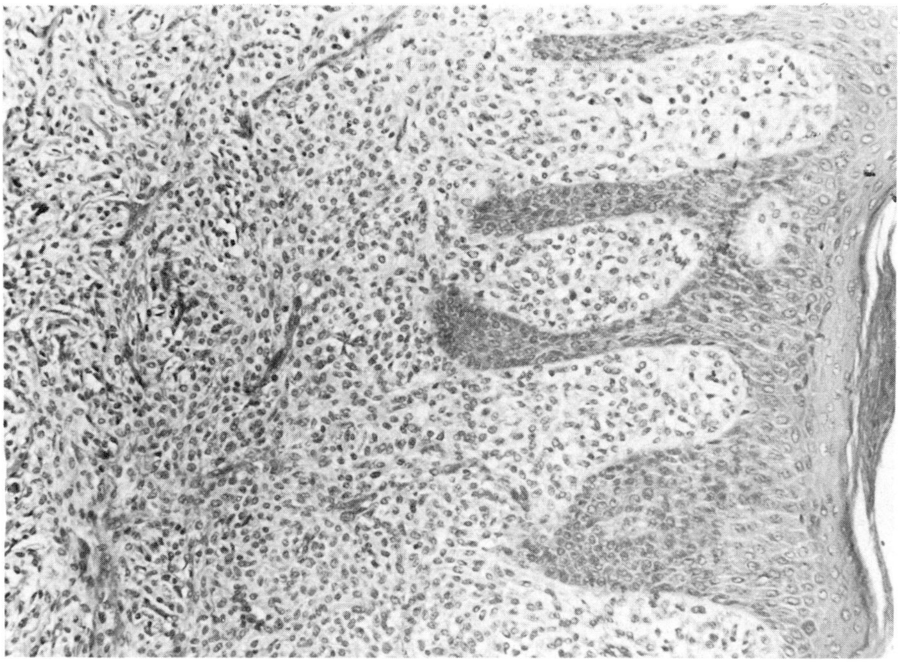

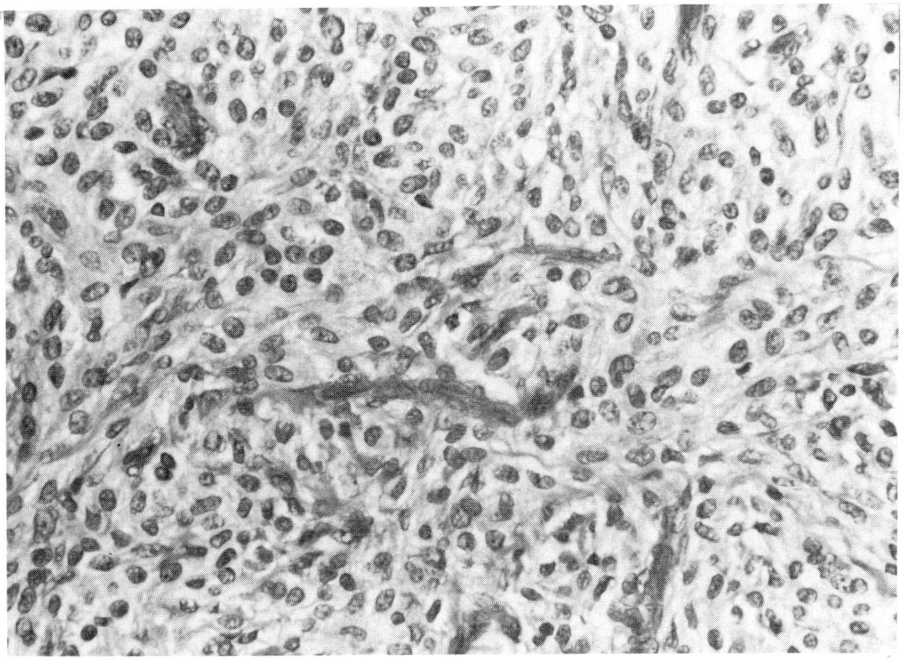

fibroblasts and may produce lesions that mimic granulomas (Fallon *et al.*, 1981). The presence of the eosinophils may alert pathologists to the diagnosis of mast cell disease. Confirmation can be obtained with special stains including metachromatic staining with toluidine blue or thionin and the naphthyl ASD chloroacetate esterase stain.

References

Fallon, M. D., Whyte, M. P. and Teitelbaum, S. L. (1981), Systemic mastocytosis associated with generalised osteopenia. Histopathological characterisation of the skeletal lesion using undecalcified bone from two patients. *Human Pathol.*, **12**, 813–20.

Janossy, G., Roberts, M. and Greaves, M. F. (1976), Target cell in chronic myeloid leukaemia and its relationship to acute lymphoid leukaemia. *Lancet*, **ii**, 1058–61.

Leder, L. D. (1964), Über die selektive fermentcytochemische Darstellung von neutrophilen myeloischen Zellen und Gewebsmastzellen im Paraffinschnitt. *Clin. Wschr.*, **42**, 553.

Lennert, K. and Parwaresch, M. R. (1979), Mast cells and mast cell neoplasia: A review. *Histopathology*, **3**, 349–65.

Nanba, K., Soban, E. J., Bowling, M. C. and Berard, C. W. (1977), Splenic pseudosinuses and hepatic angiomatous lesions: distinctive features of hairy cell leukemia. *Am. J. Clin. Pathol.*, **67**, 415–26.

Neiman, R. S., Barcos, M., Berard, C. *et al.* (1981), Granulocytic sarcoma: A clinicopathologic study of 61 biopsied cases. *Cancer*, **48**, 1426–37.

Palutke, M., Tabaczka, P., Mirchandani, I. and Goldfarb, S. (1981), Lymphocytic lymphoma simulating hairy cell leukemia: A consideration of reliable and unreliable diagnostic features. *Cancer*, **48**, 2047–55.

Rappaport, H. (1966), *Tumours of the Hematopoietic System. Atlas of Tumor Pathology* (Sect. 3, Fasc. 8), Armed Forces Institute of Pathology, Washington, D.C.

Stewart, D. J. and Bodey, G. P. (1981), Infections in hairy cell leukemia: (leukaemic reticuloendotheliosis). *Cancer*, **47**, 801–5.

Webb, T. A., Li, C-Y. and Yam, L. T. (1982), Systemic mast cell disease: A clinical and hematopathologic study of 26 cases. *Cancer*, **49**, 927–38.

13 Extranodal malignant lymphomas

Malignant lymphomas often involve sites that are not primary organs of the lymphoreticular system. This involvement may be part of a disseminated lymphomatous process and in such cases even when an extranodal tumour dominates the clinical presentation staging procedures will reveal lymphoma elsewhere. The organ distribution of disseminated lymphoma is rarely totally random but probably reflects the physiological circulation of the normal counterparts of the tumour cells; thus involvement of the jaws in Burkitt's lymphoma is an age-dependent phenomenon (Wright, 1971) possibly related to dental development, and the remarkable involvement of the breasts in this disease during pregnancy and lactation (Shepherd and Wright, 1967) may be related to the physiological migration of B-lymphocytes to the breast at these times.

Some lymphomas present as primary tumours in extranodal sites and remain localized at these sites for varying periods of time. Long-term remissions may be obtained in patients with such tumours by local surgery and/or radiotherapy alone. These lymphomas arise in sites of extranodal lymphoid tissue that may be physiological, as in the gastrointestinal tract, or pathological, as in Hashimoto's disease of the thyroid.

The differentiation between some of these extranodal lymphomas and reactive or inflammatory lesions can be difficult and is a cause of considerable confusion. The term pseudolymphoma has been applied to proliferations that do not fall clearly into either a reactive or a neoplastic category, yet which sometimes appear to evolve into lymphoma after a variable period of time. In recent years it has been shown that distinctive circulation pathways and homing patterns exist for the mucosal lymphoid cells of the gastrointestinal tract (Parrot, 1976) and the bronchial tree (Bienenstock *et al.*, 1973a, b). We believe that the clinical behaviour and pathological features of lymphomas arising at these sites and in the thyroid and salivary glands can only be understood in relation to the circulation and homing patterns of mucosa-associated lymphoid tissue.

The development of lymphomas from cells that home to specific mucosal and glandular tissues probably accounts for the localization of these tumours and their slow evolution over a long period of time. This concept as applied to the B-cell lymphomas of the mucosal and epithelial sites is relatively new, although the relationship between the cutaneous T-cell lymphomas and the epidermotropism of T-cell subsets has been recognized for longer. These cutaneous T-cell lymphomas also show a long period of evolution in which the infiltrations have many inflammatory features before frank tumour develops. Little is understood about the circulation pathways of cells of the monocyte/macrophage system. The condition we have categorized as malignant histiocytosis of the intestine may arise from a subgroup of macrophages that usually resides in, or homes to, the gut mucosa. This lymphoma may also exhibit long latent periods during which non-specific intestinal ulcers dominate the clinical picture before macroscopic tumour develops.

13.1 Gastrointestinal lymphoma

Lymphoid nodules, consisting of B-cell follicles and surrounding T-cell areas, are distributed throughout the gastrointestinal tract and it is, therefore, not surprising that this is the commonest site of primary extranodal lymphoma. Distinction between primary and secondary gastrointestinal lymphoma is not always easy since malignant lymphoma arising elsewhere often involves the gastrointestinal tract late in its course. Primary gastrointestinal lymphoma is best defined simply as lymphoma that presents in the gastrointestinal tract necessitating the direction of diagnostic investigations and treatment to that site (Isaacson, 1981). Primary gastrointestinal lymphoma is not a common disease. In Western countries it is estimated that lymphoma accounts for approximately 3% of gastric tumours and 20% of small intestinal tumours (Lee and Spratt, 1974). In the Middle East, however, lymphoma is the commonest intestinal malignancy.

While any type of lymphoma can arise in the gastrointestinal tract, the great majority of cases consist of one or other of the categories listed in Table 13.1 which also shows their geographic incidence. It is particularly important to be aware that Hodgkin's disease, while sometimes involving the gastrointestinal tract late in its course, only rarely occurs as a primary gastrointestinal tumour (Henry and Farrer-Brown, 1977; Isaacson *et al.*, 1979). Tumours derived from follicle centre cells (centrocytic, centroblastic/centrocytic and centroblastic) account for the majority of gastrointestinal lymphomas both in the West and in the

Middle East. Like nodal lymphomas varying numbers of immunoblasts may be found in these tumours and when they are the predominant cell the term immunoblastic lymphoma is justified. Undifferentiated (Burkitt-like) lymphoma is predominantly a tumour of childhood and occurs principally in the ileocaecal region. It is a particularly common tumour in children in the Middle East (Al-Attar *et al.*, 1979). There are two types of lymphoma which are exclusive to the gastrointestinal tract and which are, with few exceptions, restricted to the small intestine. These are malignant histiocytosis of the intestine (MHI) (Isaacson and Wright, 1978; 1980), which occurs in the West and Mediterranean lymphoma (MTL) (World Health Organization, 1976) which occurs predominantly in the Middle East. This latter tumour is, in our opinion, a variety of follicle centre lymphoma.

Table 13.1 Primary gastrointestinal lymphoma

	Western	Middle Eastern
Follicle centre cell derived	Stomach and small intestine	Stomach and small intestine
Mediterranean lymphoma (MTL)	–	Small intestine
Undifferentiated (Burkitt-type)	Small intestine and ileocaecal region	Small intestine and ileocaecal region
Malignant histiocytosis of the intestine (MHI)	Small intestine (coeliac disease)	–

13.1.1 Primary gastrointestinal lymphomas of follicle centre cell (FCC) origin

These tumours present in the stomach and small intestine with primary colorectal cases occurring less frequently. They are rarely follicular in type but a mixed follicular and diffuse pattern may be seen. Reactive follicles are often found surrounding these lymphomas which can lead to confusion. The often perplexing histology of this group of tumours becomes clearer if they are interpreted in the context of the normal histology and physiology of gut-associated lymphoid tissue (GALT) (Parrot, 1976).

In the gut lymphoid follicles are present in the form of mucosal nodules. The FCCs of these nodules are intimately related to and focally infiltrate the specialized epithelium which covers them. It is here that they encounter luminal antigens following which they leave the follicle and migrate through the lymphatics, the mesenteric lymph nodes and thoracic duct into the systemic circulation. From the circulation these B-cells home back to the lamina propria of that part of the intestine from which they were originally derived where they appear as plasma cells or small lymphocytes, so-called B2 memory cells, which can later transform into plasma cells. In this context it is not surprising that in lymphomas that arise from these mucosal lymphoid follicles the neoplastic FCCs tend to localize close to mucosal epithelium and invade epithelial structures. Circulating FCCs return to the gut mucosa as B2 memory cells and on exposure to antigen some transform into plasma cells. When this occurs, there is, at least in the early stages, a striking anatomic separation between the plasma cells which, representing the differentiated portion of the neoplasm, tends to be non-invasive and the invasive FCCs. Because of the homing proclivities of lymphocytes derived from GALT gastrointestinal FCC lymphoma tends to remain localized to the gastrointestinal tract for long periods of time.

(a) *Histology*

The histology of these tumours is essentially similar to that of their nodal counterparts (see Chapter 7). Certain patterns produced as the malignant centrocytes and centroblasts invade the mucosa are, however, distinctive and helpful in the diagnosis and differential diagnosis of this group of tumours. These lymphomas invade the lamina propria between the glands and isolated glands may remain within solid sheets of tumour (Fig. 13.1). The invasion of individual glands by centrocytes and centroblasts results in a highly characteristic lesion which, when seen, is pathognomonic of FCC lymphoma (Figs 13.2 and 13.3). Plasmacytic differentiation occurs in a minority of cases usually as a band-like infiltrate of mature plasma cells beneath the surface epithelium which pushes apart mucosal glands without invading them. Within this plasma cell infiltrate, which can be shown to be monotypic with immunohistochemical stains, invasive crypt lesions may be seen standing out in contrast to surrounding plasma cells (Fig. 13.4). This dimorphic appearance reflects the normal anatomic separations between FCCs of mucosal lymphoid nodules and lamina propria plasma cells derived from them following antigenic stimulation (Parrot, 1976).

(b) *Differential diagnosis*

Florid reactive lymphoid hyperplasia (sometimes called pseudolymphoma) is a condition that occurs most often in the stomach where it is

---

Fig. 13.1 Follicle centre cell (FCC) lymphoma of the stomach centroblastic/centrocytic diffuse. Residual and partially destroyed glands can be seen within the tumour infiltrate, × 100.

Fig. 13.2 High power view of the tumour illustrated in Fig. 13.1. FCCs can be seen focally invading two gastric glands, × 400.

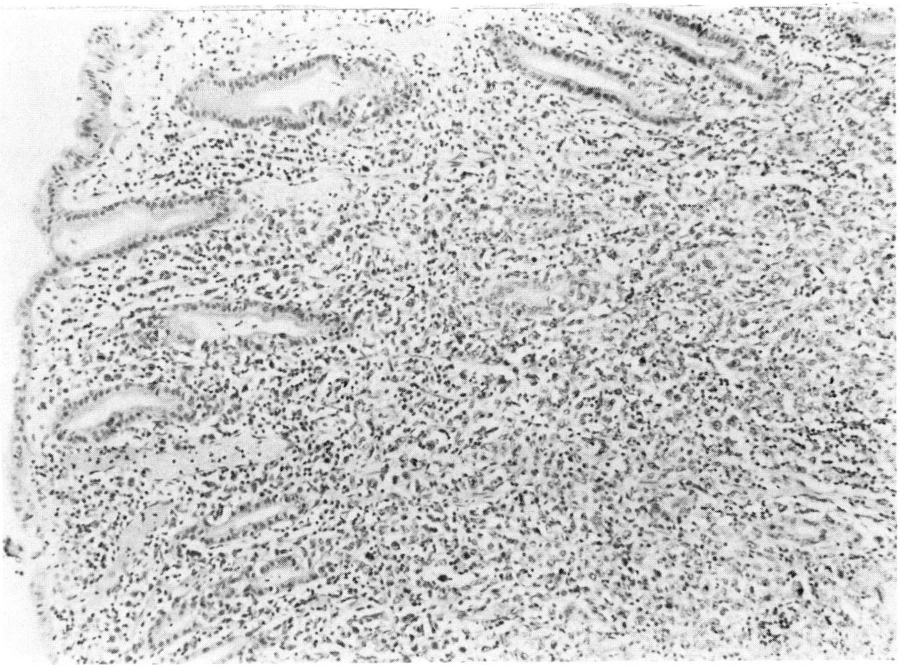

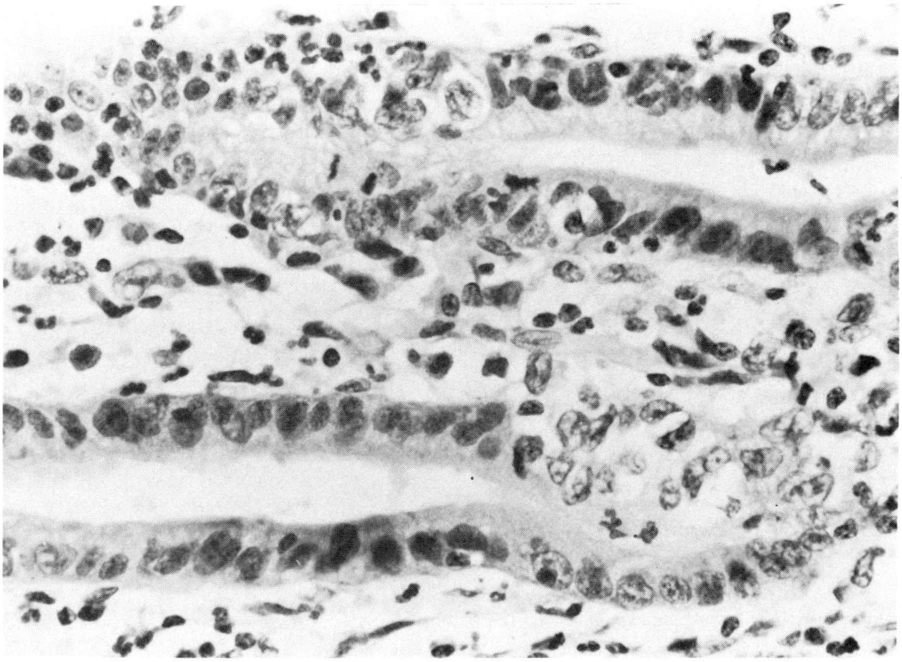

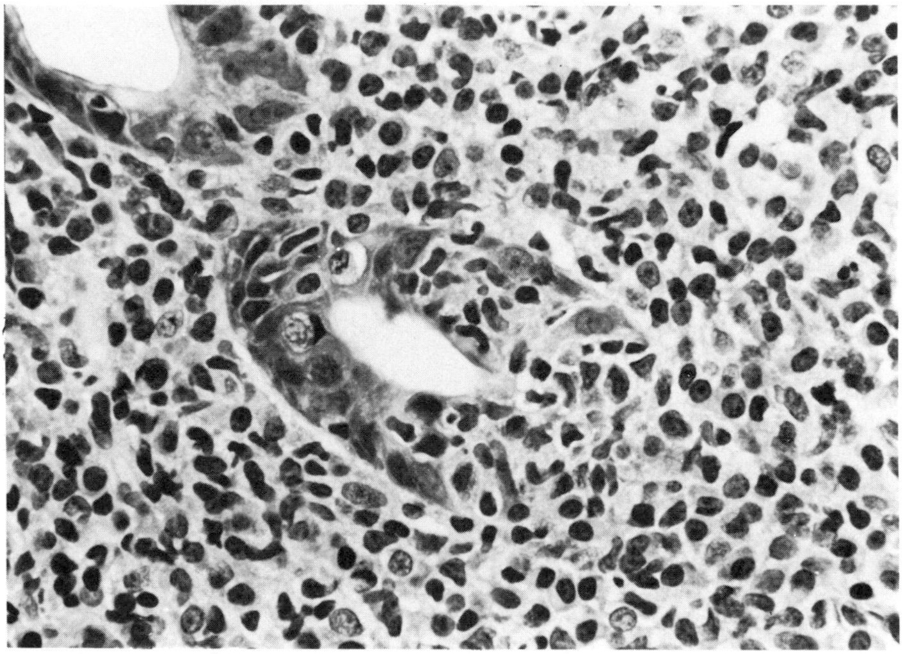

Fig. 13.3 Individual gland invasion in a FCC lymphoma of the stomach. This lesion is pathognomonic of this type of lymphoma, × 400.

usually associated with a peptic ulcer. Reactive follicles are prominent in this condition (Fig. 13.5) but the lymphocytes which infiltrate between the crypts are never seen invading them (Fig. 13.6). The cytology of these small lymphocytes is quite different from that of centrocytes and centroblasts.

In FCC lymphomas in which centroblasts or immunoblasts predominate, differentiation from poorly differentiated carcinoma can be difficult. Mucin stains are not always helpful since they may be negative in some undifferentiated carcinomas. Carcinoma tends to invade in solid masses producing an expanding lesion in contrast to lymphoma which infiltrates between glands (Fig. 13.7). The cytology and the distinctive pattern of glandular invasion seen in FCC lymphomas are important distinguishing features.

Fig. 13.4 In this FCC lymphoma of the stomach extreme plasma cell differentiation is present. Centrally the malignant centrocytes and centroblasts are invading a gland in characteristic fashion, × 250.

Fig. 13.5 Florid reactive lymphoid hyperplasia of the stomach. Note the prominent reactive follicle centres amidst the lymphoid infiltrate, × 40.

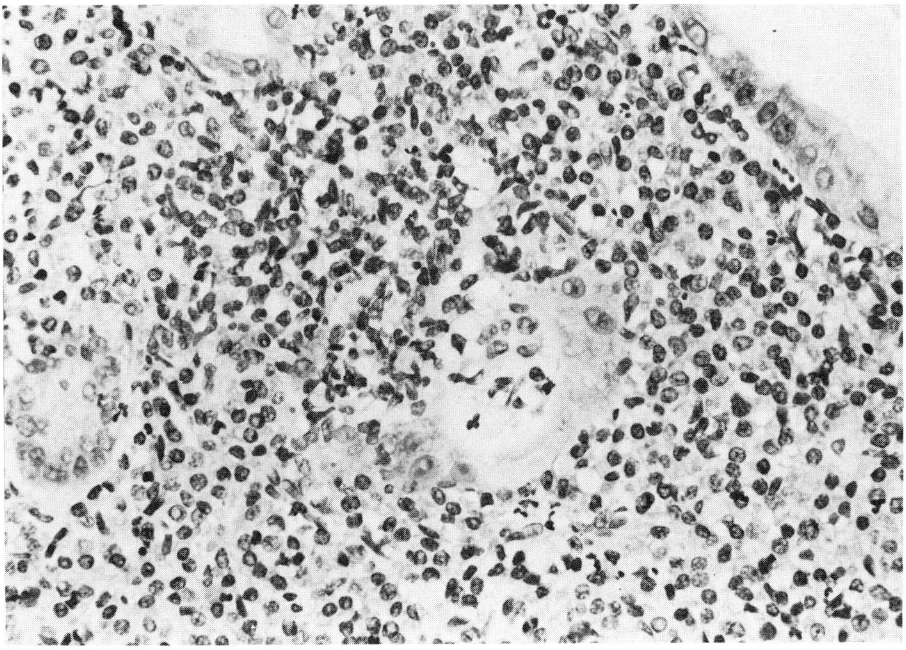

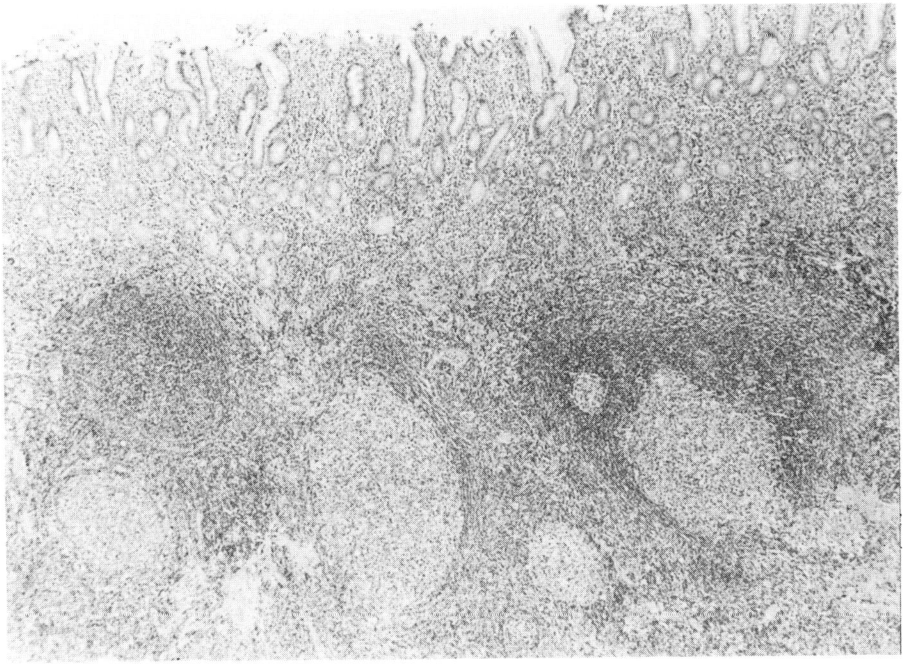

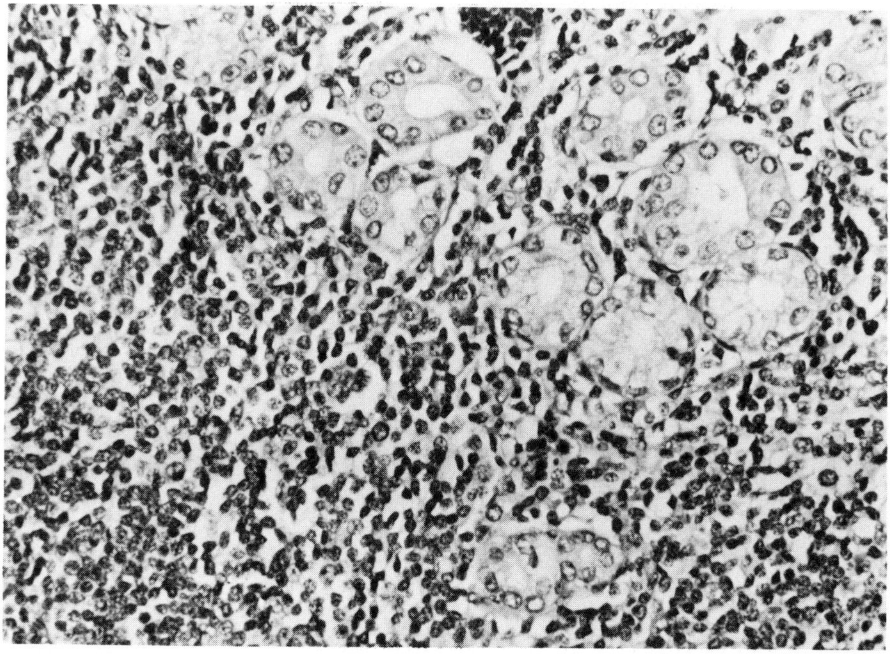

Fig. 13.6 High power view of Fig. 13.5 showing lymphocytes and plasma cells infiltrating between gastric glands without glandular invasion, × 400.

In rectal biopsies from patients with Crohn's disease invasion of single glands by epithelioid macrophages may result in lesions resembling those of lymphoma. The surrounding polymorphic infiltrate of Crohn's disease is, however, quite different from that of lymphoma.

13.1.2 Mediterranean lymphoma

Among the large numbers of cases of gastrointestinal lymphoma occurring in the Middle East a proportion is characterized by malabsorption and a diffuse plasmacytic infiltrate of the small intestine. To this group the terms Mediterranean lymphoma (MTL) or immunoproliferative small intestinal disease (IPSID) have been applied (World Health Organization, 1976). In some of these cases an abnormal α-heavy chain is produced by the plasma cells and can be detected in the blood or

---

Fig. 13.7 Poorly differentiated carcinoma (a) showing well-defined pushing edge and absence of gastric glands within the tumour. In contrast (b) malignant lymphoma, composed largely of centroblasts, infiltrates between glands and lacks an expanding edge, × 100.

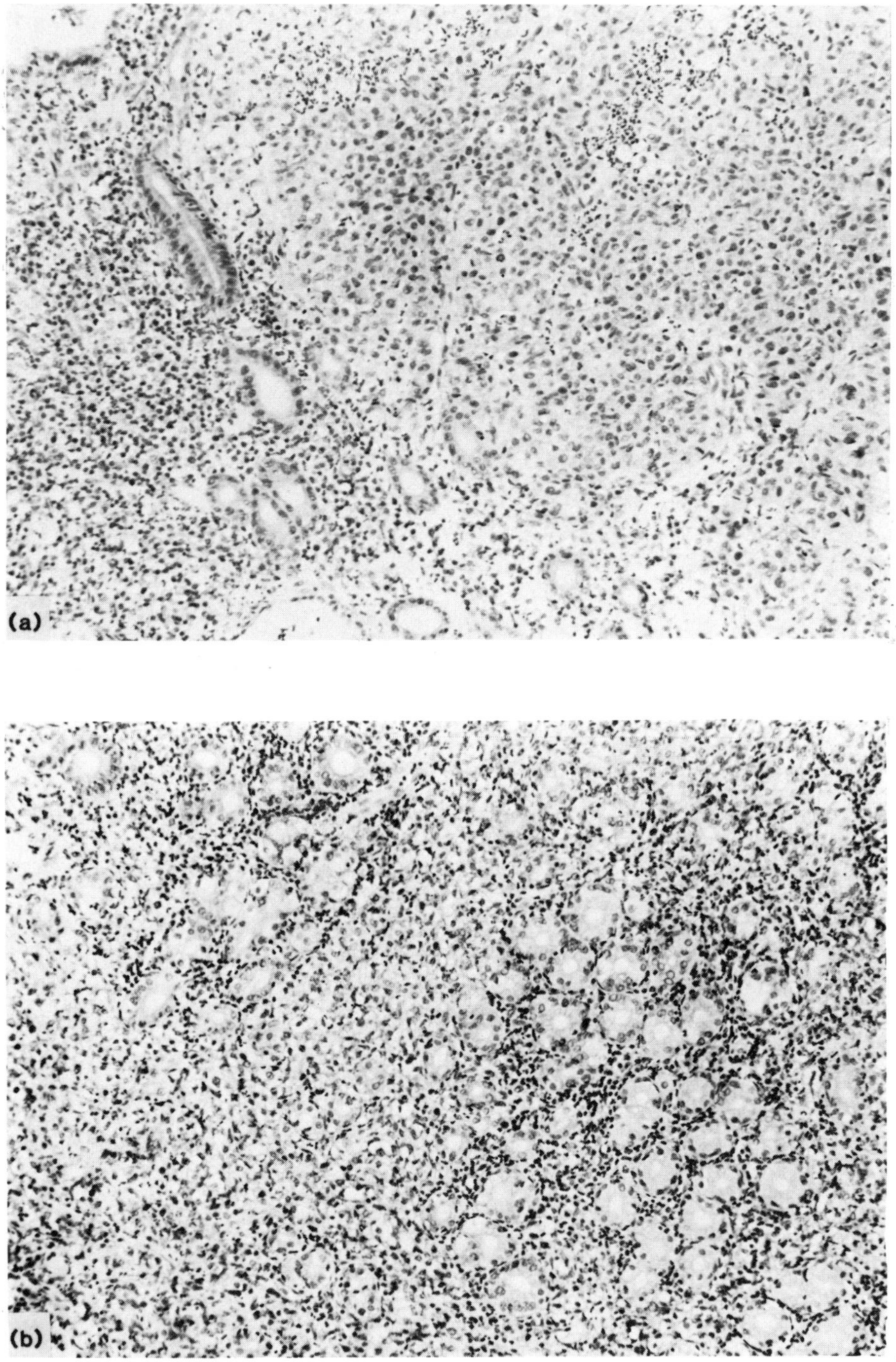
(a)
(b)

duodenal juice, giving rise to the term α-chain disease (ACD) (Seligmann *et al.*, 1968). We regard Mediterranean lymphoma essentially as a type of FCC lymphoma with extreme plasmacytic differentiation. In the early stages the non-invasive plasma cells dominate the histological picture but with time the invasive FCCs emerge and eventually form the bulk of the neoplasm (Isaacson, 1979).

(a) *Histology*

A diffuse plasma cell infiltrate is present in the small intestine which pushes the crypts apart and broadens the villi (Fig. 13.8). In this setting

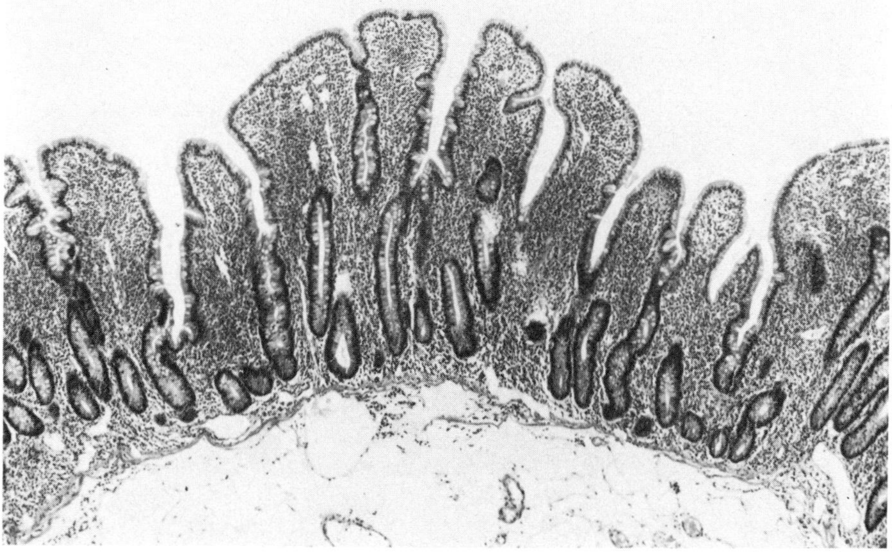

Fig. 13.8 Mediterranean lymphoma of small intestine. The villi are broadened and the crypts pushed apart by an infiltrate of mature plasma cells, × 40.

destructive infiltrates of centrocytes and centroblasts occur producing the characteristic leasion of FCC lymphoma already described (Figs 13.9 and 13.10). As the disease progresses confluent masses of centroblastic/centrocytic lymphoma arise which may contain pleomorphic cells and

---

Fig. 13.9 Mediterranean lymphoma of small intestine. A band-like and nodular infiltrate of lymphoid cells is present and destructive infiltrates of individual crypts are apparent, × 40.

Fig. 13.10 Mediterranean lymphoma. Individual small intestinal crypts are infiltrated by centrocytes. Compare with Figs 13.2, 13.3 and 13.4, × 400.

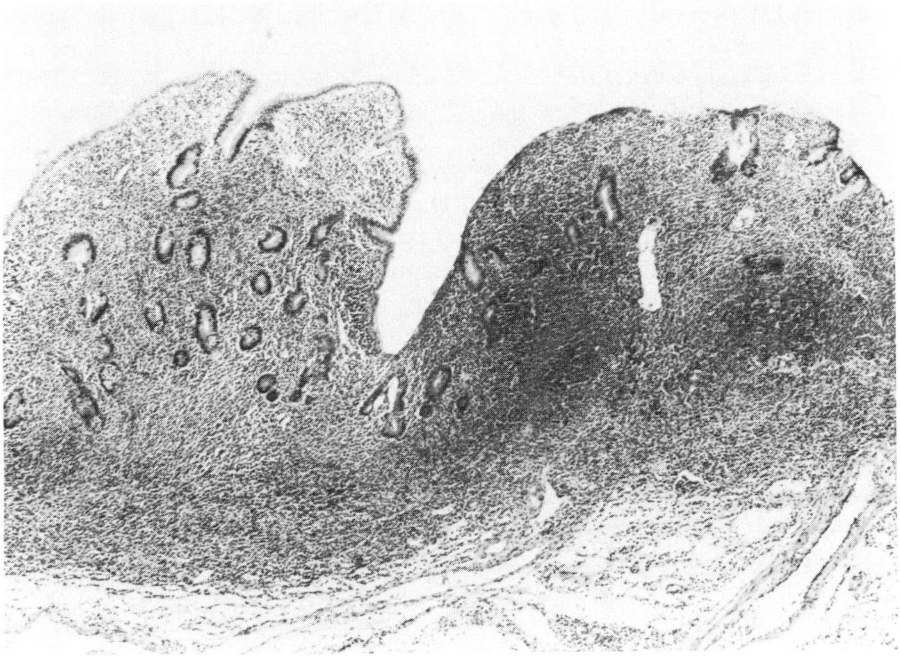

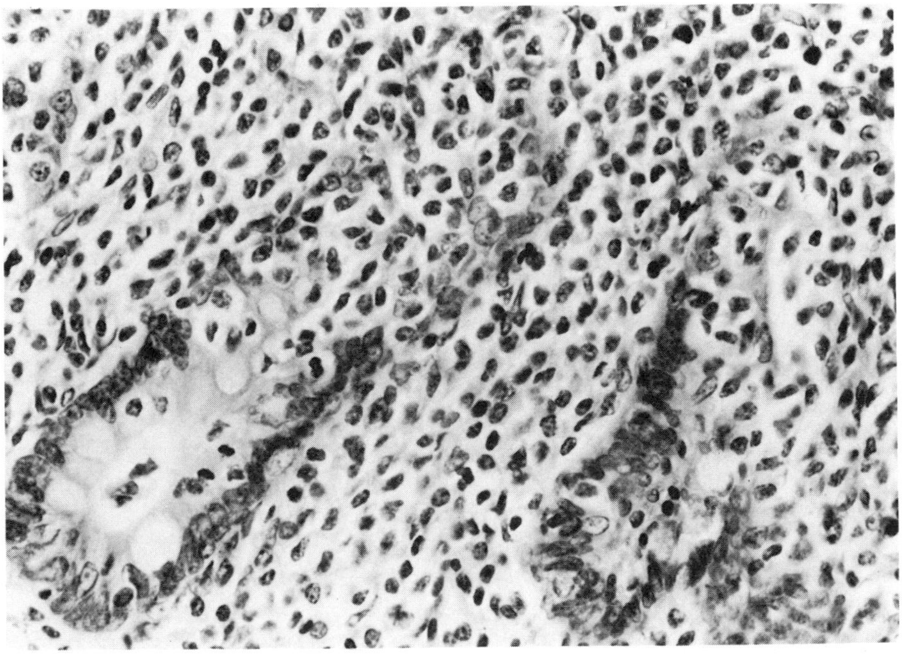

varying numbers of immunoblasts. The histology of MTL is thus very similar to those cases of 'Western' FCC lymphoma in which there is plasmacytic differentiation. Spread of MTL beyond the intestine and mesenteric lymph nodes is rare except in the terminal stages of the disease.

(b) *Differential diagnosis*

The plasmacytic infiltrate in MTL should not be mistaken for coeliac disease. In contrast to coeliac disease there is no crypt hyperplasia and the surface epithelium does not show degenerative changes or a significant increase of intraepithelial lymphocytes.

13.1.3 *Undifferentiated (Burkitt-like) lymphoma*

The histological appearances of this type of lymphoma are the same whether it occurs in the lymph nodes or the gastrointestinal tract and have already been described in Chapter 8. Although very common in the Middle East it should not be regarded as a form of MTL from which it is quite different. In particular, the mucosal plasma cell population is quite normal in this disease and there is no associated malabsorption.

13.1.4 *Malignant histiocytosis of the intestine*

A significant proportion of small intestinal malignant lymphomas in the United Kingdom occurs as a complication of coeliac disease (Holmes *et al.*, 1976). This type of lymphoma has been characterized as a form of malignant histiocytosis which appears to originate in the macrophages of the small intestinal lamina propria (Isaacson and Wright, 1978; 1980). The name malignant histiocytosis of the intestine (MHI) has been given to this disease in order to distinguish it from classical malignant histiocytosis (see Chapter 11).

Patients who develop MHI may have a history of coeliac disease or alternatively the onset of MHI may be the first indication that they have coeliac disease. They are usually over 50 years of age but cases have been recorded in patients in their 20's. The onset of MHI is heralded by abdominal pain and weight loss and often recurrence of steatorrhoea in patients previously responsive to a gluten-free diet. Finger clubbing and a skin rash may be present and acute intestinal obstruction, perforation or haemorrhage leads to a laparotomy, often under emergency conditions. Resection of the macroscopically involved segment of small intestine may be followed by remission but this is usually of short duration and death from a repeated gastrointestinal catastrophe is the rule. The prognosis of this disease is, with few exceptions, very poor.

The appropriate investigations in a patient in whom the diagnosis of

MHI is suspected includes a bone marrow aspirate (the malignant histiocytes are more likely to be seen in an aspirate smear than in a trephine section), a liver biopsy and, if these are negative, a laparotomy. At laparotomy intestinal lesions, if present, should be resected. In the absence of identifiable disease a full thickness jejunal biopsy should be performed together with generous biopsies of mesenteric lymph nodes and wedge biopsy of the liver.

(a) *Histology*

The intestinal lesion of MHI may consist of circumscribed solid tumours or ulcers. These are frequently multiple. Small lesions, not visible macroscopically, may be present, and in some cases the intestinal lesion is restricted to 'benign' ulcers or focal macrophage aggregates with crypt destruction, the so-called early lesion (Isaacson, 1980) (Fig. 13.11). There is considerable variation in the histology of MHI both between cases and within the same case. The tumour may be monomorphic either consisting of recognizable histiocytes (Fig. 13.12) or of cells resembling immunoblasts (Fig. 13.13). In many instances there is marked pleomorphism with

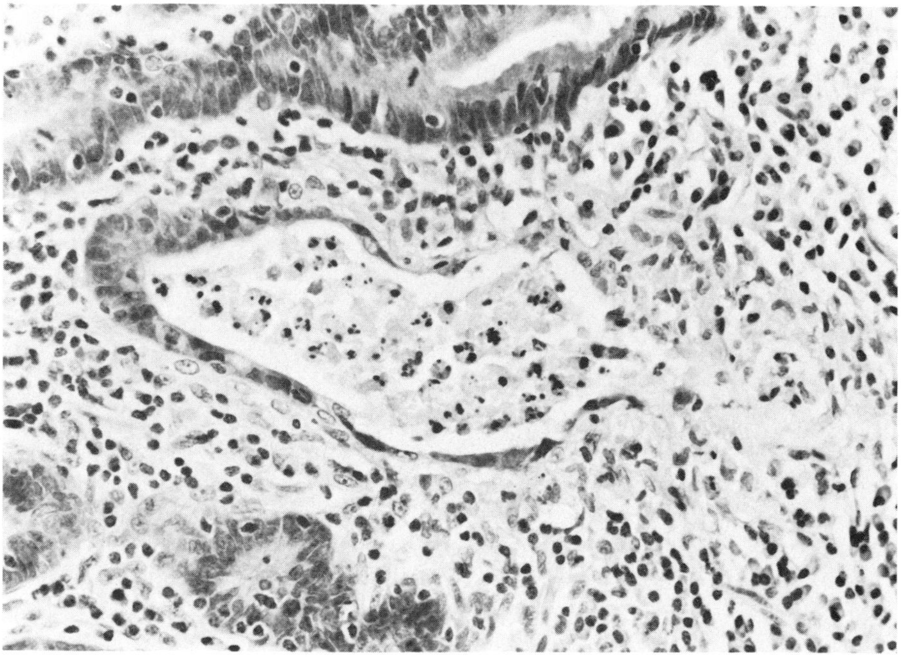

Fig. 13.11 Malignant histiocytosis of the intestine (MHI). In this jejunal biopsy taken five years before overt malignancy was diagnosed the characteristic early lesion is present. A partially destroyed crypt is surrounded by an aggregate of macrophages. The biopsy was otherwise characteristic of coeliac disease, × 250.

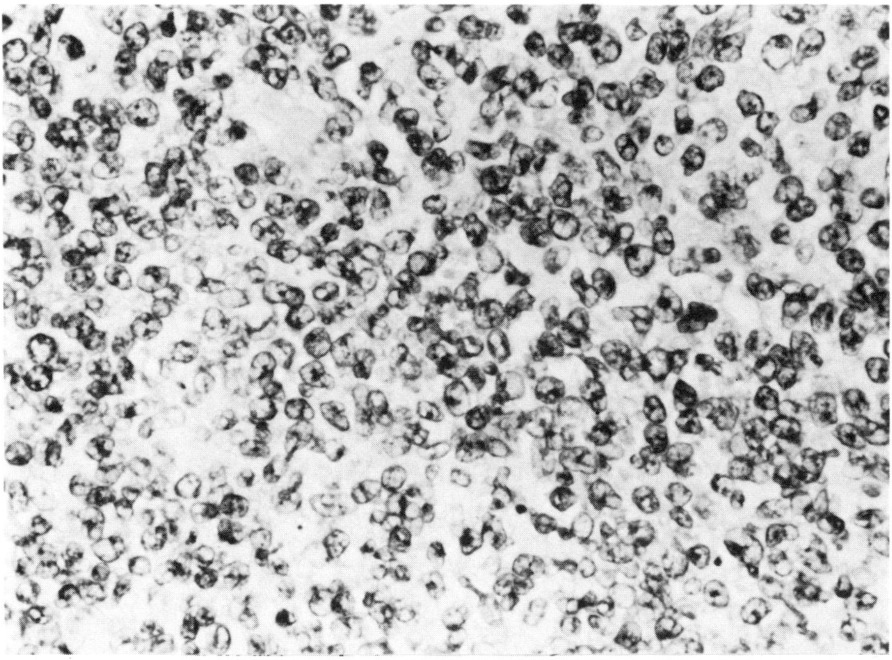

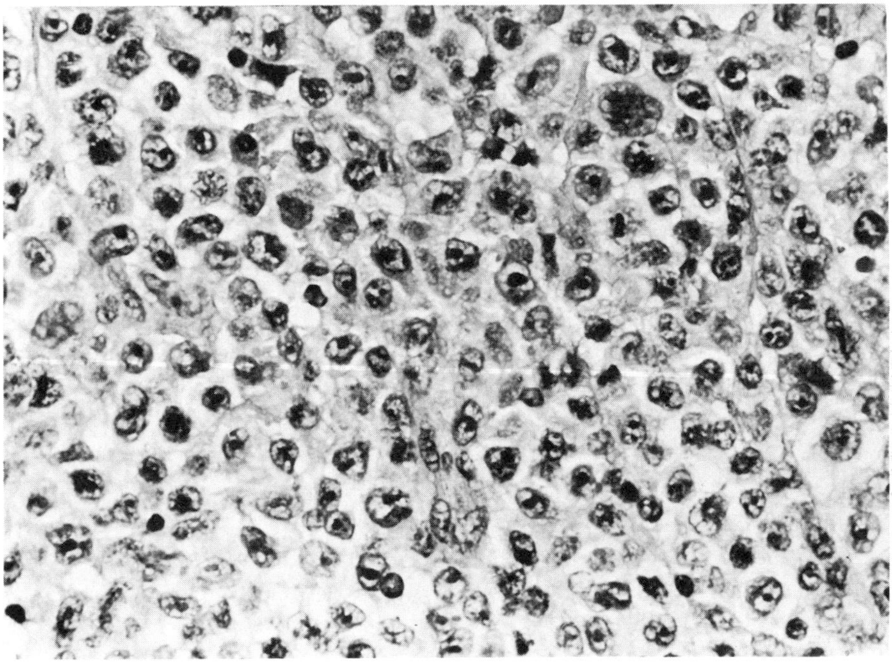

multinucleated giant cells (Fig. 13.14). Dissemination produces histological appearances in lymph nodes, liver, spleen and other organs which are identical to those of classical malignant histiocytes (Figs 13.15 and

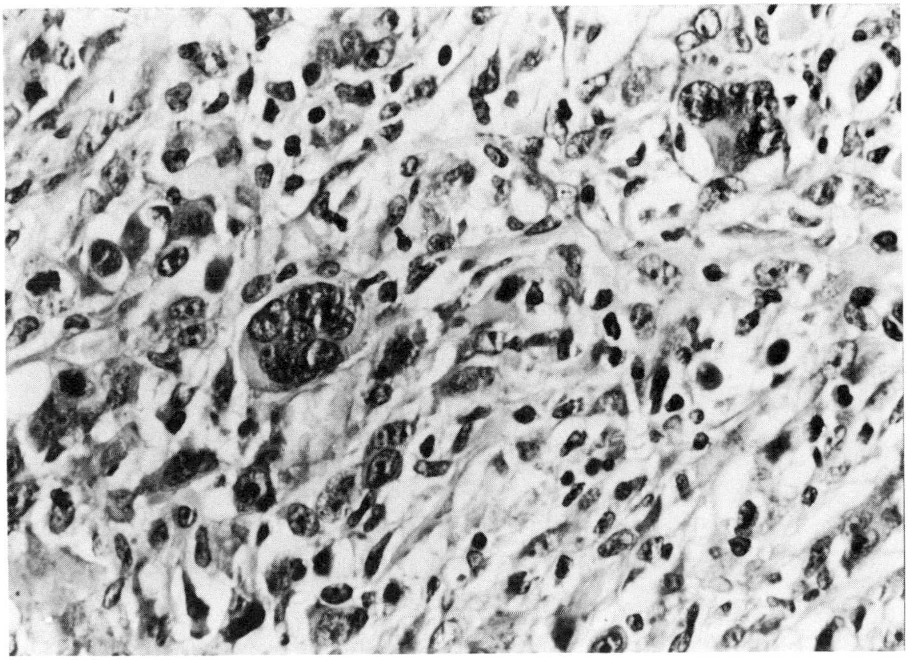

Fig. 13.14 MHI. In this pleomorphic tumour the large multinucleated giant cells are characteristic, × 400.

13.16). In contrast to classical malignant histiocytosis the spleen in MHI is not significantly enlarged and frequently is atrophic. In the latter case clusters of malignant histiocytes may be seen between broad connective tissue bands.

Immunohistochemical findings are characteristic. The malignant cells contain granules of alpha-1-antitrypsin (Fig. 13.17) and stains for immunoglobulin either give negative results or demonstrate polytypic

---

Fig. 13.12 MHI. The tumour in this case is composed of small uniform cells many of which have indented nuclei resembling mature histiocytes. In many of the cells prominent nucleoli are situated in apposition to the nuclear indentation, × 400.

Fig. 13.13 MHI. The cells comprising this monomorphic tumour are larger than those in Fig. 13.12. The nuclei are characterized by large nucleoli which are often centrally situated resulting in a resemblance to immunoblasts, × 400.

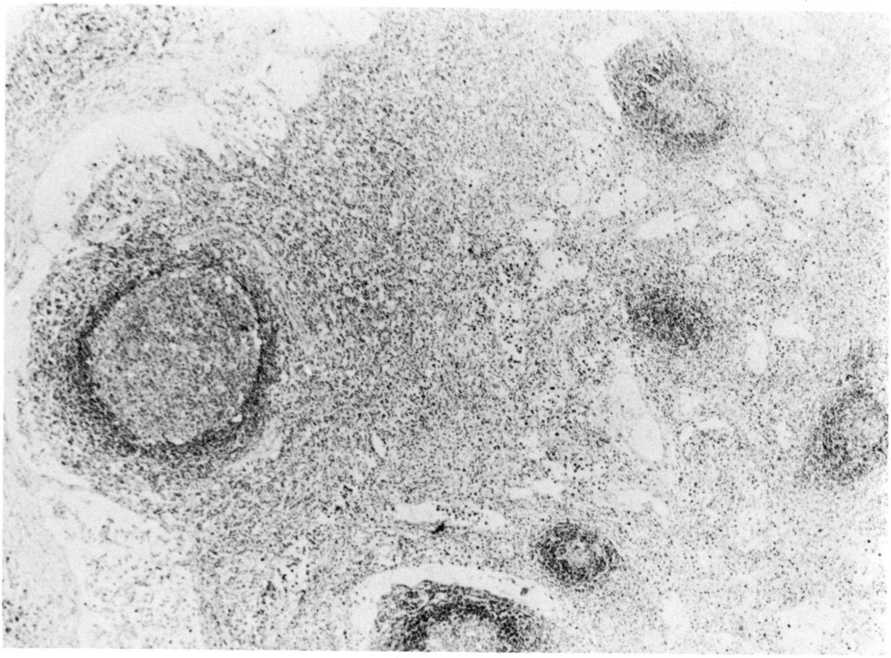

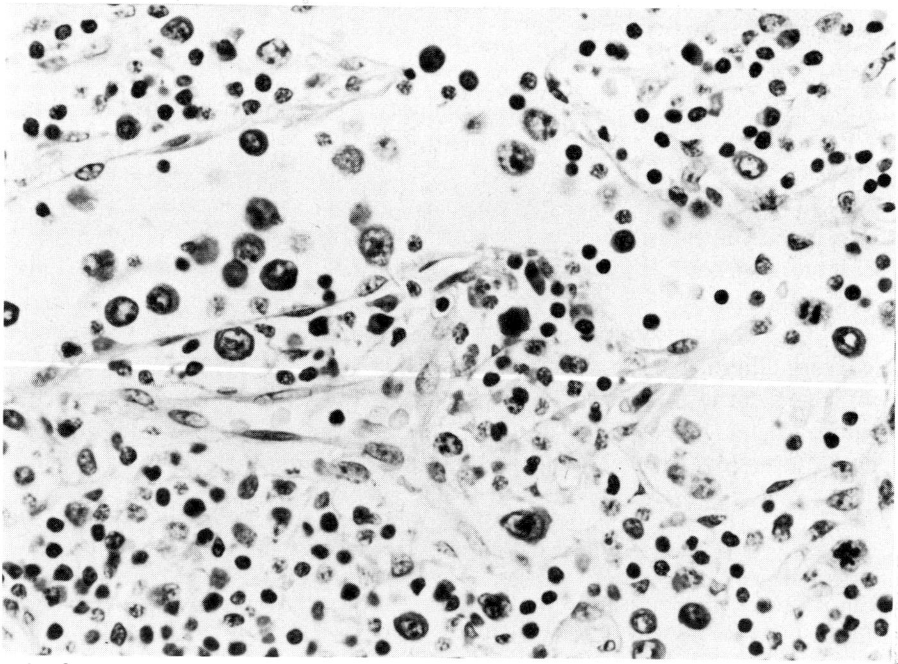

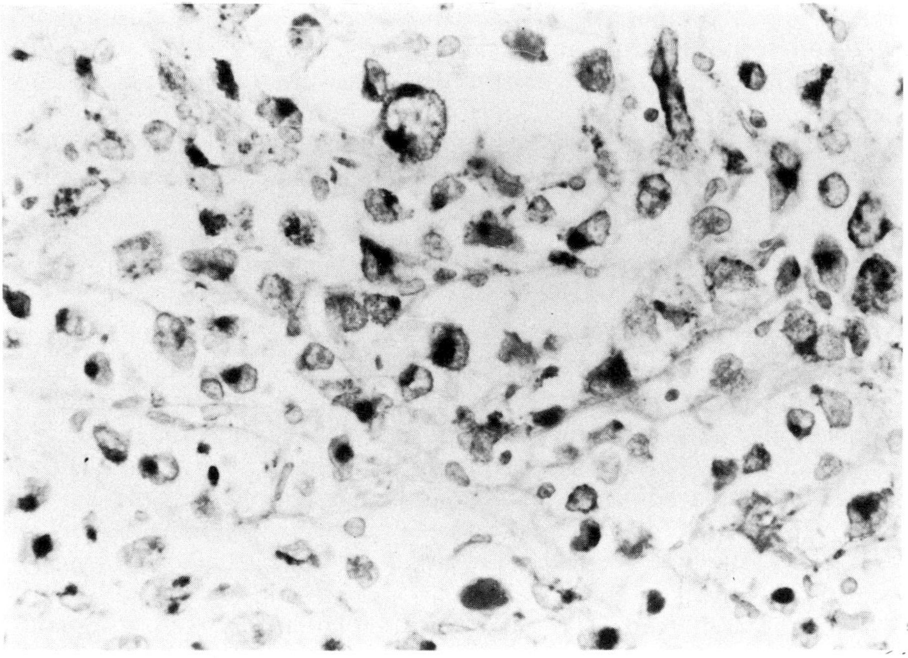

Fig. 13.17 Pleomorphic variety of MHI stained by the immunoperoxidase technique for alpha-1-antitrypsin. Positive staining is mostly confined to the cytoplasm close to the nuclear indentation, × 1000.

immunoglobulin (usually IgG), which has been taken up by the tumour cells. Histochemical studies show non-specific esterase and acid phosphatase in the tumour cells (Isaacson *et al.*, 1982).

(b) *Differential diagnosis*

Because of the frequent occurrence of multinucleate giant cells cases of MHI were frequently misdiagnosed as Hodgkin's disease in the past. The setting of these cells is quite wrong for Hodgkin's disease which, in any event, rarely involves the gastrointestinal tract.

The malignant cells in MHI often bear a close resemblance to immunoblasts. Resemblance to immunoblastic lymphoma is compounded by a plasmacytoid appearance that can be induced by inadequate fixation. The sinusoidal pattern of spread in mesenteric

---

Fig. 13.15 Mesenteric lymph node from a case of MHI. There is follicular hyperplasia and even in this low power photomicrograph abnormal cells can be seen in the dilated sinuses, × 30.

Fig. 13.16 High power view of the intrasinusoidal malignant histiocytes shown in Fig. 13.15, × 400.

lymph nodes, liver and spleen and immunohistochemical features serve to distinguish MHI from immunoblastic lymphoma.

Non-specific benign ulceration of the small intestine is described in coelic disease. This condition, known as ulcerative jejunitis, bears a close resemblance to MHI and is often complicated by its onset after a variable latent period. In our opinion ulcerative jejunitis and MHI are the same disease.

13.2 Salivary gland lymphoma

Infiltration of the salivary glands by lymphoid cells accompanied by acinar atrophy and proliferation of the ductular cells to form epimyoepithelial islands is a characteristic of Sjogren's syndrome. Similar changes may be seen in biopsies of salivary gland lesions, often solitary, from patients without other evidence of Sjogren's syndrome. These proliferations have been designated as 'benign lymphoepithelial lesion' (Godwin, 1952). For several years the presence of epimyoepithelial islands was thought to connote a benign lesion (Morgan and Castleman, 1953; Cruikshank, 1965; Evans and Cruikshank, 1970). However, Azzopardi and Evans (1971) reported the occurrence of malignant lymphoma in five patients with lymphoepithelial lesion of the parotid and four of the 33 malignant lymphomas of salivary gland reported by Hyman and Wolff (1976) were associated with this lesion. Using immunohistochemical techniques Zulman *et al.* (1978) showed that six of nine lymphomas developing in patients with Sjogren's syndrome were monoclonal B-cell lymphomas. The term 'benign lymphoepithelial lesion' is clearly no longer acceptable and has been replaced by myoepithelial sialadenitis (MESA) (Schmid *et al.*, 1982).

Schmid *et al.* (1982) investigated 45 cases of MESA, 16 of whom had Sjogren's syndrome or other autoimmune diseases. In 26 of these confluent areas of monotypic lymphoplasmacytoid cells or immunoblasts were present and these cases were designated 'manifest malignant lymphomas'. Fourteen of these patients later developed extrasalivary malignant lymphoma of the same histology. Lesser, but equally convincing, evidence of lymphoma was present in 16 cases, four of which later progressed to extrasalivary lymphoma. The interval between the onset of salivary gland enlargement and the diagnosis of malignant lymphoma (usually lymphoplasmacytic but occasionally immunoblastic lymphoma) ranged from 1.5–12 years. The authors concluded that there is close histogenic relationship between MESA with or without autoimmune disease and lymphoplasmacytic immunocytoma and B-immunoblastic lymphoma.

We agree with this concept but interpret the malignant lymphomas as a

FCC lymphoma of salivary gland-associated lymphoid tissue showing varying degrees of plasmacytic differentiation similar to that described in the gastrointestinal tract. We regard the lymphoid infiltrates of the epimyoepithelial islands seen in these salivary gland lymphomas as analogous to the lesions produced by glandular invasion in gastrointestinal FCC lymphoma. The small irregular cells in these epimyoepithelial islands are thus centrocytes and not T-cells as proposed by Lennert (Schmid *et al.*, 1982).

Malignant lymphomas of salivary gland not showing features of MESA usually arise in intrasalivary lymph nodes. The surrounding salivary tissue may be compressed or invaded by lymphoma but it does not show acinar atrophy or epimyoepithelial islands. These lymphomas show the same histological features as other nodal lymphomas and are not further discussed here. Burkitt's lymphoma frequently involves the salivary glands (but not the intrasalivary lymph nodes) and is not associated with MESA (Wright, 1971).

13.2.1 *Histology*

A characteristic feature of primary malignant lymphoma of the salivary gland is the presence of epimyoepithelial islands infiltrated by small tortuous centrocytes either singly or in groups (Figs 13.18 and 13.19). The epimyoepithelial islands are surrounded by broad swathes of lymphoid cells. These may consist predominantly of lymphocytes usually larger and with more irregular nuclei than those seen in lymphocytic lymphomas. These cells are probably closely related to centrocytes and possibly represent the B2 memory cells described above. More typical centrocytes and centroblasts may occur focally or in sheets. Lymphoplasmacytoid and plasma cells are present in variable numbers and may dominate the histological picture (Fig. 13.20). Epithelioid histiocytes often occur singly or in groups and occasionally outnumber lymphoid cells.

13.2.2 *Differential diagnosis*

In the past there has been considerable debate on the differentiation between benign lymphoepithelial lesion of salivary gland (MESA) and malignant lymphoma. We believe that most, if not all, cases of MESA that occur as solitary tumours should be regarded as slowly progressive primary lymphoma of salivary tissue. Most of these patients do not have other features of Sjogren's syndrome (Cruikshank, 1965). The lesions of Sjogren's syndrome involve minor as well as major salivary glands and are more obviously inflammatory with a greater range of reactive cells,

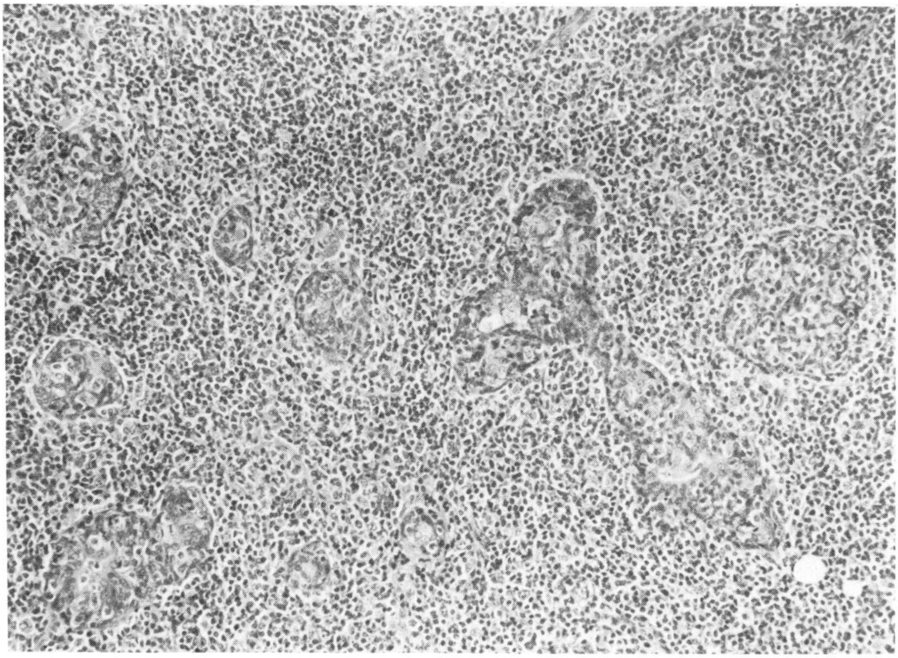

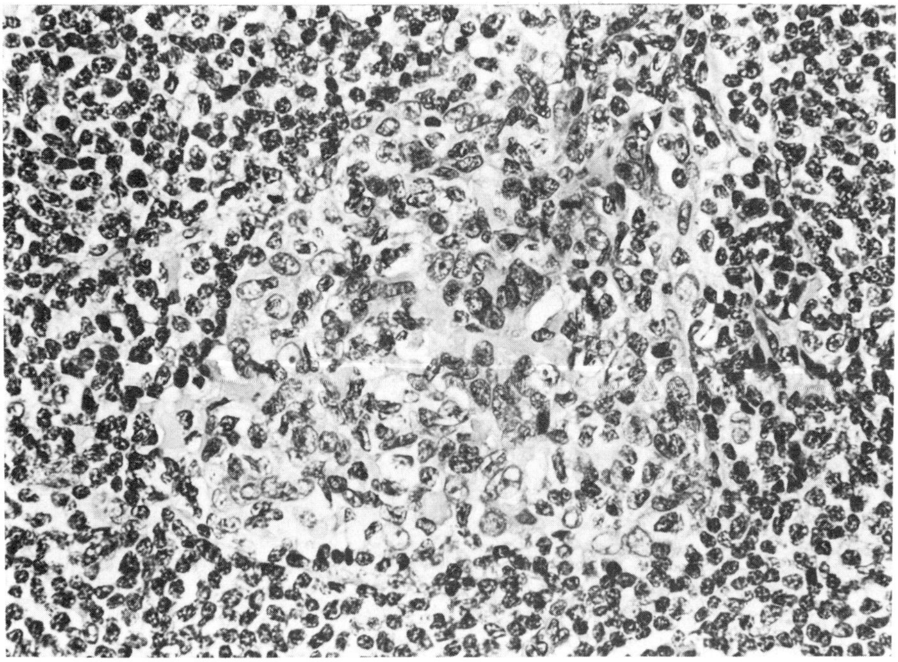

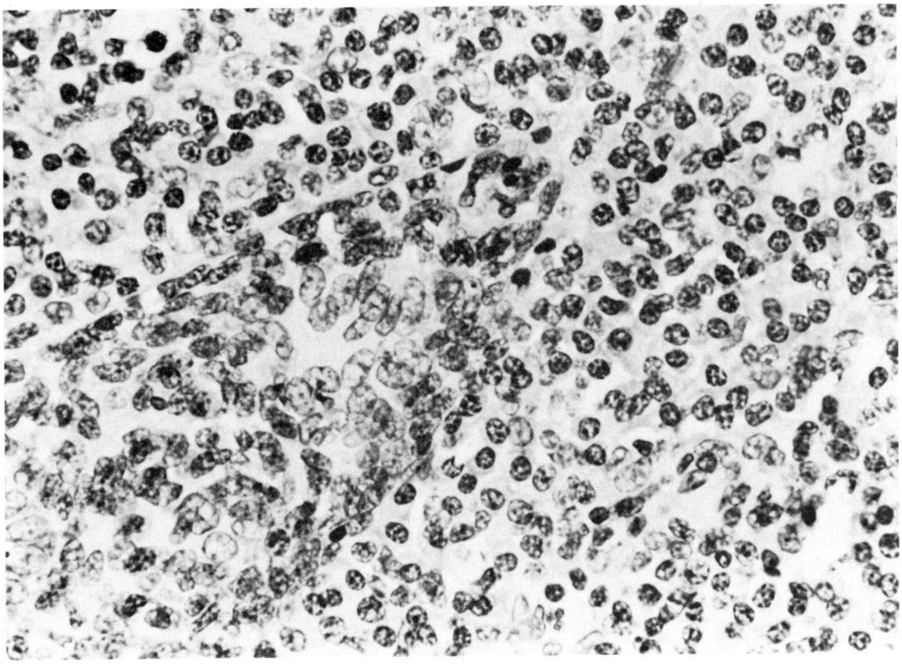

Fig. 13.20 In this primary salivary gland lymphoma the epimyoepithelial island infiltrated by centrocytes is surrounded by mature plasma cells which proved to be monotypic when stained for immunoglobulin. Compare with Fig. 13.4, × 400.

prominent reactive lymphoid follicles and progressive fibrosis. An increased incidence of malignant lymphoma has been reported in patients with Sjogren's syndrome (Zulman *et al.*, 1978; Kassan and Gardy, 1978) but it is not clear how many of these had the full syndrome rather than localized MESA.

In non-specific sialadenitis, often associated with sialolithiasis, the ducts are dilated, contain inflammatory cells and do not form epimyoepithelial islands. The reactive lymphoid tissue in these glands does not form the broad swathes seen in most malignant lymphomas.

Fig. 13.18 Primary malignant lymphoma of salivary gland showing prominent epimyoepithelial islands surrounded by lymphoid cells, × 120.
Fig. 13.19 High power view of an epimyoepithelial island infiltrated by centrocytes. The surrounding lymphocytes have slightly irregular nuclei similar but not identical to centrocytes. Compare with Fig. 13.3, × 300.

13.3 Malignant lymphoma of the thyroid gland

Generalized malignant lymphomas may involve the thyroid gland either as subtle infiltrates detectable only by histological examination or rarely as a cause of goitre which may be the presenting clinical feature. Thus, 37% of children with Burkitt's lymphoma have involvement of the thyroid gland at autopsy and 4.3% have a clinically manifest goitre (Wright, 1971). Secondary lymphomas of the thyroid are much less of a diagnostic problem than primary lymphomas because they are not superimposed on a pre-existing thyroiditis and the nature of the disease is usually apparent from biopsies taken at other sites.

The recognition of primary lymphoma of the thyroid and its differentiation from Hashimoto's disease on the one hand, and small cell carcinoma of the thyroid on the other, can be one of the most difficult problems in diagnostic histopathology. This difficulty is frequently compounded by the poor quality of the histological material available for study. Fixatives penetrate thyroid tissue slowly and in resection specimens the tissue at the centre of the thyroid is poorly preserved unless the organ is sliced before placing into fixative or soon after it is received in the laboratory. Needle biopsies are usually well fixed but may suffer from traction artefact and, in any event, present only a small sample of tissue from what may be a very heterogeneous histological lesion.

Primary lymphoma of the thyroid is predominantly a disease of females with a peak incidence in the sixth and seventh decades of life. Burke *et al.* (1977) recorded a five-year survival of 54%. In many reported series and in our unpublished cases long survival of patients with FCC lymphoma of the thyroid have been recorded following local therapy alone. Although thyroid-associated lymphoid tissue is not described the nature of FCC lymphomas of the thyroid bears a close resemblance to those of the gastrointestinal tract and salivary glands. This probably reflects the embryological relationship of the thyroid gland to the gastrointestinal tract.

13.3.1 Histology

Almost all primary lymphomas of the thyroid are of FCC origin (Burke *et al.*, 1977; Maurer *et al.*, 1979). The tumours are frequently diffuse and often contain a high proportion of centroblasts. Follicular and diffuse tumours are seen but purely follicular tumours are uncommon. Eight of the 29 cases reported by Maurer *et al.* (1979) were categorized as immunoblastic sarcomas. Most primary lymphomas of the thyroid gland arise in a setting of Hashimoto's disease or lymphocytic thyroiditis and sections of residual thyroid gland will show evidence of this. Residual acinar within the lymphoma usually show eosinophilic change and varying degrees of cytological atypia suggestive of previous involvement of thyroiditis. A pathognomonic feature of FCC lymphoma is invasion of the thyroid acini by centrocytes (Figs 13.21 and 13.22). Sometimes these accumulate in acini or in the attenuated remains of acini producing a highly characteristic histological appearance (Compagno and Oertel, 1980). This lesion is strikingly similar to that produced by lymphomatous invasion of individual glands in the gastrointestinal tract and epimyoepithelial islands in salivary glands. The residual acini are surrounded by FCCs showing varying proportions of centroblasts and centrocytes and by small lymphocytes similar to those seen in salivary gland lymphomas. Plasma cells and plasmacytoid cells are often present in large numbers. These sometimes represent residual reactive plasma cells associated with the preceding thyroiditis but can often be shown to be monotypic indicating that they are part of the neoplastic population. Such cases may be designated as lymphoplasmacytic or plasmacytic

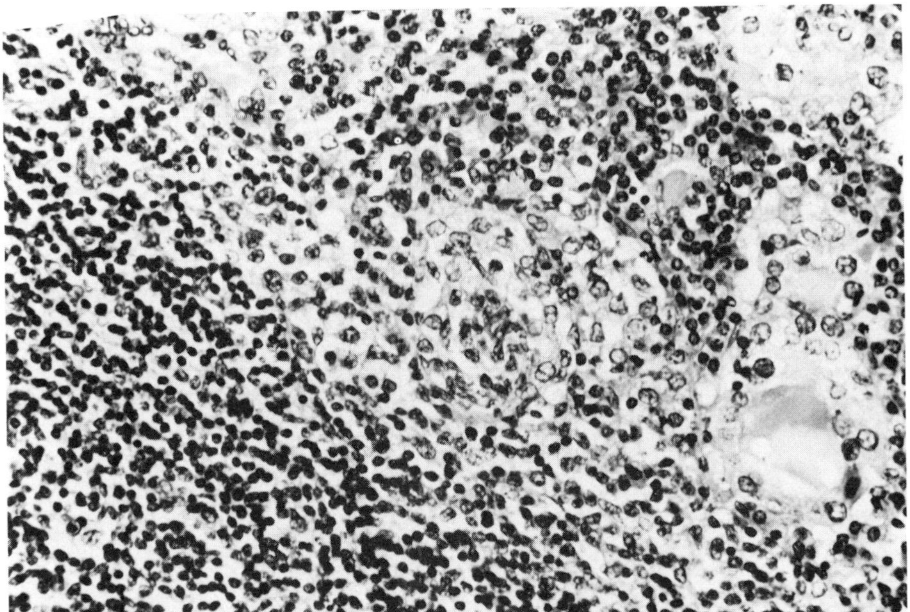

Fig. 13.21 Primary malignant lymphoma of the thyroid. Lymphocytes (lower left) and plasma cells (upper right) infiltrate between thyroid acini, one of which shows invasion by centrocytes, × 250.

tumours but as in the gastrointestinal tract and salivary gland, we believe they are a manifestation of FCC lymphoma.

Other histological features that are of value in the diagnosis of malignant lymphoma of the thyroid are the presence of vascular invasion and invasion outside the gland (Compagno and Oertel, 1980). The latter feature may also have prognostic significance (Woolner *et al.*, 1966). The presence of areas of necrosis is a feature that may help to differentiate between malignant lymphoma and Hashimoto's disease. Areas of sclerosis are common within FCC lymphomas of the thyroid. It is difficult to determine whether this is a feature of the tumour or represents residual sclerosis from preceding Hashimoto's disease.

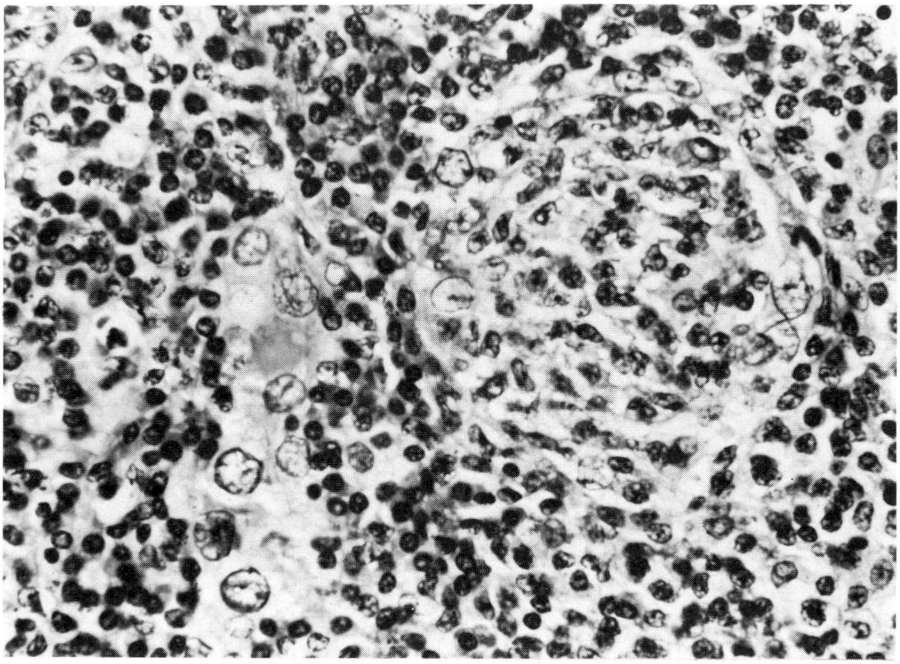

Fig. 13.22 High power view of a primary thyroid lymphoma showing the characteristic acinar invasion by centrocytes with a surrounding (monotypic) plasma cell infiltrate. Compare with Figs 13.4 and 13.20, × 400.

13.3.2 Differential diagnosis

Most cases of primary lymphoma of the thyroid develop on the basis of Hashimoto's disease or lymphocytic thyroiditis and the differentiation of these conditions can be difficult. In those lymphomas in which there are broad swathes of monomorphic lymphoid cells the problem does not arise but many primary follicle centre cell lymphomas of the thyroid show a confusing mixture of atypical epithelial cells, follicle centre cells with varying numbers of plasma cells, as well as residual areas of thyroiditis. The presence of acinar invasion by centrocytes is pathognomonic of lymphoma and invasion outside the capsule of the gland and of blood vessel walls are useful supporting features when present. The immunoperoxidase technique is particularly valuable in distinguishing between the polytypic plasma cell proliferation seen in Hashimoto's disease and the monotypic cells of malignant lymphoma.

The differentiation between malignant lymphoma of the thyroid and small cell anaplastic carcinoma has been a subject of great debate in the past but it is now generally agreed that most small cell tumours are lymphomas (Woolner *et al.*, 1966; Heimann *et al.*, 1978). These two conditions can usually be separated on the basis of their cell morphology and the presence of the characteristic acinar lesion in lymphoma but the presence of abnormal epithelial cells in malignant lymphoma can cause confusion. A PAS stain may prove useful in such cases since it stains both thyroglobulin and basement membrane and may assist in the delineation of residual acini. Lymphomas tend to have a more infiltrative growth pattern than carcinomas and this pattern of infiltration is particularly well seen in the walls of veins and the extraglandular tissues. Carcinomas of the thyroid are often infiltrated by polymorphs particularly around areas of necrosis. This is not a feature of lymphomas even when necrosis is present.

13.4 Malignant lymphoma of the lung

Pulmonary involvement by malignant lymphoma may result from direct extension of mediastinal disease, seen most commonly in patients with Hodgkin's disease, or by haematogenous dissemination. T-cell lymphomas including cutaneous T-cell lymphomas show a predilection for pleuropulmonary involvement (Rappaport and Thomas, 1974; Wolfe *et al.*, 1980; Waldron *et al.*, 1977) Histopathological examination may be necessary to distinguish these secondary lymphomas from opportunistic infection or pulmonary fibrosis due to chemotherapeutic agents. They show similar histopathological features to the primary tumours and will not be further discussed here.

Primary lymphomas of the lung have been the cause of considerable confusion for many years. Liebow *et al.* (1972) described an angiocentric lymphoproliferative lesion of the lung that they designated lymphomatoid granulomatosis. They noted that many of these cases had been interpreted initially as malignant lymphoma. Vascular invasion is a feature of both primary and secondary malignant lymphoma of the lung and it is now apparent that most cases of lymphomatoid granulomatosis are in fact malignant lymphomas (Colby and Carrington, 1982). Vascular invasion may lead to tumour necrosis with resultant infiltration by reactive and inflammatory cells. The differentiation of these tumours from inflammatory lesions such as Wegener's granulomatosis must be made on basic histopathological principles, in particular the cytology and homogeneity of the lymphoma cells.

The nature of so-called 'pseudolymphoma' of the lung and its relationship to malignant lymphoma has been debated for over two decades. This condition occurs over a wide range (Greenberg *et al.*, 1972) and may be detected by routine chest radiology in patients who are asymptomatic. The lesion is usually unilateral involving one lobe or it may be bilateral. Grossly the cut surface of the lung has an homogenous grey colour and the edges of the lesion are ill-defined. Many patients with 'pseudolymphoma' of the lung remain asymptomatic following local resection (McNamara *et al.*, 1969; Gwynne-Jenkins and Salm, 1971), although disseminated malignant lymphoma may develop after a period of many years (Greenberg *et al.*, 1972). This slow progression to malignant lymphoma led Gibbs and Seal (1978) to prefer the term 'premalignant lymphoma' to 'pseudolymphoma'. Saltzstein (1963) attempted to define those features that separate 'pseudolymphoma' from malignant lymphoma. The features he considered characteristic of 'pseudolymphoma' were a proliferation of mature lymphocytes and other inflammatory cells, the presence of germinal centres and the absence of involvement of the hilar lymph nodes. Other authors (McNamara *et al.*, 1969; Gwynne-Jenkins and Salm, 1971) suggest that it is not possible to distinguish between 'pseudolymphoma' and lymphoma of the lung. However these lesions are designated it is difficult to reconcile a lesion composed of large sheets of small lymphoid cells with an inflammatory or reactive condition and conversely, it would appear unusual for a lymphoma composed predominantly of small lymphocytes to remain as a localized tumour for many years. Recognizing this problem Al-Saleem and Peale (1969) suggested that the tumours represent a proliferation of immunologically incompetent lymphocytes.

We believe that 'pseudolymphoma' of the lung is a malignant lymphoma of FCC origin with the same pathogenesis as those already described arising in other sites of mucosa-associated lymphoid tissue. It can, therefore, be best understood in relationship to the normal physiology of the bronchus-associated lymphoid tissue (BALT) (Bienenstock *et al.*, 1973a, b). All cases that we have been able to study by immunological or immunohistochemical techniques have shown monotypic surface or cytoplasmic immunoglobulin indicating that this is a neoplastic proliferation (unpublished observations). If this neoplasm develops from bronchus-associated FCCs the progeny of these cells would home back to the mucosal site of origin. It is our opinion that the lymphoid cells that accumulate into these tumours are B2 memory cells which in some tumours show differentiation towards plasma cells. Since these cells are differentiated products of the neoplastic B-lymphocytes they accumulate locally but do not replicate. The parent neoplastic FCCs as in other lymphomas of mucosa-associated lymphoid tissue localize around and invade epithelial structures, in this case bronchioles, only later extending into the lung parenchyma where they are mixed with the small lymphoid cells and, occasionally, plasma cells. On the basis of our immunological studies and the above hypothesis, we suggest that the term 'pseudolymphoma' should be abandoned and that these tumours should be grouped with the other FCC lymphomas of mucosa-associated lymphoid tissue.

13.4.1 Histology

At low power mucosa-associated lymphoma shows what appears to be a monomorphic infiltration of small lymphocytes within which can be seen entrapped blood vessels, bronchi and bronchioles (Fig. 13.23). At the periphery of the tumour lymphoma cells infiltrate into the lung along bronchovascular bundles and alveolar septae giving an appearance reminiscent of lymphocytic interstitial pneumonia (Fig. 13.24). Higher power examination shows that these lymphoma cells are not typical small lymphocytes but show small degrees of nuclear irregularity. Tumour cells can also be seen infiltrating bronchiolar epithelium and filling out bronchioles. These cells are slightly larger, have more irregular nuclei and resemble small centrocytes or occasionally centroblasts (Fig. 13.25). Secondary obstructive features may be seen at the periphery and within the tumour. These consist of collections of intraalveolar foamy macrophages or cholesterol crystals, the latter usually inducing a giant cell reaction. In our experience follicles, either reactive or neoplastic, occur uncommonly in these lymphomas. Lymphoma cells typically invade the walls of veins and bronchi often leaving islands of cartilage isolated in a sea of lymphoid cells. Invasion of hilar lymph nodes can be difficult to detect histologically. They usually show reactive follicular hyperplasia only but in such cases we have detected monotypic B-cell populations using immunological techniques. A minority of tumours show plasmacytic differentiation and have an appearance similar to a lymphoplasmacytic lymphoma.

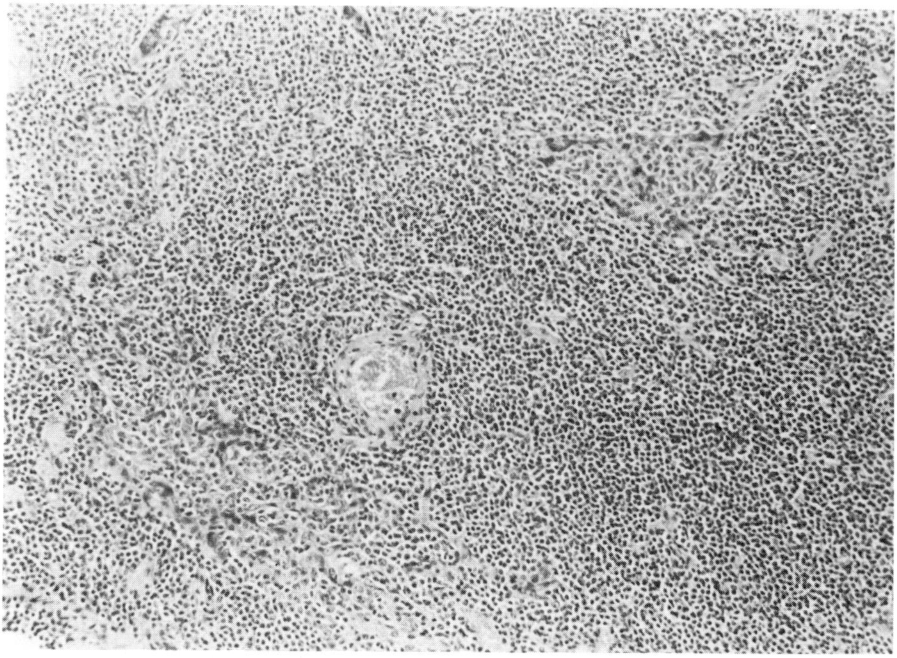

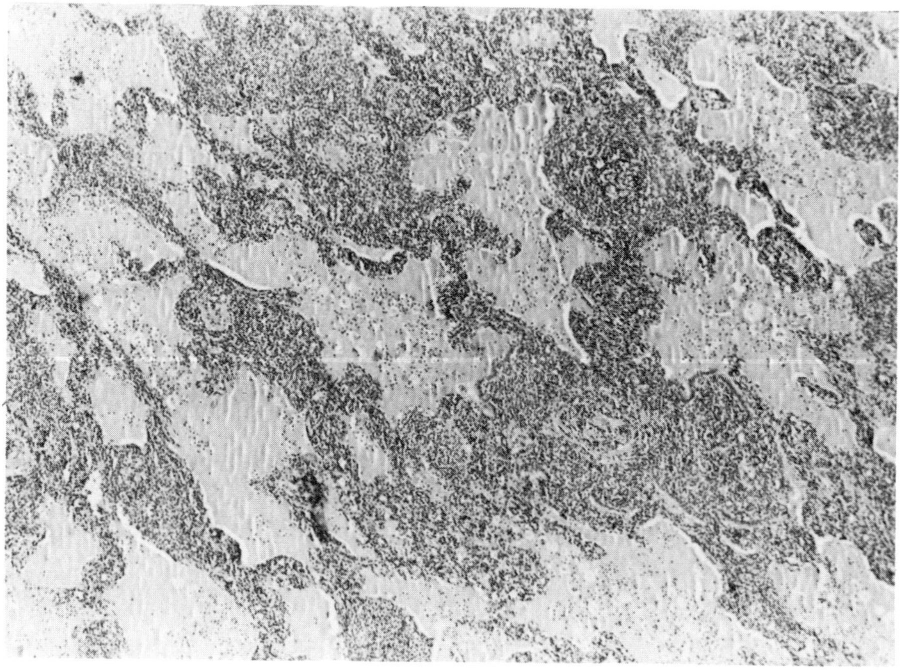

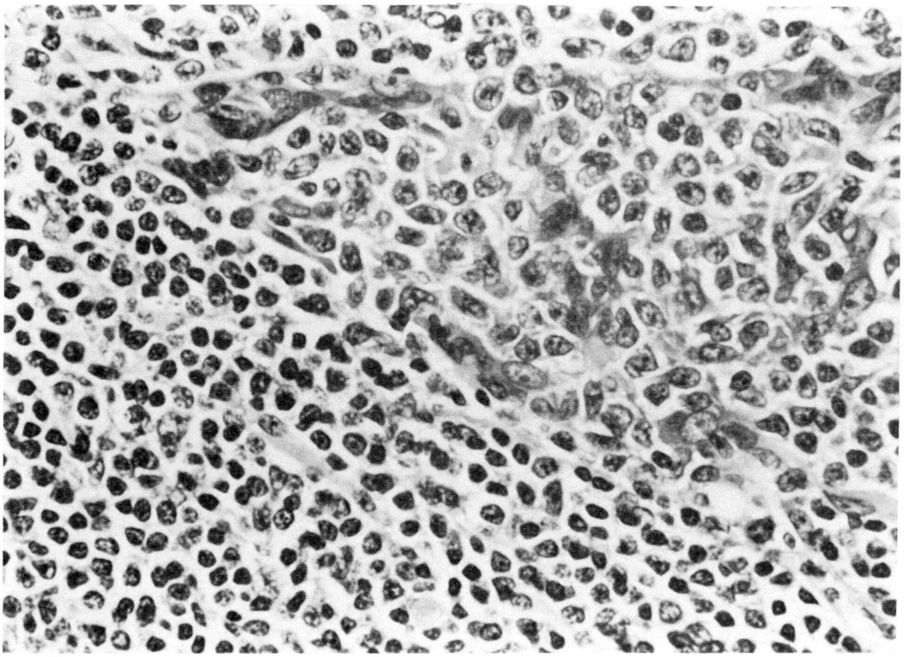

Fig. 13.25 A bronchiole in this primary lung lymphoma is invaded and filled out by centrocytes. The nuclei of the surrounding lymphoid cells are larger and more irregular than those of small lymphocytes. Compare with Fig. 13.19, × 400.

13.4.2 Differential diagnosis

Pulmonary lymphoma must be distinguished from a large number of reactive and inflammatory conditions that may occur in the lung. The monomorphism of the tumour cell population and their invasive properties as described above will usually identify malignant lymphoma. Immunological marker studies on dispersed cells or frozen sections are invaluable for identifying monotypic neoplastic lymphoid cells. In those cases showing plasmacytic differentiation, immunoperoxidase staining of paraffin sections is of value.

13.5 Cutaneous malignant lymphomas

Skin infiltration may occur during the course of almost any disseminated

Fig. 13.23 Primary malignant lymphoma of lung. Entrapped bronchioles at lower left and upper right are seen within a monomorphic lymphoid infiltrate, × 100.

Fig. 13.24 Periphery of primary lymphoma of the lung showing widening of bronchovascular bundles and alveolar septae by the lymphocytic infiltrate, × 40.

malignant lymphoma or leukaemia. Malignancies of T-lymphocytes and of the monocyte/macrophage system have a greater predilection for the skin than neoplasms of B-lymphocytes. Nevertheless, because of their overall preponderance, B-cell lymphomas, and follicle centre cell lymphoma in particular, are the most common skin lymphomas encountered.

Occasional malignant lymphomas appear to be primary within the skin; that is to say lymphoma is not apparent elsewhere at the time of presentation. Many of these patients will exhibit evidence of extracutaneous dissemination within five years (Evans *et al.*, 1979). Doubt has recently been cast on some of the reported cases of primary cutaneous lymphoma on the grounds that these may be examples of 'rhythmic paradoxical eruptions' such as lymphomatoid papulosis (Macauley, 1978). It is clear that any putative primary skin lymphoma should be subjected to critical histological examination and clinicopathological correlation together with appropriate staging procedures before treatment. Some authors have cautioned against making a diagnosis of malignant lymphoma on skin biopsy alone (Clark *et al.*, 1974). We share that caution but believe that malignant lymphoma can be separated from reactive lesions in the majority of cases, provided adequate histological material is available.

13.5.1 T-cell lymphomas

The cutaneous T-cell lymphomas, mycosis fungoides and Sezary's syndrome arise from skin-associated lymphocytes. They remain localized in the skin over periods of many years and only manifest extracutaneous tumours later in the disease. T-lymphocytic lymphoma (TCLL) and some of the node-based T-cell lymphomas also show a predilection for the skin with infiltration of the epidermis (Leong *et al.*, 1980). These tumours are discussed in Chapter 9.

(a) *Differential diagnosis*

Any dermatosis that causes lymphoid infiltration in the epidermis may have to be considered in the differential diagnosis of T-cell lymphoma. In many instances the differentiation will be based on the characteristics of the lymphoid cells (see Chapter 9). There is, however, a group of conditions designated by Macauley (1966) as 'lymphomatoid papulosis' and by Black and Wilson Jones (1972) as a 'lymphomatoid pityriasis lichenoides' that appear to be histologically malignant but clinically benign. These patients have single or multiple recurrent skin nodules and in a later publication Macauley (1978) refers to them as rhythmic paradoxical eruptions. Most run a benign course, although one of the cases reported by Black and Wilson Jones (1972) developed disseminated malignant lymphoma after a 16-year history of recurrent eruptions. Histologically these lesions are characterized by infiltration of the dermis and epidermis by cells with hyperchromatic cerebriform nuclei (Fig. 13.26). It would appear that these lesions cannot be separated from T-cell lymphoma except by taking into account the clinical features. It may be that they are in fact self limiting or slowly progressive neoplasms.

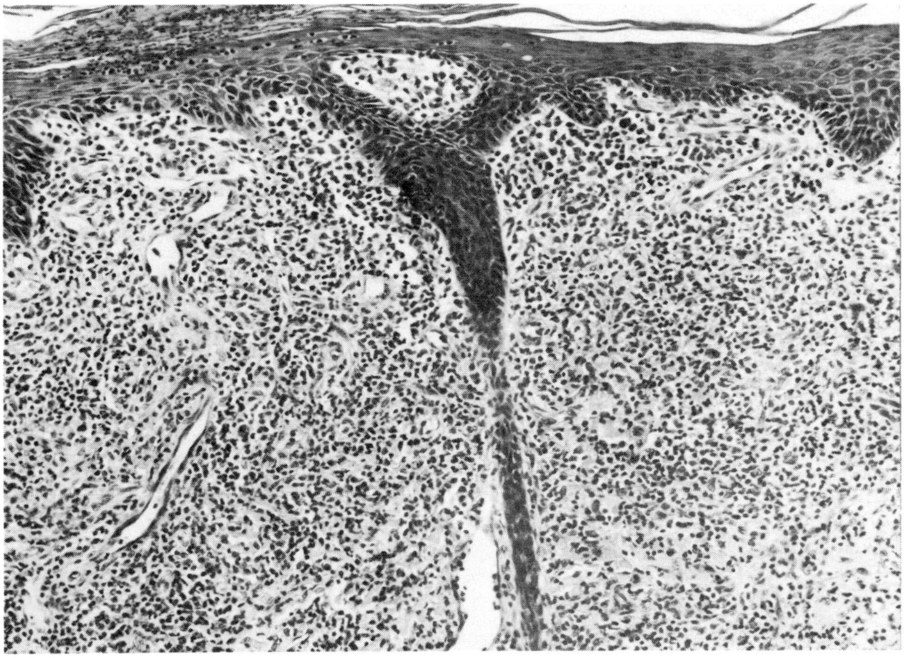

Fig. 13.26 Lymphomatoid papulosis. There is invasion of the dermis and, to a lesser extent, the epidermis by pleomorphic lymphoid cells, × 120.

Actinic reticuloid (Ive *et al.*, 1969) is a chronic dermatosis associated with severe photosensitivity that shows dense dermal lymphoid infiltrates, cellular atypia and epidermal invasion resembling malignant lymphoma. This condition also illustrates the need to take cognisance of clinical features before making a diagnosis of cutaneous lymphoma.

13.5.2 B-cell lymphomas

Skin involvement accounts for approximately 20% of the extranodal manifestations of most B-cell lymphomas (Lennert, 1981). The majority of these are of follicle centre cell origin, although a distinct subgroup of lymphoplasmacytic/cytoid lymphomas designated oculocutaneous by Lennert (1978) shows a predilection for the skin and orbit. Follicle centre cell lymphomas may involve the skin in patients with widely disseminated disease or present as apparently primary cutaneous lymphomas. Of the 25 primary lymphomas of the skin reported by Long *et al.* (1976), 22 developed extracutaneous lymphoma after periods ranging from six months to five years.

(a) *Histology*

In contrast to the cutaneous T-cell lymphomas, follicle centre cell lymphomas show a perivascular distribution predominantly in the reticular dermis, sparing the most superficial papillary dermis (Fig. 13.27). The tumour frequently extends through the full thickness of the dermis into the subcutaneous fat, a feature that may be helpful in differentiating lymphoma from many reactive and inflammatory lesions. Infiltration and destruction of blood vessels, nerves and skin appendages may also be helpful in making this distinction (Long *et al.*, 1976). Evans *et al.* (1979) claimed that follicle centre cell lymphomas did not exhibit a follicular structure in the skin, whereas Long *et al.* (1976) found 24% of their series to be follicular. In our experience follicle centre cell

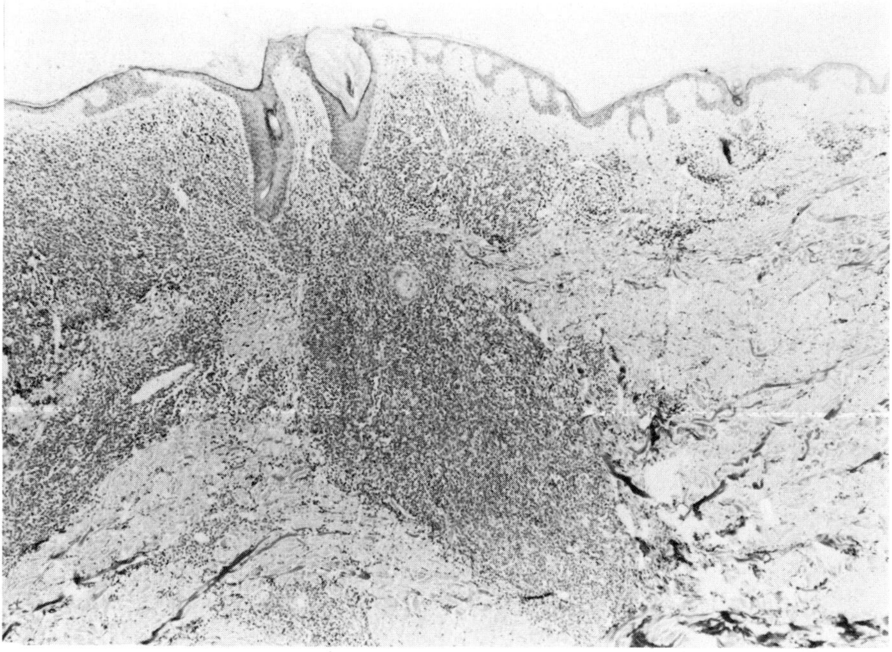

Fig. 13.27 Malignant lymphoma of skin B-cell (follicle centre cell) type. Note the sparing of the papillary dermis and epidermis, × 30.

lymphomas of the skin are frequently diffuse but may exhibit a follicular structure (Fig. 13.28). Essentially, the identification of follicle centre cell lymphomas in skin biopsies is based on the recognition of the characteristic cytological features of the tumour cells (Fig. 13.29). Tumours containing a high proportion of centroblasts are usually easily recognized. Those with a high proportion of centrocytes and many reactive small lymphocytes may be more difficult to separate from inflammatory and reactive proliferations.

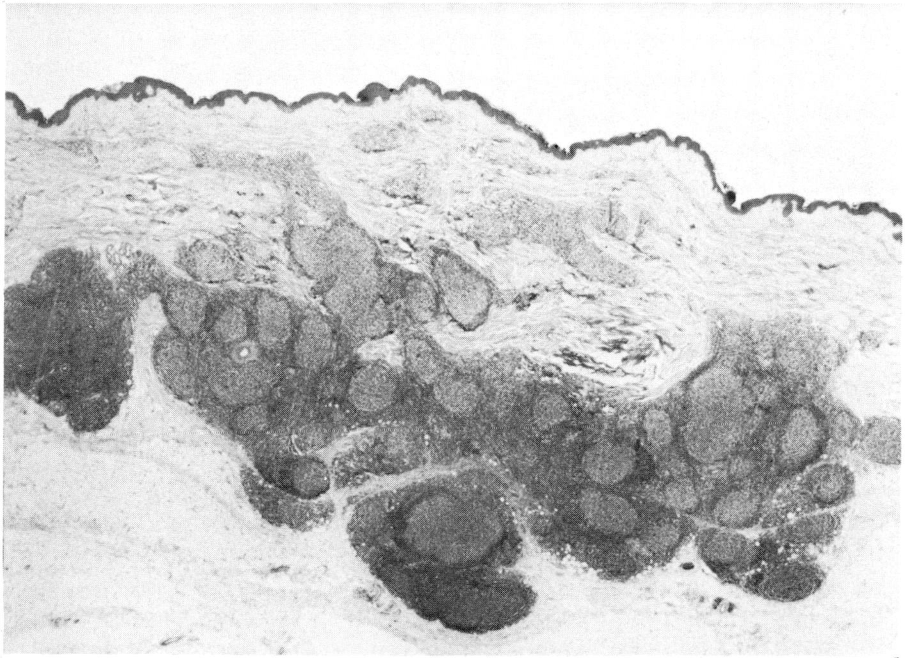

Fig. 13.28 Malignant lymphoma of the skin, centroblastic/centrocytic follicular. The malignant follicles infiltrate the subcutaneous fat, × 12.

(b) *Differential diagnosis*

Many dermatoses are associated with lymphoid infiltrates of the skin and enter into the differential diagnosis of malignant lymphoma. In a study of 225 biopsies, Caro and Helwig (1969) concluded that the features that differentiate benign lesions are epidermal, stromal and vascular abnormalities and an infiltrate composed of polymorphous well-differentiated cells. Fisher *et al.* (1976) however, found that the criteria for separating reactive from lymphomatous infiltrations of the skin were unreliable. The more precise recognition of the cellular characteristics of malignant

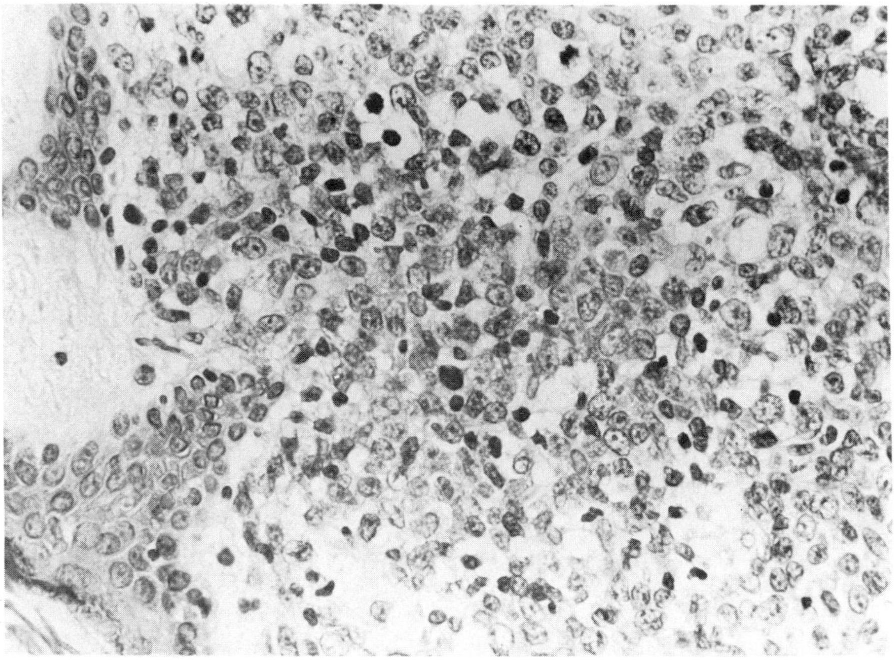

Fig. 13.29 High power of Fig. 13.27. The cytological features of the cells are those of centroblasts and centrocytes, × 300.

lymphomas in recent years should allow a more positive identification of these tumours, although clearly considerable caution must be exercised before diagnosing malignant lymphoma on a skin biopsy alone.

The term pseudolymphoma of Spiegler–Feldt (lymphocytoma cutis) has been applied to a follicular lesion that may occur as single or multiple skin nodules. This lesion has a predilection for the face and histologically has a follicular structure. Lever and Shaumburg–Lever (1975) note that these lesions may be difficult to distinguish from follicular lymphoma and that some of the patients with multiple nodules eventually develop frank lymphoma. It seems probable that many of these lesions were lymphomatous from the outset. The slow evolution of some of these cases with eventual development of lymphoma is reminiscent of the pseudolymphomas discussed elsewhere in this chapter, and it may be that these cases evolve from skin-associated follicle centre cells. In individual biopsies the same criteria must be applied to distinguish between reactive and neoplastic follicles, as is used at other sites and described in Chapter 7.

13.6 Lymphoma of the breast

Although the breast may be involved in disseminated malignant lymphoma, primary malignant lymphoma of the breast is uncommon, accounting for 0.12% of all primary malignant breast tumours in the large series reported by Mambo *et al.* (1977). These tumours may clinically resemble carcinoma of the breast and it is important that they should be recognized at the time of frozen section if unnecessarily radical surgery is to be avoided. We have found imprint cytology to be a rapid and reliable means of differentiating lymphoma from carcinoma. Many subtypes of malignant lymphoma may involve the breast (Lennert, 1981) but the commonest primary lymphomas are of follicle centre cell origin, usually with a diffuse growth pattern. The tumour infiltrates in a characteristically interstitial manner leaving isolated ducts within the tumour mass.

Granulocytic sarcoma may occur in the breast (Pascoe, 1970; Sears and Reid, 1976) and sometimes precedes the onset of leukaemia. It can be identified by the naphthol-ASD-chloroacetate esterase stain or by immunohistochemistry (see Chapter 12). Massive bilateral breast enlargement is a characteristic manifestation of Burkitt's lymphoma during pregnancy and lactation (Shepherd and Wright, 1967). This feature is of interest in relation to the known migration of B-lymphocytes into the breast in late pregnancy.

13.7 Lymphoma of the ovary

Ovarian tumour is an uncommon presenting manifestation of malignant lymphoma (Chorlton *et al.*, 1974). In contrast to malignant lymphoma of the testis which occurs predominantly in the sixth, seventh and eighth decades of life, lymphoma of the ovaries is uncommon after the fifth decade (Chorlton *et al.*, 1974; Paladugu *et al.*, 1980). The majority of tumours appear to be of follicle centre cell derivation and five of the cases reported by Chorlton *et al.* (1974) had a follicular growth pattern. The tumours show a similar infiltrative growth pattern and morphology to follicle centre cell lymphomas at other sites. Bilateral ovarian tumours often massive, are a characteristic feature of Burkitt's lymphoma (Wright, 1971).

13.8 Malignant lymphoma of the testis

Testicular tumour is a presenting feature of approximately 4% of African children with Burkitt's lymphoma and is found in 10% of the patients at autopsy (Wright, 1971). Approximately one-third of the patients have concomitant bilateral tumours. Relapse of lymphoblastic leukaemia is sometimes accompanied by infiltration of the testis (Kuo *et al.*, 1976) and in some treatment protocols biopsy of the testis is performed at the end of chemotherapy to look for residual leukaemic cells. These may be difficult to detect using routine stains but can be highlighted by immunohistochemical techniques using antibodies to terminal transferase (Greaves, 1981).

The cases of malignant lymphoma of the testis submitted to the British Testicular Tumour Panel showed a peak age incidence in the 60–80 year age group (Gowing, 1976). Of the 128 cases reviewed in this series, six had bilateral tumours at presentation and 21 subsequently developed involvement of the opposite testis. Lymphoma of the testis is usually part of more widespread disease, although half the patients reported by Turner *et al.* (1981) were considered to have Stage I disease and a small number of patients have had long survivals following orchidectomy alone or orchidectomy and regional radiotherapy (Gowing, 1976; Turner *et al.*, 1981). The majority of cases of lymphoma of the testis reported in the literature and in our own experience are follicle centre cell lymphomas with a diffuse growth pattern. A small number of plasmacytomas of the testis have been reported (Gowing, 1976).

13.8.1 Histology

Malignant lymphoma infiltrates the testis in a diffuse interstitial pattern infiltrating around and into seminiferous tubules (Fig. 13.30). Residual tubules are usually lined by Sertoli cells without evidence of spermatogenesis. The peritubular reticulin is expanded by the infiltrating lymphoma (Fig. 13.31) cells giving an appearance quite different from seminoma of the testis which compresses the peritubular reticulin (Gowing, 1976). Invasion of the walls of veins is also a characteristic of malignant lymphoma. The identification of individual lymphomas is based on the same cytological criteria as those used at other sites. Immunohistochemistry may be of value in identifying immunoglobulin production in lymphoma cells and in distinguishing between monotypic neoplastic plasma cells and reactive plasma cell proliferations.

Fig. 13.30 Malignant lymphoma of testis, centroblastic/centrocytic diffuse. The tumour cells can be seen infiltrating in and around a seminiferous tubule, × 300.
Fig. 13.31 Section of the testicular lymphoma shown in Fig. 13.30 stained for reticulin. The peritubular reticulin is expanded by the tumour infiltrate, × 120.

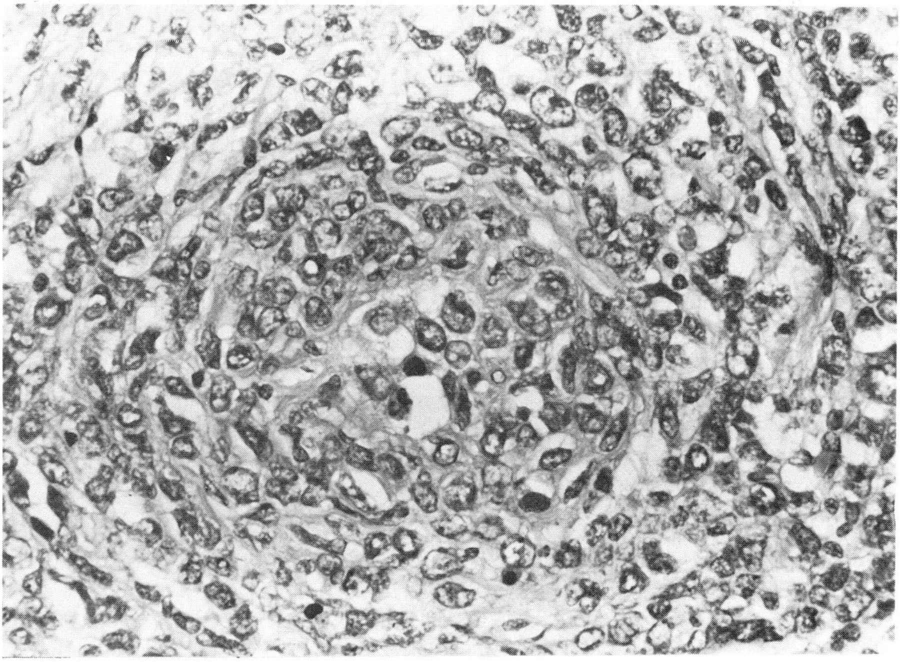

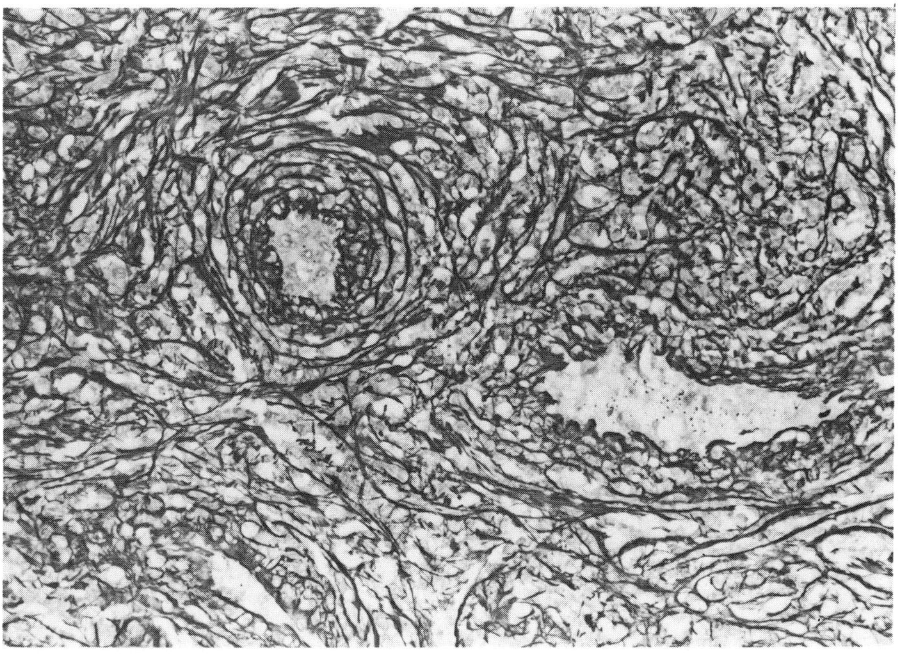

13.9 Malignant lymphoma of the central nervous system

Advanced malignant lymphoma may secondarily involve the brain. In a study of 24 cases Law *et al.* (1975) found that large cell lymphomas tend to invade the substance of the brain whereas small cell lymphomas show leptomeningeal seeding. The meninges are a common site of relapse for lymphoblastic and Burkitt's lymphoma. Paraplegia in patients with malignant lymphoma may result from spinal epidural deposits. Burkitt's lymphoma and other lymphomas that give rise to massive retroperitoneal tumours may compromise the blood supply to the lower thoracic cord causing infarction and irreversible paraplegia (Wright, 1971).

Primarily malignant lymphomas of the brain have been variously categorized as microgliomas and reticulum cell sarcomas. They are often multifocal within the brain but do not usually show dissemination outside the CNS even when these patients come to autopsy (Henry *et al.*, 1974). The tumours form solid nodules invading the surrounding brain along perivascular spaces (Fig. 13.32). Sampling and fixation problems have confused the detailed histopathological study of these lymphomas. Immunohistochemical studies have shown that many are of the B-cell

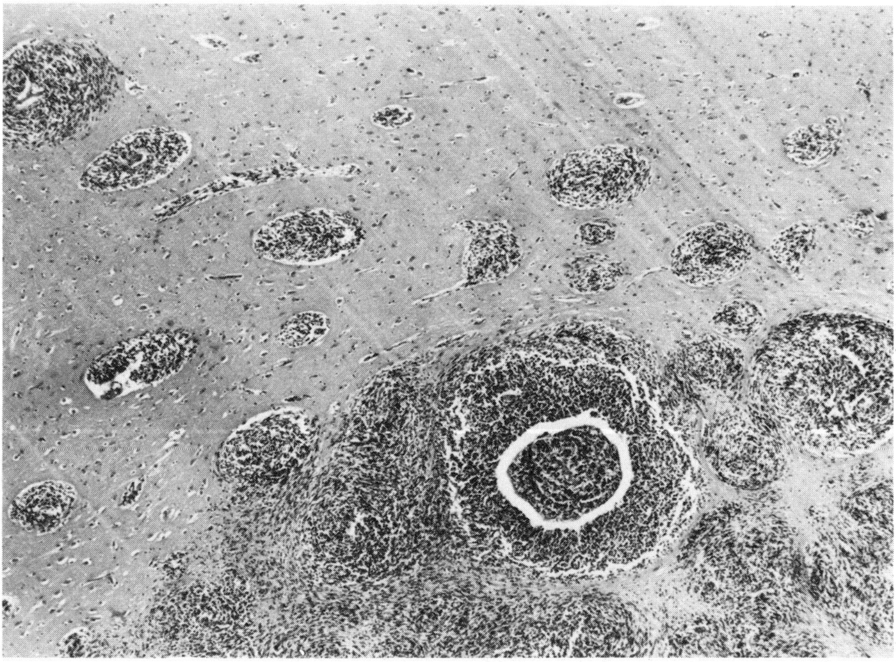

Fig. 13.32 Primary malignant lymphoma of the brain showing invasion along perivascular spaces, × 30.

lineage (Taylor *et al.*, 1978). In a study of 24 cases these workers categorized 12 as immunoblastic sarcoma and 12 as follicle centre cell or plasmacytoid lymphomas. These tumours may show considerable pleomorphism with giant cell formation which probably accounts for some of the cases categorized as Hodgkin's disease in the older literature. Primary brain lymphoma has a markedly increased incidence in renal transplant and other immunosuppressed patients (Hoover and Fraumeni, 1973; Hanto *et al.*, 1981).

13.10 Malignant lymphoma of bone

Parker and Jackson (1939) recognized reticulum cell sarcoma as a distinct primary bone sarcoma separate from other bone tumours. In a study of 179 patients presenting with malignant lymphoma of the bone, Boston *et al.* (1974) found 81 patients had disease elsewhere but that 98 had primary bone tumours without evidence of dissemination. The former group had a five-year survival of 23% and the latter of 44%, Shoji and Miller (1971) also found a five-year survival of 44% in 47 patients with primary malignant lymphoma of bone. The same group had a ten-year survival of 36.6%. There does not appear to be a predilection for any part of the skeleton. Many authors have noted that reticulum cell sarcoma of the bone have a similar morphology to reticulum cell sarcomas in extraosseous sites but there have been few detailed studies of the histopathology of these tumours. The description of Mahoney and Alexander (1980) based on a light microscope and ultrastructural study of four cases suggests that the tumours are centroblastic or centroblastic/centrocytic lymphomas with a diffuse growth pattern. Our own observations support this view.

Malignant lymphoma of bone must be differentiated from Ewing's sarcoma, neuroblastoma, alveolar rhabdomyosarcoma and other small cell tumours. This should be based on the positive identification of the morphological characteristics of follicle centre cell lymphoma, although the histological artefacts associated with bone biopsies may make this difficult. In general, the cells of Ewing's sarcoma are smaller and more regular than those of malignant lymphoma. Several authors have stressed the value of demonstrating cytoplasmic glycogen as a means of identifying Ewing's sarcoma and differentiating it from malignant lymphoma.

References

Al-Attar, A., Al-Mondhirg, H., Al-Bahrani, Z. and Al-Saleem, J. (1979), Burkitt's lymphoma in Iraq. Clinical and pathological study of forty-seven patients. *Int. J. Cancer*, **23**, 14–17.

Al-Saleem, T. and Peale, A. R. (1969), Lymphocytic tumors and pseudo tumors of the lung. Report of five cases with special emphasis on pathology. *Am. Rev. Resp. Dis.*, **99**, 767–72.

Azzopardi, J. G. and Evans, D. J. (1971), Malignant lymphoma of parotid associated with Mikulicz disease (benign lymphoepithelial lesion). *J. Clin. Pathol.*, **24**, 744–52.

Bienenstock, J., Johnston, M. and Perey, D. Y. E. (1973a), Bronchial lymphoid tissue. I. Morphologic characteristics. *Lab. Invest.*, **28**, 686–92.

Bienenstock, J., Johnston, N. and Perey, D. Y. E. (1973b), Bronchial lymphoid tissue. II. Functional characteristics. *Lab. Invest.*, **28**, 693–8.

Black, M. M. and Wilson Jones, E. (1972), 'Lymphomatoid' pityriasis lichenoides; a variant with histological features simulating a lymphoma. A clinical and histopathological study of 15 cases with details of long-term follow-up. *Br. J. Dermatol.*, **86**, 329–47.

Boston, H. C., Dahlin, D. C., Ivins, J. C. and Cupps, R. E. (1974), Malignant lymphoma (so-called reticulum cell sarcoma) of bone. *Cancer*, **34**, 1131–7.

Burke, J. S., Butler, J. J. and Fuller, L. M. (1977), Malignant lymphomas of the thyroid: A clinical pathologic study of 35 patients including ultrastructural observations. *Cancer*, **39**, 1587–1602.

Caro, W. A. and Helwig, E. B. (1969), Cutaneous lymphoid hyperplasia. *Cancer*, **24**, 487–502.

Chorlton, I., Norris, H. J. and King, F. M. (1974), Malignant reticuloendothelial disease involving the ovary as a primary manifestation. A series of 19 lymphomas and 1 granulocytic sarcoma. *Cancer*, **34**, 397–407.

Clark, W. H., Mihm, M. C., Reed, R. J. and Ainsworth, A. M. (1974), The lymphocytic infiltrates of the skin. *Human Pathol.*, **5**, 25–43.

Colby, T. V. and Carrington, C. B. (1982), Pulmonary lymphomas simulating lymphomatoid granulomatosis. *Am. J. Surg. Pathol.*, **6**, 19–32.

Compagno, J. and Oertel, J. E. (1980), Malignant lymphoma and the lymphoproliferative disorders of the thyroid gland. A clinicopathologic study of 245 cases. *Am. J. Clin. Pathol.*, **74**, 1–11.

Cruickshank, A. H. (1965), Benign lymphoepithelial salivary lesion to be distinguished from adenolymphoma. *J. Clin. Pathol.* **18**, 391–400.

Evans, H. L., Winkelmann, R. R. and Banks, P. M. (1979), Differential diagnosis of malignant and benign cutaneous lymphoid infiltrates. A study of 57 cases in which malignant lymphoma had been diagnosed or suspected in the skin. *Cancer*, **44**, 699–717.

Evans, R. A. and Cruickshank, A. H. (1970), *Epithelial Tumours of the Salivary Glands*, W. B. Saunders Co., Philadelphia, London, Toronto, pp. 279–95.

Fisher, E. R., Park, E. J. and Wechsler, H. L. (1976), Histologic identification of malignant lymphoma cutis. *Am. J. Surg. Pathol.*, **65**, 149–58.

Gibbs, A. R. and Seal, R. M. E. (1978), Primary lymphoproliferative conditions of lung. *Thorax*, **33**, 140–52.

Godwin, T. (1952), Benign lymphoepithelial lesion of the parotid gland. *Cancer*, **5**, 1089–103.

Gowing, N. F. C. (1976), Malignant lymphoma of the testis. In *Pathology of the Testis* (ed. R. C. B. Pugh), Blackwell Scientific Publications, Oxford, pp. 334–355.

Greaves, M. F. (1981), Analysis of the clinical and biological significance of lymphoid phenotypes in acute leukemia. *Cancer Res.*, **41**, 4752–66.

Greenberg, S. D., Heisler, J. G., Gyorkey, F. and Jenkins, D. E. (1972), Pulmonary lymphoma versus pseudolymphoma: A perplexing problem. *South Med. J.*, **65**, 775–84.

Gwynne-Jenkins, B. A. and Salm, R. (1971), Primary lymphosarcoma of the lung. *Br. J. Dis. Chest.*, **65**, 225–37.

Hanto, D. W., Frizzera, G., Purtilo, D. T. *et al.* (1981), Clinical spectrum of lymphoproliferative disorders in renal transplant recipients and evidence for the role of Epstein–Barr virus. *Cancer Res.*, **41**, 4253–61.

Heimann, R., Vanninheuse, A., DeSloover, C. and Dor, P. (1978), Malignant lymphomas and undifferentiated small cell carcinoma of the thyroid: A clinicopathological review in the light of the Kiel classification for malignant lymphomas. *Histopathology*, **2**, 201–13.

Henry, J. M., Heffner, R. R., Dillard, S. H. *et al.* (1974), Primary malignant lymphomas of the central nervous system. *Cancer*, **34**, 1293–1302.

Henry, K. and Farrer-Brown, G. (1977), Primary lymphomas of the gastro-intestinal tract. I. Plasma cell tumours. *Histopathology*, **1**, 53–76.

Holmes, G. K. T., Stokes, P. L., Soraham, J. M. *et al* (1976), Coeliac disease, gluten free diet and malignancy. *Gut*, **17**, 612–19.

Hoover, R. and Fraumeni, J. F. (1973), Risk of cancer in renal-transplant recipients. *Lancet*, **ii**, 55–7.

Hyman, G. A. and Wolff, M. (1976), Malignant lymphomas of the salivary glands. Review of the literature and report of 33 new cases, including four cases associated with the lymphoepithelial lesion. *Am. J. Clin. Pathol.*, **65**, 421–38.

Isaacson, P. (1979), Middle East lymphoma and α-chain disease. An immuno-histochemical study. *Am. J. Surg. Pathol.*, **3**, 431–41.

Isaacson, P. (1980), Malignant histiocytosis of the intestine: the early histological lesion. *Gut*, **21**, 381–6.

Isaacson, P. (1981), Primary gastrointestinal lymphoma. *Virchows Arch. (Pathol. Anat.)*, **391**, 1–8.

Isaacson, P., Jones, D. B., Sworn, M. J. and Wright, D. H. (1982), Malignant histiocytosis of the intestine. Report of 3 cases with immunological and cytochemical analysis. *J. Clin. Pathol.*, **35**, 510–16.

Isaacson, P. and Wright, D. H. (1978), Malignant histiocytosis of the intestine: its relationship to malabsorption and ulcerative jejunitis. *Human Pathol.*, **9**, 661–77.

Isaacson, P. and Wright, D. H. (1980), Malabsorption and intestinal lymphomas. In *Recent Advances in Gastrointestinal Pathology* (ed. R. Wright), W. B. Saunders, London, pp. 193–212.

Isaacson, P., Wright, D. H., Judd, M. A. and Mepham, B. L. (1979), Primary gastrointestinal lymphomas: A classification of 66 cases. *Cancer*, **43**, 1805–19.

Ive, F. A., Magnus, I. A., Warin, R. P. and Wilson Jones, E. (1969), 'Actinic reticuloid'. A chronic dermatosis associated with severe photosensitivity and the histological resemblance to lymphoma. *Br. J. Dermatol.*, **81**, 469–85.

Kassan, S. S. and Gardy, M. (1978), Sjögen's syndrome: An update and overview. *Am. J. Med.*, **64**, 1037–45.

Kuo, T. T., Tschang, T. P. and Chu, J. Y. (1976), Testicular relapse in childhood acute lymphocytic leukaemia during bone marrow remission. *Cancer*, **38**, 2604–12.

Law, I. P., Dick, F. R., Blom, J. and Bergevin, P. R. (1975), Involvement of the central nervous system in non-Hodgkin's lymphoma. *Cancer*, **36**, 225–31.

Lee, Y-TN. and Spratt, J. S. (1974), Gastrointestinal malignant lymphomas. In *Malignant Lymphoma Nodal and Extranodal Diseases* (Modern Surgical Monograph), Grune and Stratton, New York, pp. 229–60.

Lennert, K. (1978), Malignant lymphomas other than Hodgkin's disease. In *Handbuch der Speziellen. Pathologischen Anatomie und Histologie*, Springer-Verlag, Berlin (in collaboration with N. Mohri, H. Stein, E. Kaiserling and H. K. Müller-Hermelink).

Lennert, K. (1981), *Histopathology of Non-Hodgkin's Lymphomas (Based on the Kiel Classification)*, Springer-Verlag, Berlin.

Leong, A. S-Y., Sage, R. E., Kinnear, G. C. and Forbes, I. J. (1980), Preferential epidermotrophism in adult T-cell leukemia–lymphoma. *Am. J. Surg. Pathol.*, **4**, 421–30.

Lever, W. F. and Schaumburg-Lever, G. (1975), *Histopathology of the Skin*, 5th edn, J. B. Lippincott Co. Philadelphia, Toronto.

Liebow, A. A., Carrington, C. B. and Friedman, P. J. (1972), Lymphomatoid granulomatosis. *Human Pathol.*, **3**, 457–58.

Long, J. C., Mihm, M. C. and Qazi, R. (1976), Malignant lymphoma of the skin. A clinicopathologic study of lymphoma other than mycosis fungoides diagnosed by skin biopsy. *Cancer*, **38**, 1282–96.

Macauley, W. L. (1966), Lymphomatoid papulosis: A continuing self-healing eruption, clinically benign, histologically malignant. *Arch. Dermatol.*, **94**, 26–32.

Macauley, W. L. (1978), Lymphomatoid papulosis. *Int. J. Dermatol.*, **17**, 204–12.

McNamara, J. J., Kingsley, W. B., Paulson, D. L. *et al.* (1969), Primary lymphosarcoma of the lung. *Ann. Surg.*, **169**, 133–9.

Mahoney, J. P. and Alexander, R. W. (1980), Primary histiocytic lymphoma of bone. A light and ultrastructural study of four cases. *Am. J. Surg. Pathol.*, **4**, 149–61.

Mambo, N. C., Burke, J. S. and Butler, J. J. (1977), Primary malignant lymphomas of the breast. *Cancer*, **39**, 2033–40.

Maurer, R., Taylor, C. R., Terry, R. and Lukes, R. J. (1979), Non-Hodgkin lymphomas of the thyroid. A clinicopathologic review of 29 cases applying the Lukes–Collins classification and an immunoperoxidase method. *Virchows Arch. (Pathol. Anat.)*, **383**, 293–317.

Morgan, W. S. and Castleman, B. (1953), Clinicopathologic study of 'Mikulicz's disease'. *Am. J. Pathol.*, **29**, 471–503.

Paladugu, R. R., Bearman, R. M. and Rappaport, H. (1980), Malignant lymphoma with primary manifestation in the gonad. A clinicopathologic study of 38 patients. *Cancer*, **45**, 561–71.

Parker, F. and Jackson, H. (1939), Primary reticulum cell sarcoma of bone. *Surg. Gynecol. Obstet.*, **68**, 45–53.

Parrott, D. M. V. (1976), The gut as a lymphoid organ. *Clin. Gastroenterol.*, **5**, 211–28.

Pascoe, H. R. (1970), Tumors composed of immature granulocytes occurring in the breast in chronic granulocytic leukaemia. *Cancer*, **26**, 697–703.

Rappaport, H. and Thomas, L. B. (1974), Mycosis fungoides: the pathology of extracutaneous involvement. *Cancer*, **34**, 1198–229.

Saltzstein, S. L. (1963), Pulmonary malignant lymphomas and pseudolymphomas: classification therapy and prognosis. *Cancer*, **16**, 928–55.

Schmid, V., Helbron, D. and Lennert, K. (1982), Development of malignant lymphoma in myoepithelial sialadenitis (Sjögren's syndrome). *Virchows Arch. (Pathol. Anat.)*, **395**, 11–43.

Sears, H. F. and Reid, J. (1976), Granulocytic sarcoma. Localised presentation of a systemic disease. *Cancer*, **37**, 1808–13.

Seligmann, M., Danon, F., Hurez, D. *et al.* (1968), Alpha chain disease: a new immunoglobulin abnormality. *Science*, **162**, 1396–7.
Shepherd, J. J. and Wright, D. H. (1967), Burkitt's tumour presenting as bilateral swelling of the breast in women of child-bearing age. *Br. J. Surg.*, **54**, 776–80.
Shoji, H. and Miller, T. R. (1971), Primary reticulum cell sarcoma of bone. *Cancer*, **28**, 1234–44.
Taylor, C. R., Russell, R., Lukes, R. J. and Davis, R. L. (1978), An immunohistological study of immunoglobulin content of primary central nervous system lymphomas. *Cancer*, **41**, 2197–205.
Turner, R. R., Colby, T. V. and MacKintosh, F. R. (1981), Testicular lymphoma: A clinicopathologic study of 35 cases. *Cancer*, **48**, 2095–102.
Waldron, J. A., Leech, J. H., Glick, A. D. *et al.* (1977), Malignant lymphoma of peripheral T-lymphocyte origin. Immunologic pathologic and clinical features in six patients. *Cancer*, **40**, 1604–17.
Wolfe, J. D., Trevor, E. D. and Kjeldsberg, C. R. (1980), Pulmonary manifestations of mycosis fungoides. *Cancer*, **46**, 2648–53.
Woolner, L. B., McConahey, W. M., Beahrs, O. H. and Black, B. M. (1966), Primary malignant lymphoma of the thyroid. Review of forty-six cases. *Am. J. Surg.*, **111**, 502–23.
Wright, D. H. (1971), Burkitt's lymphoma: A review of the pathology, immunology and possible etiologic factors in *Pathology Annual*. (ed. S. C. Sommers), Appleton-Century Crofts, New York, pp. 337–63.
Zulman, J., Jaffe, R. and Talal, N. (1978), Evidence that the malignant lymphoma of Sjögren's syndrome is a monoclonal B-cell neoplasm. *New Engl. J. Med.* **299**, 1215–20.

14 Technical methods for lymphoreticular biopsies

From a surgical point of view the diagnostic lymph node biopsy may be regarded as a minor operation. The repercussions of this biopsy, particularly in a young patient, may, however, be of far greater consequence than the heroics of the major operations' list. Ideally the enlarged node to be biopsied should be identified, avoiding the upper cervical and inguinal nodes if possible, although this is not of great importance if there are definite pathological changes in the node. Once identified, the node should be excised with its capsule intact and without undue traction. When lymph node biopsies are relegated to the end of the list to be performed often by inexperienced surgeons, two mistakes are commonly made. The first of these is the removal of the most accessible node irrespective of its size. Such nodes frequently show only non-specific reactive changes despite the presence of specific infection or neoplasm in deeper nodes. This mistake can frequently be recognized by the discrepancy between the size of the nodes described in the clinical summary on the request form and the size of the specimen received. In such circumstances the pathologist should ask for a repeat biopsy. The second common mistake arising from the timidity of inexperienced surgeons is to avulse the lymph node piecemeal through an inadequate skin incision. Unless the diagnosis is clear cut in such a specimen the pathologist should request a further biopsy.

Once excised the further handling of the lymph node biopsy will depend upon local custom. Poor fixation is probably the greatest single problem in the accurate diagnosis of lymph node biopsies and care should be taken over this procedure. As with other tissues, the biopsy should be placed in at least ten times its own volume of fixative. This, however, is not by itself sufficient. An enlarged lymph node with an intact capsule will never be adequately fixed in any volume of fixative. It is necessary, particularly with markedly enlarged nodes to cut the biopsy into approximately 0.2 cm thick slices to obtain satisfactory fixation. Ideally the slices should go almost through the node retaining a small portion of capsule intact so that the specimen can be folded together again in order to ascertain the original size and shape of the node. Histology of the spleen will be quite unsatisfactory unless it is sliced before being placed in fixative. We routinely slice the spleen at approximately 1 cm intervals before immersing it in a large volume of formol saline. When dealing with staging laparotomy specimens further sectioning can be performed after fixation.

The fixative used for biopsies of lymphoreticular tissues varies in different laboratories. We use neutral buffered formol saline (NBFS) almost exclusively and would recommend fixation for a minimum of 24 hours. Many workers advocate mercurial fixatives for haematopathology and Zenker's and Bouin's solutions are widely used. In the United States a fixative designated B5 (Bouin's solution without picric acid) is widely used. The appearances of the tumour cytology varies with the type of fixative used. Mercury-based fixatives give very crisp nuclear features but tend to disrupt cytoplasmic structure. We have also found that critical immunohistochemical studies are less satisfactory on mercury-fixed than on formalin-fixed tissue.

If it is logistically possible we would recommend that biopsies are not placed in fixative in the operating theatre but sent immediately in a sterile, dry container to the laboratory. The node should then be sliced cleanly at right angles to its long axis with a razor blade or new scalpel blade. Representive slices of the node may then be examined utilizing the following procedures (Table 14.1).

14.1 Routine histology

Light microscopy of H and E stained sections of paraffin embedded tissue remains the foremost means of diagnosing lymphoreticular disease. Since cytological characteristics of the tissue often have a major diagnostic role efforts should be made to obtain high quality sections cut at a thickness of not more than 5 μm. It is impossible to overemphasize the need for good fixation of this tissue. In addition to H and E a number of special stains may be of value. The reticulin stain has been traditionally used for biopsies of lymphoreticular tissues. It is valuable as a means of outlining normal lymph node structure and of identifying distortions or loss of that structure. Arising from the use of the term reticulum cell sarcoma there is a widespread, but erroneous, belief that tumours in this category produce reticulin and are associated with a dense reticulin framework. Reticulin is in fact not produced by lymphoma cells but by fibroblasts or fibroblast-like cells associated with them. In practice many large cell lymphomas that would have been categorized as reticulum cell sarcomas contain very little reticulin. Abundant reticulin formation with

Table 14.1 The lymph node biopsy

NBFS fixed tissue (0.2 cm slices 24 hours)		Touch preparations	Minced tissue in tissue culture fluid	Snap frozen tissue (liquid nitrogen)	Tissue into sterile container
Process into paraffin	Process into plastic	Cytology (Romanowsky stains)	Dispersed cells for:	Frozen sections for:	Microbiology
Routine stains	1 μm sections				Virology
			Immunology	Histochemistry	
H and E	Thin sections for EM	Cytochemistry	Cytochemistry	Immunohistochemistry (membrane antigens)	
PAS			Cytogenetics		
MGP			Tissue culture		
Reticulin					
Immunohistochemistry (cytoplasmic antigens)					

packaging of tumour cells is characteristic of some large centrocytic lymphomas and some true histiocytic tumours.

The PAS technique should be included in the profile of routine stains used for biopsies of lymphoreticular tissues. It stains basement membranes and is particularly useful for outlining blood vessels in such conditions as angioimmunoblastic lymphadenopathy and in T-cell lymphomas. Most immunoglobulin-synthesizing lymphomas secrete IgM and when this accumulates intracytoplasmically it may be detected as a PAS-positive, diastase-resistant blush in the cytoplasm of plasma cells or as intracytoplasmic or intranuclear inclusions. Such inclusions are characteristic of lymphoplasmacytoid lymphomas and distinguish them from small lymphocytic lymphomas. Large B-cell lymphomas may contain immunoglobulin inclusions and the application of the PAS stain followed by a careful search for inclusions will often assist in the separation of these tumours from other large cell lymphomas. Reactive histiocytes in lymphoma tissue frequently show focal cytoplasmic PAS positivity particularly in the region of the Golgi apparatus. The PAS stain may be of value in differentiating other anaplastic tumours from malignant lymphomas by virtue of their cytoplasmic content of muco-substances or glycogen.

The methyl green pyronin stain is of value in the diagnosis of lymphoreticular disease but is particularly susceptible to technical variation and fixation artefacts. Methyl green has an affinity for DNA and stains nuclei green. In practice methyl green is invariably contaminated by methylene blue which can only be removed by exhaustive extraction procedures, as a result nuclei usually stain blue rather than green. Pyronin has an affinity for RNA and within the cell may be regarded as a specific stain although a number of extracellular materials, such as osteoid and thyroid colloid are pyroninophilic. Cells that contain large amounts of cytoplasmic RNA either as rough endoplasmic reticulum or as polyribosomes will exhibit strong pyroninophilia. Traditionally the stain has been used to identify plasma cells which show uniform strong cytoplasmic pyroninophilia except at the nuclear hof where the Golgi apparatus pushes aside the rough endoplasmic reticulum to give a clear zone. Immunoblastic sarcomas and Burkitt's lymphomas are always strongly pyroninophilic and should not be diagnosed in the absence of this feature. Basophilia in Giemsa-stained preparations is related to the RNA content of cells and is equivalent to pyroninophilia in the methyl green pyronin stain.

14.2 Plastic sectioning

We have found that 1 μm sections of formol saline-fixed tissue embedded in resin are a most valuable adjunct to other techniques. The thinness of the sections obtained with this method permits the use of oil immersion objectives and the visualization of cytological detail that is not apparent in conventional paraffin sections. Furthermore, this technique preserves cytoplasmic structure and does not induce the 10–20% shrinkage caused by paraffin embedding. Plastic embedding cannot, of course, overcome the changes induced by bad fixation or autolysis although even here it may assist in the study of such tissues.

In our laboratory we embed tissues in Spurr resin and stain the 1 μm sections with toluidine blue. This permits us to go on to electron microscopy if we wish. Many cellular organelles can be visualized by this technique and others can be directly related to the staining characteristics of the cell. The darkness of cytoplasmic staining relates to the content of RNA either as rough endoplasmic reticulum or as polyribosomes. If there is no facility or desire to proceed to electron microscopy larger fragments of tissue may be embedded in other media, such as methyl methacrylate, and sections stained by most conventional histological stains.

14.3 Electron microscopy

Electron microscopy has a limited role in the diagnosis of lymphoreticular disease. When interpreting electron micrographs it should be borne in mind that most lymphomas consist of a mixture of neoplastic and reactive cells in which the latter may predominate. Since electron microscopy is a somewhat selective technique care should be taken not to interpret reactive cells as neoplastic cells. Electron microscopy should not be interpreted in isolation but always in conjunction with the overall light microscopic appearances. Few electron microscopic features are entirely specific. In the lymphoreticular system only eosinophil granules, mast cell granules and Langerhan's granules fall into this category. The presence of stacks of rough endoplasmic reticulum does not necessarily mean that a cell is of the plasma cell lineage and lysosomes are not in themselves diagnostic of histiocytes.

Despite these cautions electron microscopy clearly has an important role in the characterization of cells of the lymphoreticular system. It may also be of value in the separation of lymphomas from anaplastic tumours simulating malignant lymphoma. In our experience good quality electron micrographs, adequate for diagnostic purposes can be obtained from surgical biopsies well fixed in buffered formalin.

14.4 Imprint cytology

Few diagnostic histopathologists are experienced in interpreting imprint cytology of lymphoid tissue and this technique is too little used. It is, however, very simply performed and can be a valuable aid to diagnosis and with experience, a means of rapid diagnosis. It may also provide a valuable comparison with cytological preparations made from effusions or haematological preparations obtained from the same patient. We would, however, caution against using imprint cytology as the sole means of diagnosis except where the findings are unequivocal e.g. a monomorphic lymphoid tumour cell population or Reed–Sternberg cells in an appropriate cellular environment. Reactive and inflammatory nodes can produce alarming cytological appearances with numerous mitotic figures and blast cells.

Imprints are made by touching a freshly cut surface of the lymph node gently against a clean glass slide. Excess pressure will cause distortion and smearing of cells and can be avoided by holding the slide vertically and allowing the slice of tissue suspended from one point of its capsule to gently touch it. Excess blood or tissue fluid should be gently blotted off the tissue before making the imprint. The slide should then be rapidly air dried. It may be stained by any of the Romanowski techniques commonly applied to haematological preparations.

The quality of imprints obtained from lymphoid tissue varies widely. In general soft, non-cohesive lymphomas such as Burkitt's lymphoma and well-differentiated lymphocytic lymphomas make good preparations. Conversely, the yield of cells from nodes that contain a large amount of reticulin or collagen may be poor, and the cells obtained often show severe traction artefacts. In such cases better cytology may often be obtained by incubating the minced tissue in tissue culture fluid for 30 minutes and depositing the cells on a slide with a cytocentrifuge. We have illustrated the cytology in this book only when we consider it to be a particularly valuable aid to diagnosis.

14.5 Surface markers

Surface markers may be used to identify lymphocyte subpopulations and as such may be a valuable adjunct to histology. This is particularly so when a population of cells monotypic for surface immunoglobulin is identified. Furthermore, marker studies may assist with staging procedures by aiding in the identification of a neoplastic population in the peripheral blood or bone marrow. If a laboratory competent to perform these techniques is available we would recommend that part of the unfixed node should routinely be sent for these investigations. Marker studies should, however, not be interpreted in isolation from the histological findings. They are performed on a suspension of cells that will often contain large numbers of reactive lymphocytes and histiocytes, and in the case of many large cell lymphomas where it is difficult to obtain suspensions of the tumour cells, the cells analysed may be unrepresentative of the original nodal population. This error will be greatest in those laboratories that count their rosettes 'wet' in a counting chamber as opposed to those that use cytocentrifuge preparations in which the morphology of the rosetting cells can be seen.

14.6 Cytochemistry and histochemistry

A large number of cytochemical/histochemical techniques have been used for the identification of, and differentiation between, cells of the lymphoreticular system. Some of the common enzymes which can be demonstrated are shown in Table 14.2. We routinely stain our imprint

Table 14.2 Histochemical reactions of myeloid and lymphoid cells

	AP	BG	ANAE	CAE	NASDA	NASDA-F
Granulocytic	D			D	D	D
Monocyte/macrophage	D	D	D	±	D	–
Immature T-cells	F	F	–	–	–	–
Mature T-cells	F	F	F	–	–	–
B-cells	±	–	–	–	–	–

D: Diffuse staining
F: Focal staining
AP: Acid phosphase
BG: β-glucuronidase
ANAE: Acid α-naphthyl acetate esterase
CAE: Naphthyl-ASD-chloro acetate esterase
NASDA: Naphthyl-ASD-acetate esterase
NASDA-F: Naphthyl-ASD-acetate esterase with sodium fluoride inhibition

preparations for acid phosphatase and alpha-naphthyl-acetate esterase which provides a relatively simple means of identifying cells of the monocyte/macrophage lineage and mature and immature T-cells. We would like, however, to make two cautionary points. Firstly, neoplastic cells frequently show less enzyme reactivity than their normal analogues. Thus, we have seen tumours that give the immunohistochemical reaction of histiocytes yet which show very weak or negative reactions for acid phosphatase and non-specific esterase. Secondly, benign histiocytes are frequently present in large numbers in malignant lymphomas and in unfixed frozen sections or imprint preparations their enzymes are spilled over other cells and the enzyme reaction product may diffuse into the surrounding tissues. This can obscure the reaction of weakly staining cells or lead to false positive interpretations.

14.7 Immunohistochemistry

The immunohistochemical demonstration and localization of immunoglobulins and a number of other proteins and enzymes has provided a valuable means of study of lymphoreticular disease. Immunohistochemical techniques are exacting and require meticulous application if consistent and reliable results are to be obtained. Some skill and experience is also needed in the interpretation of these preparations. Immunohistochemistry may be performed using fluorochromes as labels and this technique is widely used by immunologists on dispersed cells. Labels such as horseradish peroxidase and alkaline phosphatase are probably slightly less sensitive in detecting small amounts of antigen but have the advantage that their reaction product can be seen with an ordinary light microscope and visualized in relation to the structure of the cells and tissues being studied. Immunohistochemical techniques can either be performed on fixed paraffin-embedded tissue (Mepham *et al.*, 1979) or on frozen sections (Stein *et al.*, 1980). Cytoplasmic immunoglobulin (CIg) and other cytoplasmic antigens are best demonstrated in paraffin sections whilst surface immunoglobulin (SIg) and other membrane antigens can only be demonstrated in frozen sections. The methods used in our laboratory for immunohistochemistry are given in Tables 14.3 and 14.4.

The demonstration of CIg in tumour cells is of value in establishing their B-cell nature and in distinguishing between monotypic neoplastic proliferations and polytypic reactive proliferations. Not all B-cell lymphomas contain CIg and in those that do the distribution may be very focal and in a minority of cells. The absence of immunoglobulin does not therefore necessarily imply that the tumour is of T-lymphocyte or histiocyte lineage.

Non-Hodgkin's lymphomas of B-cell type are always monotypic with respect to immunoglobulin light chain synthesis. Occasional lymphomas are found to contain tumour cells that are polytypic in their immunoglobulin content. This could be due to the cells having leaky membranes and taking up serum proteins non-specifically or more specifically to uptake of immunoglobulin via Fc receptors (Isaacson *et al.*, 1980). Table 14.5 shows how the staining reactions to a battery of proteins and enzymes may be used to distinguish between these possibilities.

J-chain is found only in early B-lymphocytes and in plasma cells synthesizing IgM or dimeric IgA. It is not found in extracellular locations. Staining for this polypeptide therefore provides a valuable means of distinguishing between cells synthesizing immunoglobulins and those that have taken it up from their environment. Staining for albumin provides a means of identifying cells that are degenerate and that are

Table 14.3 Immunoperoxidase technique for demonstration of antigens in paraffin sections

1.	Deparaffinize for 10 min × 2 in Xylol and take to alcohol
2.	Inhibit endogenous peroxidase by treating with freshly prepared 0.5% H_2O_2 in methanol for 10 min
3.	Wash well in tap water
4.	Place in distilled water at 37° C for 10 min
5.	Treat with 0.1% trypsin in 0.1% $CaCl_2$ (adjust to pH 7.8 with N/10 NaOH) for 15–30 min at 37° C*
6.	Rinse in cold distilled water 2–3 min with agitation
7.	Wash in Tris buffered saline (TBS) 10 min × 2
8.	Normal swine serum diluted $\frac{1}{5}$ with TBS, 10 min. Drain off. (Use to reduce excessive background staining – an optional step)
9.	Rabbit antihuman serum (at current dilution in TBS)† 30 min
10.	TBS wash 10 min × 3
11.	Swine antirabbit IgG (at current dilution in TBS)† 30 min
12.	TBS wash 10 min × 3
13.	PAP (peroxidase/rabbit antiperoxidase), (at current dilution in TBS)† 30 min
14.	TBS wash 10 min × 3
15.	Diaminobenzidine (DAB)
16.	Wash in TBS followed by a wash in running tap water 5 min
17.	Counterstain with haematoxylin, wash well 2–3 min. Differentiate in 1% acid alcohol, blue by washing in tap water for at least 10 min
18.	Dehydrate, clear and mount

* Time may vary with batch of trypsin
† Determined by titration

non-specifically absorbing plasma proteins. Diffuse staining for alpha-1-antitrypsin (αlantiT) and alpha-1-antichymotrypsin (αlantiCT) is also an indicator of cells with damaged or leaky membranes. Granular staining for these antiproteases is found in some cells of the monocyte/macrophage series and provides a useful marker for these cells.

We would stress the need to observe the distribution of antigen staining in cells rather than to merely record whether they are positive or negative. Immunoglobulin synthesizing cells may show a variety of staining patterns. Immunoglobulin inclusions may be present in the cytoplasm or indenting the nucleus. Staining in the perinuclear space and Golgi regions is frequently seen in early cells of the B-lymphocyte series and granular cytoplasmic staining corresponds to protein within dilated profiles of endoplasmic reticulum. Diffuse cytoplasmic staining usually signifies uptake of antigen from the cellular environment. Such staining is most marked at the periphery of the cell with less intense staining around the nucleus; the reverse of the pattern seen in synthetic cells.

Lysozyme is widely used as a marker for histiocytes but we have not found it entirely reliable either for benign or malignant histiocytes. This

Table 14.4 Immunoperoxidase technique for demonstration of membrane antigens

1. Cut cryostat sections at 6 μm
2. Air dry 30 min at room temperature (18–20° C)
3. Freeze dry at −63° C and 10^{-2} torr for 18 hours
4. Wrap slides in aluminium foil and seal
5. Store at −20° C until required
6. Bring wrapped slides to room temperature
7. Fix in acetone for 20 min at room temperature
8. Transfer to tris buffered saline (TBS) without allowing sections to dry
9. Rinse in TBS

Monoclonal antibodies

10. Apply mouse anithuman serum (at current dilution in TBS*) 30 min
11. Wash in TBS 2 min × 3
12. Apply rabbit antimouse Ig peroxidase conjugated (at current dilution in TBS*) 30 min
13. Wash in TBS 2 min × 3
14. Apply DAB 10 min
15. Rinse in TBS followed by a wash in running tap water 5 min
16. Counterstain in Harris's haematoxylin 5 min
17. Wash in tap water, differentiate in 1% acid alcohol. Blue in running tap water
18. Dehydrate clear and mount

Surface immunoglobin

10. Apply rabbit antihuman serum (at current dilution in TBS*) 30 min
11. Wash in TBS 2 min × 3
12. Apply goat antirabbit IgG (at current dilution in TBS*) 30 min
13. Wash in TBS 2 min × 3
14. Apply rabbit peroxidase antiperoxidase (at current dilution in TBS*) 30 min
15. Wash in TBS 2 min × 3
16. Apply DAB 10 min
17. Rinse in TBS followed by a wash in running tap water 5 min
18. Counterstain in Harris's haematoxylin
19. Wash in tap water
    Differentiate in 1% acid alcohol.
    Blue in running tap water
20. Dehydrate, clear and mount

* Determined by titration

Table 14.5 Immunoglobulin-containing cells in malignant lymphoma

	Cells synthesizing Ig	Cells taking up Ig
Pattern of staining	Granular	Smooth
	Concentration in Golgi region	Concentration at periphery of cytoplasm
	Staining of perinuclear space	Diffuse, cytoplasmic staining
Immunoglobulin	Monotypic	Polytypic
J chain	+	−
Other plasma proteins	−	±

Table 14.6 Immunohistochemistry of malignant lymphomas

		Lymphocytic	Lymphoplasmacytic/ lymphoplasmacytoid	Plasmacytic	Follicle centre cell	Immunoblastic	T-cell	Histiocytic	Hodgkin's disease (RS cells)
Frozen sections	SIg	Monotypic	Monotypic on lymphoid cells	–	Monotypic	Monotypic	–	–	–
	Membrane antigens	+*	+*	–	+*†	+*	+‡	+*	–
Paraffin sections	CIg	–	Monotypic in plasma cells and plasmacytoid cells	Monotypic	Monotypic in up to two-thirds of cases	Monotypic	–	– or polytypic (IgG)	Polytypic (IgG)
	J chain	–	+ in plasma cells and plasmacytoid cells	+	+ in CIg +ve cells	+	–	–	–
	Lysozyme	–	–	–	–	–	–	Occasionally +ve	–
	αlantiT αlantiCT	–	–	–	–	–	–	+	±

* HLADR antigens
† drc = dendritic reticulum cell antigen as defined by monoclonal antibodies
‡ T-cell antigens as defined by monoclonal antibodies

may reflect inadequacies of fixation or technique but may also be related to the fact that this enzyme although synthesized by the cell is not stored in sufficient quantities to be visualized. We find that granular staining for αlantiT and αlantiCT are more reliable histiocytic markers (Isaacson *et al.*, 1981).

Using frozen sections it is possible to demonstrate SIg and a wide variety of membrane antigens including those defined by monoclonal antibodies. The immunohistochemical reactions of both frozen and paraffin sections of malignant lymphoma are summarized in Table 14.6. It is likely that as more monoclonal antibodies become available frozen section immunohistochemistry will become increasingly important in the characterization of malignant lymphomas.

References

Isaacson, P., Wright, D. H., Judd, M. A. *et al.* (1980), The nature of the immunoglobulin-containing cells in malignant lymphoma. *J. Histochem. Cytochem.*, **28**, 761–70.

Isaacson, P., Jones, D. B., Sadler, G. H. M. *et al.* (1981), Alpha-1-antitrypsin in human macrophages. *J. Clin. Pathol.*, **34**, 982–90.

Mepham, B. L., Frater, W. and Mitchell, B. S. (1979), The use of proteolytic enzymes to improve immunoglobulin staining by the PAP technique. *Histochem. J.*, **11**, 345–57.

Stein, H., Bonk, A., Tolksdorf, G. *et al.* (1980), Immunohistologic analysis of the organisation of normal lymphoid tissue and non-Hodgkin's lymphomas. *J. Histochem. Cytochem.*, **28**, 746–60.

Appendix

National Cancer Institute Sponsored Study of Classifications of Non-Hodgkin's Lymphomas Working Formulation

The National Cancer Institute of the National Institutes of Health, Bethesda, sponsored an international multi-institutional clinicopathological study comparing six major classifications of the non-Hodgkin's lymphomas (*Cancer*, **49**, 2112–35, 1982). It was concluded that all six classifications were valuable and comparable in reproducibility and clinical correlations. A 'Working Formulation' was proposed which separates non-Hodgkin's lymphomas into ten major groups using morphological criteria only. The purpose of this formulation is not to supplant any of the currently utilized classifications but to provide a means for translation of terminology from one classification to another and for the comparison of clinical therapeutic trials. The relationship between the Working Formulation and the Kiel classification is shown in Table A.1.

Table A.1. A Working Formulation of non-Hodgkin's lymphomas for clinical usage (equivalent or related terms in the Kiel classification are shown)

Working Formulation	Kiel equivalent or related terms
Low grade	
A. Malignant lymphoma	
Small lymphocytic	
consistent with CLL	ML lymphocytic, CLL
plasmacytoid	ML lymphoplasmacytic/ lymphoplasmacytoid
B. Malignant lymphoma, follicular	ML centroblastic/centrocytic (small), follicular ± diffuse
Predominantly small cleaved cell	
diffuse areas	
sclerosis	
C. Malignant lymphoma, follicular	
Mixed, small cleaved and large cell	
diffuse areas	
sclerosis	

Working Formulation	Kiel equivalent or related terms
Intermediate grade	
D. Malignant lymphoma, follicular	
Predominantly large cell	
diffuse areas	ML centroblastic/centrocytic (large),
sclerosis	follicular ± diffuse
E. Malignant lymphoma, diffuse	
Small cleaved cell	ML centrocytic (small)
sclerosis	
F. Malignant lymphoma, diffuse	ML centroblastic/centrocytic (small),
Mixed, small and large cell	(small)
sclerosis	ML lymphoplasmacytic/cytoid,
epithelioid cell component	polymorphic
G. Malignant lymphoma, diffuse	ML centroblastic/centrocytic (large),
Large cell	diffuse
cleaved cell	ML centrocytic (large)
noncleaved cell	ML centroblastic
sclerosis	
High grade	
H. Malignant lymphoma	
Large cell, immunoblastic	ML immunoblastic
plasmacytoid	
clear cell	
polymorphous	T-zone lymphoma
epithelioid cell component	Lymphoepithelioid cell lymphoma
I. Malignant lymphoma	
Lymphoblastic	
convoluted cell	ML lymphoblastic, convoluted cell type
nonconvoluted cell	ML lymphoblastic, unclassified
J. Malignant lymphoma	
Small noncleaved cell	
Burkitt's	
follicular areas	ML lymphoblastic, Burkitt type and other B-lymphoblastic
Miscellaneous	
Composite	–
Mycosis fungoides	Mycosis fungoides
Histiocytic	–
Extramedullary plasmacytoma	ML plasmacytic
Unclassifiable	–
Other	–

In his comments on the Working Formulation, Professor Lennert noted his reservations which were that it separates entities that are histologically related and groups together unrelated lymphomas. This is mainly because the Formulation takes no account of the immunological identity of lymphomas. We would like to stress therefore, that although the Formulation may prove to be useful for the comparison of clinical trials it does not provide a satisfactory conceptual basis for the understanding and classification of malignant lymphomas.

Index

Italic page numbers refer to illustrations